D1206737

BETTER HEARING WITH COCHLEAR IMPLANTS

BETTER HEARING WITH COCHLEAR IMPLANTS

Studies at the Research Triangle Institute

Blake S. Wilson
Michael F. Dorman

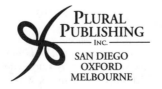

PLURAL
PUBLISHING
— INC. —
SAN DIEGO
OXFORD
MELBOURNE

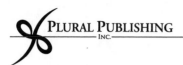

5521 Ruffin Road
San Diego, CA 92123

e-mail: info@pluralpublishing.com
Web site: http://www.pluralpublishing.com

49 Bath Street
Abingdon, Oxfordshire OX14 1EA
United Kingdom

FSC
www.fsc.org

MIX
Paper from
responsible sources

FSC® C011935

Copyright © by Plural Publishing, Inc. 2012

Typeset in 11/13 Garamond by Flanagan's Publishing Services, Inc.
Printed in the United States of America by McNaughton & Gunn

All rights, including that of translation, reserved. No part of this publication may be reproduced, stored in a retrieval system, or transmitted in any form or by any means, electronic, mechanical, recording, or otherwise, including photocopying, recording, taping, Web distribution, or information storage and retrieval systems without the prior written consent of the publisher.

For permission to use material from this text, contact us by
Telephone: (866) 758-7251
Fax: (888) 758-7255
e-mail: permissions@pluralpublishing.com

Every attempt has been made to contact the copyright holders for material originally printed in another source. If any have been inadvertently overlooked, the publishers will gladly make the necessary arrangements at the first opportunity.

Library of Congress Cataloging-in-Publication Data

Wilson, Blake S., 1948-
  Better hearing with cochlear implants: studies at the Research Triangle Institute / Blake S. Wilson, Michael F. Dorman.
     p. ; cm.
  Includes bibliographical references and index.
  ISBN-13: 978-1-59756-253-9 (alk. paper)
  ISBN-10: 1-59756-253-X (alk. paper)
  I. Dorman, Michael F. II. Title.
  [DNLM: 1. Research Triangle Institute. 2. Cochlear Implants. WV 274]
  LC Classification not assigned
  617.8'9—dc23
                            2011051397

The cover art is reproduced with permission from K. B. Hüttenbrink, T. Zahnert, C. Jolly, & G. Hofmann. (2002). Movements of cochlear implant electrodes inside the cochlea during insertion: An x-ray microscopy study. *Otology and Neurotology, 23,* 187–191. Copyright © 2002 Lippincott Williams & Wilkins.

CONTENTS

PART III
Combined Electric and Acoustic Stimulation (EAS) of the Auditory System
Introduction 271

Chapter 17
Psychophysical Studies Relating to Combined EAS 275

Chapter 18
Speech Reception With Combined EAS 307

PART IV
Representations of Temporal Information With Cochlear Implants
Introduction 327

Chapter 19
Temporal Representations With Cochlear Implants 331

Chapter 20
Strategies for the Repair of Deficits in Temporal Representations With Cochlear Implants 345

Chapter 21
High Rate Studies, Subject SR2 361

ACKNOWLEDGMENTS

An exceptionally large number of organizations and highly talented and dedicated investigators contributed to the research described in this book. In addition, the research would not have been possible without the generous contributions of time by the many cochlear implant users who participated in the studies.

The research was supported primarily by the National Institutes of Health (NIH), through its Neural Prosthesis Program (NPP). The first project began in September 1983 and the final of the seven contiguous projects ended in March 2006. Funding for our particular projects within the NPP was provided by the National Institute of Neurological Disorders and Stroke (NINDS) for the first two projects and by the National Institute on Deafness and Other Communication Disorders (NIDCD) for the remaining projects. Funding by the NIDCD began on May 1, 1989.

In addition, a study involving subjects fitted with an experimental version of the Nucleus cochlear implant device was jointly supported by the NIH and Cochlear Americas Corp. This study began in the spring of 1994.

Travel expenses for visiting subjects and guest scientists also were generously covered by the MED-EL GmbH for studies involving: (1) recipients of bilateral MED-EL implants; (2) users of combined electric and acoustic stimulation of the auditory system; (3) users of the newly introduced MED-EL PULSAR implant system; and (4) a subject implanted on one side for amelioration of intractable tinnitus and who had nearly normal hearing on the other side. MED-EL additionally provided important technical assistance in these studies.

Most of the work was conducted at the Research Triangle Institute (RTI) in the Research Triangle Park in North Carolina. RTI is a large, not-for-profit research institute that was created in 1958 by the three largest research universities in the area, Duke

University, North Carolina State University, and the University of North Carolina at Chapel Hill. The present staff at the RTI includes more than 2,800 people at multiple locations in the United States and in other countries. The RTI is also known as RTI International, a trade name for RTI.

In addition, a substantial fraction of the research was conducted at the Duke University Medical Center in Durham, North Carolina. The great majority of patient studies were conducted there until the fall of 1995, when two new laboratories were built at the RTI. Use of the laboratory at Duke was tapered down to zero over the ensuing two years and, ultimately, all studies were conducted in the RTI laboratories.

At the outset of our work in 1983, and up until mid-1985, studies with research subjects were conducted at the University of California at San Francisco (UCSF). The projects required collaboration with a tertiary care center that was active in the clinical application of cochlear implants. When the projects began, the only such centers in the United States were at UCSF, Stanford University in Palo Alto, California, and the House Ear Clinic in Los Angeles, California. UCSF graciously agreed to be our collaborating clinical center.

A cochlear implant program was created at Duke in early 1985. Soon thereafter, the laboratory was created at Duke for cochlear implant studies, and space and funding for the laboratory were generously provided by David C. Sabiston Jr., MD, who was the Chair of the Department of Surgery. Once the laboratory was operational, most studies were transferred from UCSF to Duke with enthusiastic technical support by—and ongoing collaboration with—UCSF.

The members of the RTI teams over the years included the people listed in Chapter 1, under the subheading "Composition of the RTI Teams." Each of the members contributed strongly to the overall effort.

A hallmark of the projects was collaboration with many investigators, universities, and companies worldwide. Lists of the collaborating investigators and their affiliations at the times of their participation in the RTI studies are presented in Appendix A. Among the investigators, special acknowledgements are due to Michael M. Merzenich, PhD, who welcomed us into his program at UCSF at the beginning of our work when we had little to offer in return, and Joseph C. Farmer Jr., MD, who asked us to conduct patient studies at Duke and supported our efforts with the highest enthusiasm thereafter.

Spectacular support also was provided by the management at the RTI. All requests for equipment were approved, and ample space and other resources were provided throughout the course of the projects. Special thanks are due to George R. Herbert, who was RTI's president during the early years of the projects; Grace C. Boddie, who was a vice president and the chief counsel for the Institute during the same period; and F. Thomas Wooten, PhD, who was the vice president of the Electronics and Systems Division within the RTI from 1983 to 1989 and became RTI's president in 1989 when Mr. Herbert retired. All of these and many other great people at the RTI supported the projects strongly.

Of course, we could not have done anything without our research subjects. We were blessed with some of the best, and we were continually amazed by their engagement in the studies and by their generosity in spending time with us.

We were blessed as well to be a part of the NPP. The heads of that program, F. Terry Hambrecht, MD, and, later, William J. Heetderks, MD, PhD, fostered a collaborative spirit among the participants in the program. For example, a Neural Prosthesis Workshop was held each year at NIH to review the progress of the many projects within the NPP and for the investigators to interact and share ideas. The cross-pollination of ideas was impressive, and advice was freely given and received. Everyone and each of the projects benefitted, and these benefits were made possible by the positive tone set by Terry and Bill.

Terry and Bill also were the project monitors for our projects. Terry and then Terry and Bill made regular site visits to our laboratories to review progress, plans, and problems that had been encountered. In addition, they read our progress reports carefully and communicated with us frequently about the work and especially about new ideas.

The site visits were both intense and rewarding. Terry and Bill never failed to offer the most insightful suggestions imaginable, including suggestions for solving problems, for new hypotheses, and for refined or new research directions. The guidance so selflessly provided by these two brilliant and dedicated leaders of the NPP was vital to our successes.

This book was made possible with the generous and highly able assistance of Susanne Stoops, Jeannie H. Cox, Callen Shutters, Dewey T. Lawson, and Stefan M. Brill. We are especially indebted to Susanne for her many efforts in helping to produce the book, including her expert transformation of the selected sections from NIH progress reports into the manuscripts for Chapters 2 through 21.

In addition, we are deeply indebted to the spectacular team at Plural for their sterling and highly professional efforts. The team members we worked with included Caitlin Thompson Mahon, Angie S. Singh, Kim White, Judy Meyer, Mandy Licata, Casey Stach, Stephanie Meissner, and Sandy Doyle. We are sad to announce that Sandy is now deceased; she helped us greatly with the graphics aspects of the book. Among the many contributions by the Plural team, Caitlin's editorial and production work stands out. She is the best of the best.

The concept for this book was suggested by Professor Michael F. Dorman many years ago. Although I thought the concept was wonderful, I kept delaying the project due to the press of ongoing activities and obligations. He persisted, however, and even offered to write the book with me. We finally began working on the book in earnest in the winter of 2011. I will forever be grateful to Michael for the concept, and for his perseverance, cheerful encouragement, and many key contributions to the writing. Indeed, those contributions and his guiding hand produced a book that is very much better than any book I could have written on my own.

Our RTI teams were privileged to have had the grand opportunity to pursue the work described herein. We were helped mightily every step of the way.

Blake Wilson, July 2011

There are only a few times in a career in science when you get goose bumps. One of mine came when one of my patients, Max Kennedy, was being tested at RTI with a version of a continuous interleaved sampling (CIS) processor. I was watching Dewey Lawson input Max's responses to the monitor program and Max's responses keep coming up "correct." Near the end of the test, everyone in the room was staring at the monitor wondering if Max was going to get 100 percent correct on a difficult test of consonant identification. He came close, and at the end of the test, Max sat back, slapped the table in front of him, and said loudly, "Hot damn, I want to take this one home with me." I am indebted to Blake, Dewey, Charlie, and Marian for the goose bumps.

Michael Dorman, August 2011

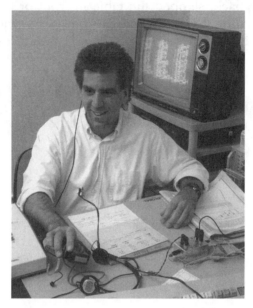

Michael L. Pierschalla, 1955–2002

This book is dedicated to Michael L. Pierschalla for his unparalleled contributions as a research subject to the development of cochlear implants, and to F. Terry Hambrecht, MD, and William J. Heetderks, MD, PhD, whose informed and inspired leadership of the Neural Prosthesis Program at the NIH led to many important advances in treatments of deafness and other sensory and neurological disorders. These great men played critical roles in making modern cochlear implants possible.

Chapter 1

OVERVIEW

Blake S. Wilson and Michael F. Dorman

As recently as the early 1980s, the success of cochlear implants (CIs) was very much in doubt. Indeed, it seemed that the more a researcher knew about auditory neurophysiology or speech acoustics, the more confident he was that implants could not provide a high (or even useful) level of speech understanding. Fortunately, pioneers in the implant field persisted in the face of doubt and, at times, intense criticism, and provided the foundation for the extremely successful CI devices that are available today.

Three large steps were needed to produce the present-day CIs: (1) the pioneering step to implant the first patients and to develop devices that were safe and had a life span of many years; (2) the development of devices that provided multiple sites of stimulation in the cochlea to take advantage of the tonotopic organization of the auditory system; and (3) the development of highly effective processing strategies that utilized the multiple sites of stimulation and supported for the first time high levels of speech recognition for most users of CIs. Findings from the landmark "Bilger study" in 1977 (Bilger et al., 1977)—and from the two consensus development conferences on cochlear implants held at the National Institutes of Health (NIH) in 1988 and 1995 (National Institutes of Health, 1988, 1995)—indicate the status of CIs at each of these steps. Principal conclusions from the Bilger study and the two consensus statements are presented in Table 1–1. As noted there, especially large gains in performance were obtained in step 3.

1

Table 1–1. *Major Indicators of Progress in the Development of Cochlear Implants*

Persons or Event	Year	Comment or Outcome
Bilger et al.	1977	"Although the subjects could not understand speech through their prostheses, they did score significantly higher on tests of lipreading and recognition of environmental sounds with their prostheses activated than without them." (This was an NIH-funded study of all 13 implant patients in the United States at the time.)
First NIH Consensus Statement	1988	Suggested that multichannel implants were more likely to be effective than single-channel implants, and indicated that about 1 in 20 patients could carry out a normal conversation without lip-reading. (The world population of implant recipients was about 3,000 in 1988.)
Second NIH Consensus Statement	1995	"A majority of those individuals with the latest speech processors for their implants will score above 80% correct on high-context sentences, even without visual cues." (The number of implant recipients approximated 12,000 in 1995, and the number exceeded 220,000 in late 2010.)

Teams at the Research Triangle Institute (RTI) in North Carolina, USA, along with their many collaborating investigators from other research organizations worldwide, contributed significantly to step 3. This book describes the program of research at the RTI and the collaborating organizations, and presents key results selected from nearly 23 years of research.

THE RTI PROJECTS AND THEIR MEMBERSHIP IN THE NEURAL PROSTHESIS PROGRAM

As noted in the Acknowledgments, the research was supported primarily by the NIH, beginning in September 1983 and continu-ing through March 2006. In all, seven projects were supported. Each project had the title "Speech processors for auditory pros-theses," but a wide range of studies and activities was included in the projects that went well beyond the design and testing of novel speech processors. A list of the projects with their terms and NIH numbers is presented in Table 1–2.

The projects were a part of the Neural Prosthesis Program (NPP) at the NIH, which supported work in the many different

Table 1–2. The Series of "Speech Processors" Projects at the Research Triangle Institute

Project	NIH Number	Term
1	N01-NS-3-2356	26 September 1983 through 25 September 1985
2	N01-NS-5-2396	26 September 1985 through 30 April 1989
3	N01-DC-9-2401	1 May 1989 through 31 July 1992
4	N01-DC-2-2401	1 August 1992 through 31 July 1995
5	N01-DC-5-2103	1 August 1995 through 29 September 1998
6	N01-DC-8-2105	30 September 1998 through 31 March 2002
7	N01-DC-2-1002	1 April 2002 through 31 March 2006

areas relating to neural prostheses, for example, reambulation of paralyzed limbs or extremities; restoration of bladder control for quadriplegics; restoration of sensory inputs to the brain including auditory, visual, and vestibular inputs; brain-machine interfaces; packaging of implanted electronics; insulation for the nonactive parts of stimulating electrodes; alternative electrode designs for various neural prostheses; alternative stimulus designs; and safety of electrical stimulation.

Our area was restoration of auditory inputs to the brain, and our projects were accompanied by others in that same area. The projects at the RTI spanned the entire period from 1983 to 2006, and each of the other projects relating to auditory prostheses spanned shorter periods within those years. At the outset, our projects were the only projects directed primarily at better speech processor designs. In later years, either two or three projects on this topic were supported at any one time up until 2006 when the projects ended and the NPP had been reorganized into smaller units across multiple institutes at the NIH. (The reorganization occurred in 2004 and followed Bill Heetderks' decision in late 2002 to resign from his position as the Head of the NPP, so that he could accept an offer to become the Director of Extramural Programs at the newly created National Institute on Biomedical Imaging and Bioengineering; the NPP ceased to exist as a single entity with the reorganization.) These other "speech processors" projects were conducted at Stanford University in Palo Alto, CA; the University of Melbourne in Melbourne, Australia; the House Ear Institute in Los Angeles, CA; and the Massachusetts Eye and Ear Infirmary (MEEI) in Boston, MA.

Among the companion projects, we had an especially close and productive relationship with the team and projects at the MEEI. We developed portable speech processors together, and Don Eddington and Bill Rabinowitz of the MEEI team made important contributions to the development at the RTI (and Duke University Medical Center) of an especially effective and enduring processing strategy for CIs: the continuous interleaved sampling (CIS) strategy. This partnership leveraged the NIH support of the projects in Boston and North Carolina, in that we could accomplish more together than separately.

QPRs—Four a Year for Over Twenty Years

Projects within the NPP were supported through the contracts mechanism, which was in accord with an integrated and coordinated program to develop better neural prostheses. Requirements of the contracts included presentations by the project teams at the annual Neural Prosthesis Workshop at the NIH; a detailed report of progress and problems encountered during each quarter for each of the projects; and a final report for each of the projects. The quarterly progress reports (QPRs) included a section on plans for the next quarter for all quarters except the final quarter, and the final reports (FRs) included a section on recommendations for future research. The progress reports provided a comprehensive record of activities and achievements for each of the projects.

In all, 91 reports were produced during the seven projects at the RTI. The authors and principal topic(s) for each of the reports are presented in Appendix B, which includes a separate table for each of the seven projects.

A Very Costly Decision

Soon after the outset of the NIH projects, the RTI team at the time recommended a policy to its management for the handling of intellectual property (IP). The recommended policy was to donate all results from the NIH-sponsored research on CIs at the RTI to the public domain. The thought was that, with the inventions and other IP in the public domain, all valuable discoveries would be applied by most or all of the major manufacturers of CIs and thereby help the greatest possible number of deaf and severely hearing-impaired people.

George R. Herbert, President of the RTI, and Grace C. Boddie, General Counsel, approved the policy after careful consideration of its implications, including the relinquishing of the Institute's rights to the IP as specified by the Bayh-Dole act, which was enacted by the United States Congress in 1980. The act specified that organizations conducting research under Federal grants or contracts would have the right to retain and pursue

IP resulting from the research, so long as the Government had a nonexclusive license to utilize the IP for its own purposes. The decision to forgo potential royalties from patents and exclusive licensing agreements proved to be important in that it greatly facilitated incorporation of discoveries from the RTI projects into commercially-available CI systems at the earliest possible times. In retrospect, the negative economic consequences of the decision to approve the policy were enormous (in the 10s of millions of dollars), both to the organization and to the individual inventors. However, the policy did what it was supposed to do, and the outcomes were most gratifying to the RTI teams and management.

Composition of the RTI Teams

Members of the RTI teams over the years included Stefan M. Brill, Lianne A. Cartee, Jeannie H. Cox, Dee Dee Davis, Charles C. Finley, Kathrinn Fitzpatrick, Dewey T. Lawson, Reinhold Schatzer, Xiaoan Sun, Christopher van den Honert, Sandra Waters, Blake S. Wilson, Robert D. Wolford, and Mariangeli Zerbi. Kathrinn Fitzpatrick, Sandra Waters, Dee Dee Davis, and Jeannie H. Cox each served as the Administrative Assistant (AA) for the projects at different times in the program, and the remaining individuals served as investigators. (Jeannie Cox also assisted in patient studies in her later years in the program.) The projects were directed by Blake Wilson until he was appointed as one of the first four Senior Fellows at the RTI in late 2002. After that, Dewey Lawson became the Principal Investigator for the remainder of the final project in the series of the seven "speech processors" projects at the RTI.

A chart showing the times of service for most members of the teams is presented in Figure 1–1. As noted in the Acknowledgments, the RTI teams were assisted by many other investigators from many other research institutions worldwide, including institutions in Australia, Austria, Canada, Germany, Poland, South Korea, Spain, Switzerland, the United Kingdom, and the United States.

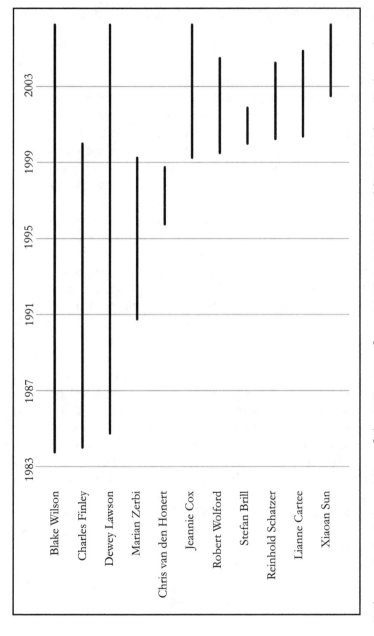

Figure 1–1. Composition of the RTI teams from 1983 to 2006. In addition to the members shown, Kathrinn Fitzpatrick, Sandra Waters, and Dee Dee Davis each served as the Administrative Assistant for the projects at different times from 1983 to 1999.

ORGANIZATION OF THIS BOOK

In the remaining chapters of this book, we present the most important sections from the most important progress reports, in part to provide a convenient access in one place to the key studies and their results. Many journal articles and book chapters also were produced as part of the projects, but they were generally brief and limited to particular studies and therefore do not provide the detail or the coverage of the progress reports. In addition, the journal articles and book chapters may be obtained easily from libraries and the web, whereas the progress reports are not as widely available.

Another reason to present material from the progress reports is that the reports convey the essence of the projects from start to finish. The journal articles fail to do that because they describe single studies only, as just mentioned, and the book chapters fail to do that because they generally integrate results from across many laboratories and areas of research to provide a tutorial for their readers. The journal articles and book chapters are cited at the appropriate places throughout the book, but the emphasis here is on the progress reports.

Following this overview chapter, the book is organized into major parts according to the principal areas of research in the RTI projects, including design and evaluation of novel processing strategies; electrical stimulation on both sides with bilateral CIs; combined electric and acoustic stimulation of the auditory system; and representations of temporal information with CIs. Multiple chapters are included in each part, and each chapter is a selected section from a progress report. In addition, each part includes a brief introduction to indicate its contents and to point to other relevant reports and findings that could not be included in the book. The references originally cited in the selected sections from the selected progress reports are now presented in the single list of references at the end of this book. Also, some of the figures have been redrafted to provide high-resolution images. Otherwise, no changes have been made in the included source material other than formatting changes in the text for a uniform style and correction of typographical and other minor errors.

In the remainder of the present chapter, we: (1) describe the role of the RTI projects in the broader context of the development of CIs; (2) indicate how we selected the sections from the NIH progress reports for inclusion in the book; and (3) offer some concluding remarks.

RTI'S ROLE IN THE DEVELOPMENT OF COCHLEAR IMPLANTS

In 1983, when the first project at RTI was underway, the first of the three steps listed near the beginning of this chapter had been taken and progress was being made in taking the second step. Dr. William F. House and a few other pioneers had implanted the first patients, and Dr. House in particular had developed single-channel devices that could be safely and usefully applied over many years. In addition, groups in the United States, Australia, and Europe had developed multielectrode arrays that could be safely inserted at surgery in the scala tympani of the cochlea and that could excite different sectors (or tonotopic regions) of the auditory nerve depending on which intracochlear electrode, or which closely spaced pair of intracochlear electrodes, was activated. However, high levels of speech recognition using hearing alone was still rare and even as late as 1988 only about one in 20 patients using any of the better multisite and multi-channel implants could carry out a normal conversation without lip-reading (National Institutes of Health, 1988; see Table 1–1). The implant systems in 1983 were mainly useful as an adjunct to lip-reading and for an awareness of environmental sounds. In the rare cases, a patient could understand high-context sentences with her or his restored hearing alone. Those best performances were far below what was to come later with some further refinements in multisite stimulation and with the completion of step 3. In addition, the completion of step 3 allowed most patients to attain high levels of sentence recognition with hearing alone, as opposed to the small fraction of patients in 1988.

Step 3 and the CIS Strategy

The largest contribution from the RTI projects was in the completion of step 3, as mentioned previously. In particular, multiple new ways to represent speech and other sounds with CIs were created in the projects, and these new ways supported high levels of sentence recognition using hearing alone for the great majority of implant users. Perhaps the best known discovery came in 1989 and was first called the "supersampler" strategy and then soon thereafter the CIS strategy (Wilson et al., 1989).

Results from the initial studies with the CIS processor were reported in *Nature* in 1991 (Wilson et al., 1991a). This paper soon became the most highly cited publication on studies with CI patients and remains as the most highly cited publication on the topic today. As of July 2011, the paper had been cited in 476 other peer-reviewed publications (Web of Knowledge, 2011).

CIS was a combination of new and prior elements, including: (1) a full representation of energies in frequency bands spanning the spectrum of speech and other sounds; (2) no further analysis of, or "feature extraction" from, this or other information, to allow the brain of the user to make the decisions about what was important or not important in the incoming stream of information; (3) nonsimultaneous stimulation with charge-balanced biphasic pulses across the electrodes in a multielectrode implant, to eliminate the component of electrode or "channel" interactions due to direct summation of overlapping electric fields from the electrodes for simultaneously presented stimuli; (4) stimulation at relatively high rates at each of the electrodes, to allow representations of fundamental frequencies for periodic sounds such as voiced speech and of distinctions between periodic versus aperiodic sounds such as unvoiced speech (again, without explicit extraction of these "features"); (5) use of cutoff frequencies in the energy (or "envelope") detectors for each of the bandpass filters that would include the fundamental frequency variations in the outputs of the detectors (cutoff frequencies in the range of 200 to 400 Hz); (6) use of current sources rather than the relatively uncontrolled voltage sources that had been used in some prior implant systems; and (7) a relatively high number of activated electrodes (at least four but generally higher and not limited in number). No assumptions about sounds in the environment, or in particular how speech is produced or perceived, were made in the way CIS was constructed. This approach allowed the brain of the user to become a far more active and important part of perception with CIs.

It is worth noting that the gains in performance produced with CIS are sometimes attributed to the non-simultaneous stimulation across electrodes. However, the gains were produced with the discovery of a unique combination of many elements, not just non-simultaneous stimulation, which had been used before (see, e.g., Doyle et al., 1964) but not in conjunction with the other elements. The breakthrough was in the combination and in exactly how the parts were put together.

Step 3 and "n-of-m" or Channel-Picking Strategies

During the late 1980s and early 1990s, the RTI teams and their collaborating investigators created multiple other ways to represent speech and other sounds with multisite and multichannel implants. These ways included the *n*-of-*m* approach that was subsequently incorporated in a line of processing strategies developed for implant devices manufactured by Nucleus Ltd. and later by Cochlear Pty. Ltd., of Lane Cove, Australia. (Nucleus was the parent company for Cochlear.) The *n*-of-*m* approach is a variation of CIS in which the envelope signals for the different bandpass channels are "scanned" prior to each frame of stimulation across the intracochlear electrodes, to identify the signals with the *n*-highest amplitudes from among a total of *m* processing channels (and associated intracochlear electrodes). Stimulus pulses are delivered only to the electrodes that correspond to the channels with those highest amplitudes. (The *n*-of-*m* approach actually was created before CIS; describing the *n*-of-*m* approach as a variation of CIS is a retrospective description.)

This channel selection or "spectral peak picking" scheme is designed in part to reduce the density of stimulation while still representing the most important aspects of the acoustic environment. The deletion of low-amplitude channels (and associated stimuli) for each frame of stimulation may reduce the overall level of masking or interference across electrode and excitation regions in the cochlea. To the extent that the omitted channels do not contain significant information, such "unmasking" may improve the perception of the input signal by the patient. In addition, for positive signal-to-noise ratios, selection of the channels with the greatest amplitudes in each frame may emphasize the primary speech (or other) signal with respect to the noise.

The *n*-of-*m* approach was first described for relatively low rates of stimulation in a QPR in 1986 (Wilson et al., 1986; also see Wilson et al., 1987, 1988a). The approach was the basis for the "spectral maxima sound processor" (SMSP) developed in Melbourne, Australia, in the early 1990s (McDermott et al., 1992; McDermott & Vandali, 1997) and later applied in slightly modified form as the "spectral peak" (SPEAK) strategy, which was used as a part of the Nucleus and Cochlear CI systems for many years thereafter. The patent for the SMSP (McDermott & Vandali, 1997) cites Wilson et al. (1987, 1988a) as the "prior art," and primarily specifies desirable values for the parameters *n* and *m*.

Soon after the creation of CIS, the RTI team at the time suggested that the relatively high rates of stimulation and other attributes of CIS might be beneficial for the *n*-of-*m* approach as well (Lawson et al., 1995; Wilson et al., 1995a, 1995b). This suggestion led to a large project at the RTI that was jointly supported by the NIH, Cochlear Pty. Ltd., and the Duke University Medical Center. An important aim of the study was to evaluate the suggestion, and the resulting data affirmed it fully (e.g., Lawson et al., 1996).

Some years later, Cochlear Pty. Ltd. introduced the "advanced combination encoder" (ACE) strategy, which used the *n*-of-*m* approach in conjunction with the relatively high rates of stimulation and other attributes of CIS. This strategy quickly became the default processing option for the Cochlear devices and remains as the default option today.

The "high rate" *n*-of-*m* strategy, as described and evaluated by the RTI team, also is used as a processing option in a series of CI systems manufactured by MED-EL GmbH of Innsbruck, Austria. The option is called the *n*-of-*m* strategy in those systems.

Step 3 and the Virtual-Channel Strategy

The RTI team also created a way to utilize virtual pitches in a multichannel processor context (e.g., Wilson et al., 1992, 1994). In that approach, pairs of adjacent intracochlear electrodes were stimulated simultaneously to produce pitches that were intermediate to the pitches produced with stimulation of either electrode in the pair alone. Each pair in the electrode array was stimulated after stimulation of the prior pair, maintaining nonsimultaneity of stimulation across the pairs (and regions of stimulation in the cochlea). Other aspects of CIS were retained as well, and these processors were called "virtual channel interleaved sampling (VCIS) processors."

The production of intermediate pitches with simultaneous stimulation of two electrodes had been described before, first by Simmons et al. in 1965 for electrodes implanted directly within the auditory nerve and then by Townshend et al. in 1987 for electrodes implanted in the scala tympani (Simmons et al., 1965; Townshend et al., 1987). The RTI group was the first to describe the use of intermediate pitches in a multichannel context and among multiple pairs of electrodes. The VCIS approach was later used in a processing strategy developed by the Advanced Bionics Corp. (ABC) of Valencia, CA, USA (e.g., Trautwein, 2006). The strategy in the ABC devices is called the "Hi-Resolution 120" or HiRes 120 strategy.

In the early development of VCIS processors, the RTI team showed that with appropriate current biasing a pitch percept could be created that was: (1) lower than the pitch percept produced by stimulation of the most apical electrode in the array or (2) higher than the pitch produced by stimulation of the most basal electrode. Signal processors were created and tested that used both between-electrode VCIS channels and a supra-apical virtual channel, which produced the lowest pitch (Dorman et al., 1996; Wilson et al., 1992). A similar concept, that is, a virtual channel with lower pitch than the most apical electrode, is now embodied in the "phantom electrode" system from ABC (Saoji & Litvak, 2010).

Step 3 and the Fine Structure Processing Strategy

The RTI team, in the early 1990s, created a way to represent the "fine structure" or "fine timing" information in channels with low center frequencies by presenting stimulus pulses at the times of detected peaks or zero crossings in the bandpass filter outputs for the channels (e.g., Wilson et al., 1990a). This approach was called a "peak picker/CIS" strategy, and all channels except the 1–3 channels with the lowest center frequencies presented CIS stimuli.

The peak picker/CIS approach was later refined by the MED-EL GmbH and utilized in its "fine structure processing" (FSP) strategies (e.g., Hochmair et al., 2006).

The processing strategies in current widespread use are shown in Table 1–3. As was the hope of the RTI teams, utilization of discoveries from the NIH projects has been excellent. All of the systems manufactured by the three largest implant companies use a version of the CIS strategy. These versions include the "CIS," "CIS+," "High Definition CIS" (HDCIS), and "Hi-Resolution" (HiRes) strategies, as named by the manufacturers. In addition, (1) the MED-EL and Cochlear systems use various implementations of the n-of-m approach, including the listed n-of-m, ACE, and SPEAK strategies; (2) the MED-EL systems use the concept of the peak picker/CIS approach in the FSP strategy; and (3) the AB systems use an implementation of the VCIS approach in their HiRes 120 strategy.

Each of these strategies and others are described in much greater detail in two chapters by Wilson and Dorman, the first on "The design of cochlear implants" (Wilson & Dorman, 2009) and the second on "Signal processing strategies for cochlear implants" (Wilson & Dorman, 2012). The first of these chapters also presents information about other aspects of the design, e.g., design considerations for the electrode array, implanted receiver/stimulator, and transcutaneous transmission link. The second of the chapters is more sharply focused on processing strategies and provides more up-to-date information on that topic. Additional relevant reviews include ones by Loizou (2006), Wilson (2004, 2006), and Zeng et al. (2008).

As of late 2010, more than 220,000 deaf or severely hearing-impaired persons had received CIs, either in one or both ears for each person. The cumulative number of implants over time is shown in Figure 1–2 (adapted and updated from Wilson & Dorman, 2008a). The rapid growth in the number beginning in the early 1990s corresponds to the introductions into standard clinical practice of new and highly effective processing strategies during the early 1990s and afterward.

Developments in Other Domains

Besides CIS and the other processing strategies mentioned previously, the RTI teams and their collaborating investigators produced or helped to enable advances in many other areas

Table 1–3. Processing Strategies in Current Widespread Use*

Manufacturer	CIS	CIS+	HDCIS	n-of-m	FSP	ACE	SPEAK	HiRes	HiRes 120
MED-EL GmbH	•	•	•	•	•				
Cochlear Ltd.	•					•	•		
Advanced Bionics Corp.	•							•	•

*Manufacturers are shown in the left column and the processing strategies used in their implant systems are shown in the remaining columns. The full names of the strategies are presented in the text.

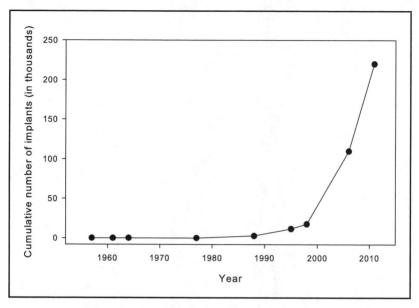

Figure 1–2. Cumulative number of cochlear implants across years. Events marked by the dots include: (1) the first implant operation by Drs. Andre Djourno and Charles Eyriès in 1957; (2) the first two implants by Dr. William F. House in 1961; (3) the first implant by Dr. F. Blair Simmons in 1964; (4) the "Bilger report" in 1977; (5) the first NIH Consensus Conference on Cochlear Implants in 1988; (6) the second NIH Consensus Conference in 1995; (7) the National Academy of Sciences report (Finn et al.) in 1998; (8) an estimate of the cumulative number published in the middle of 2006; and (9) an estimate of the number published in late 2010. Multichannel devices began to supplant single-channel devices in the early 1980s, and highly effective processing strategies were first introduced into widespread clinical use in the early 1990s, as described in the text. These large steps forward fueled the increasing acceptance and applications of cochlear implants. (Adapted with permission from Wilson, B. S., & Dorman, M. F. [2008a]. Interfacing sensors with the nervous system: Lessons from the development and success of the cochlear implant. *IEEE Sensors Journal, 8*, 131–147. Copyright 2008 IEEE.)

including but not limited to: (1) building of tools for research on CIs such as highly flexible and real-time processing systems; (2) design and application of some of the first portable processors for CIs that were based on digital signal processing and could support high numbers of processing channels and stimulus sites; (3) development of additional processing strategies for unilateral implants, for example, the "closer mimicking" strategies described in Schatzer et al. (2003) and Wilson et al. (2003, 2006, 2010); (4) evaluation and further development of bilateral CIs and processing strategies for them; (5) evaluation and further development of combined electric and acoustic stimulation of the auditory system for persons with at least some residual hearing at low frequencies; (6) development and application of mathematical models of the electrically stimulated cochlea; (7) recording and interpretation of intracochlear evoked potentials in response to a wide range of electrical stimuli; (8) elucidation of temporal patterns of neural responses in CI patients; (9) evaluation of possible relationships between the temporal patterns and pitch percepts for the same patients; (10) development of processing strategies for the Auditory Brainstem Implant or ABI; (11) psychophysical measures of responses to many different types of electrical stimuli; and (12) design of inexpensive but nonetheless highly effective CI systems primarily for use in low- and mid-income countries.

Technology Transfer

An important aspect of the work at the RTI was a program of active technology transfer to accelerate or otherwise facilitate the incorporation of inventions and other new concepts or findings into commercially available implant systems. (This program was in addition to the policy on IP described previously; both the program and the policy were designed to facilitate the incorporation of advances into commercially available systems.) We believe this active transfer was far more effective than the alternative passive approach of simply presenting some of the necessary information in publications and the progress reports. We did present the information in those ways, but we also made ourselves available to answer questions and to work directly with the design teams at the manufacturers to move research results into products that people could use. This additional effort was most unusual at the time and in retrospect was an early example of what now is called "translational research" or "translational medicine." The teamwork promoted by the effort was beneficial to all concerned.

Of course, the active technology transfer was only a small fraction of the overall effort needed to produce new or substantially modified CI devices. For that, the companies deserve the greatest credit by far.

Contributions by Others

Many teams worldwide contributed significantly to the CI systems we have today. The RTI contributions are important, but they are only a part of the story. The fascinating history of CIs is recounted in Eisen (2006, 2009), Finn et al. (1998), Hannaway (1996), Levitt (2008), Niparko and Wilson (2000), Seitz (2002), and Wilson and Dorman (2008b).

One thread that runs through the histories is the remarkable courage and perseverance of the pioneers in laying the foundations for the present devices. Another thread is that no one person or group is primarily responsible for the development of the CI. Many contributions from many sources were needed. For example, different groups contributed most strongly to each of the three major steps listed near the beginning of this chapter.

SELECTIONS FROM THE NIH PROGRESS REPORTS

Extraordinarily difficult decisions were made in selecting the sections from the NIH progress reports for inclusion in this book. At the outset, we made the easy decision to exclude sections that had been published as journal articles or book chapters, for the reasons mentioned previously. However, that decision did not produce enough of a reduction for a book-length exposition of the projects. We therefore decided to sharpen the focus for the book by excluding all sections from the remaining sections on tool building; portable processors; development of models of the electrically stimulated cochlea; and parametric and longitudinal studies with CIS and other processors. This second (and much more difficult) decision winnowed the list considerably, but did not shorten it enough. Thus, as a final step we selected what we thought to be the most important sections from among the sections still in the list. The ultimate selections included 20 sections from 18 of the 91 reports.

Guides to the excluded material are presented in Appendices C and D. Appendix C lists the journal articles and book chapters that were published during the projects and also as a result of the projects afterward. Appendix D presents the contents of the RTI progress reports sorted by topic, as opposed to the sorting by project and chronological order in Appendix B. Reference to Appendix D would allow one to identify all reports on any of the many topics, areas, and activities included in the projects.

All of the NIH progress reports are in the public domain and all can be requested from the NIH. In addition, the reports are posted at http://www.rti.org/capr/caprqprs.html, which is a daughter page within the website for the prior Center for Auditory Prosthesis Research at the RTI. This website has been maintained since the closing of the Center in 2008 and may continue to be maintained for the foreseeable future.

In the remainder of this book, the QPRs are referenced by their project number and report number in the format QPR X:Y, where X is the project number (1 through 7; see Table 1–2) and Y is the report number. Similarly, the FRs are referenced by their project number, in the format FR X. The references include: (1) citations to the reports within the text for each chapter, and (2) identification of the report from which the material is drawn for each chapter, in the title and running heading for the chapter.

NOT A MIRACLE, JUST HARD WORK

In an interview in 1998, a reporter suggested to our long-time research patient Michael Pierschalla (SR2 in the QPRs) that it must seem like a miracle that his hearing had been restored. Michael, remembering the thousands of hours he spent in the laboratory, said quietly, "It is no miracle at all. It is the result of long, long hours of very hard work by researchers around the world." The members of the RTI teams are proud to have been part of that effort and we are grateful to the sponsors, research subjects, administrators, collaborating investigators, and colleagues at companies who made our work possible. The work was exhilarating and among the greatest adventures of our lives.

Part I

DESIGN AND EVALUATION OF NOVEL PROCESSING STRATEGIES

The projects at the Research Triangle Institute (RTI) started small. The staff was small and the scope was small—largely limited to tool building. The main purpose of the first project was to design and build a speech processing system that could deliver up to eight channels of information to as many as eight stimulation sites in the implants of cochlear implant (CI) subjects. The tools developed were to be used by the clinical collaborator for the project, which was the implant team at the University of California at San Francisco (UCSF).

Tool building continued throughout the projects and was always an important element in our research. The tools enabled many new lines of investigation and provided many new capabilities for research including:

1. Rapid simulation of processor designs with a "block diagram compiler," which was based on earlier but less flexible designs developed at the Bell Laboratories in Murray Hill, NJ, USA, and which preceded by many years the advent of tools we use today for similar purposes, such as MATLAB®;

2. Real-time implementations of a wide range of novel processing strategies;
3. Psychophysical and speech reception studies with implant patients using any of almost all of the existing devices at any one time during projects 2 through 7, through the design and construction of custom interface systems that allowed either real-time laboratory control of the implanted receiver/stimulators of the devices or real-time stimulation of the implanted electrodes via percutaneous connectors;
4. Recordings of intracochlear evoked potentials in response to a wide range of electrical stimuli, using the percutaneous access available in subjects with the Ineraid or experimental Nucleus devices for both stimulation and recording;
5. Portable sound processors capable of implementing many different processing strategies and useful for evaluating changes in performance as subjects gained experience in "take-home" field trials with the processors;
6. Sophisticated software for speech testing and automated analyses of the results;
7. Studies with new speech test material that provided sensitive measures even for the best-performing CI subjects;
8. A "streaming mode" tool that allowed implementation and evaluation of especially complex strategies, by processing speech or other inputs in less than real time and then streaming the outputs to the implants of the subjects in real time and under laboratory control;
9. New measures of music reception with implants;
10. The addition of head-related transfer function (HRTF) information to speech and other sounds that allowed sound localization and other studies primarily with recipients of bilateral CIs; and
11. Mathematical models of the electrically stimulated cochlea and auditory nerve that provided important insights into the mechanisms of electrical stimulation in the environment of the cochlea and also informed the design of new processing strategies to maximize the transmission of sound information via a CI.

These tools made our work—and some of the studies at our collaborating institutions—possible. In addition, the designs for the portable sound processors provided the starting points for the ultimate designs used in sound processors manufactured by MiniMed Inc. in Sylmar, CA, USA, and by the MED-EL GmbH in Innsbruck, Austria. A detailed listing of the tools and the reports in which they are described is presented in Appendix D.

Toward the end of the first project, our colleagues at UCSF granted us testing time with some of their research subjects. At about this same time, we also built a laboratory at Duke for studies with CI patients. Once these studies at both sites were underway, the greatest emphasis in our work shifted from tool building to the studies. Over time, progressively more studies were conducted in the Duke laboratory. In 1995 we built two laboratories at the RTI, one for evoked potential studies and the other for psychophysical and speech reception studies. The first studies were conducted in the RTI laboratories in November 1995 and almost all of the later studies were conducted in those laboratories as well.

With the increase in the scope of work by the RTI team, and with some clear opportunities for improving the performance of CIs, the National Institutes of Health (NIH) increased funding for the projects. The increases in funding supported a larger staff and allowed many more studies than would otherwise be possible. In addition, the requirement to have a clinical collaborator was dropped after project 1, and the focus of the projects shifted from engineering support to the design of novel sound processing strategies and tests of those strategies in laboratory and field-trial studies.

In addition to the availability of powerful tools, we were fortunate to have access to subjects who had percutaneous connections to their implanted electrodes. The percutaneous connectors were critical in that they provided a completely transparent interface between the stimuli generated under laboratory control and the electrodes. Also, in the other direction, the connectors allowed direct recording of intracochlear evoked potentials (EPs) from unstimulated electrodes in the implant. Evaluations of many novel sound processor designs were made possible with the connectors, as were sensitive and high-fidelity recordings of the intracochlear EPs. These evaluations and recordings would not have been possible with the transcutaneous transmission links at the times of the studies, as those links were highly limited in the types of stimuli they could specify and in the amount and quality of information that could be sent in a "reverse telemetry" mode from the implant to receiving and processing equipment outside of the head. Indeed, the links for some of the implant systems did not include a reverse telemetry mode.

We were also fortunate to have wonderful colleagues and extraordinarily motivated subjects. As mentioned in the Acknowledgments and Chapter 1, we were helped in our research by colleagues at many institutions worldwide. In addition, our subjects were highly engaged in the research and many of them spent multiple one- or two-week sessions with us. One of the subjects, to whom this book is dedicated, spent well over an accumulated person year with us, over the span of more than a decade. This subject also spent considerable time in other laboratories in the United States and Europe, most notably in the laboratory directed by Don Eddington at the Massachusetts Eye and Ear Infirmary in Boston.

Our successes were the result of these advantages: powerful tools, percutaneous connectors, motivated subjects, and wonderful colleagues. In addition, we benefited tremendously from our membership in the Neural Prosthesis Program at the NIH and the highly informed and able guidance of our projects by Terry Hambrecht and Bill Heetderks.

The emphasis in this first part of the book is on work that has not been described or fully described in publications from the projects. The material is drawn from the progress reports. Chapter 2 provides a comprehensive summary of the design and evaluation of novel processing strategies up until the spring of 1989. Those strategies included two variations of "interleaved pulses" strategies, one of which was the first implementation of what later became known as the n-of-m strategy. Chapter 3 describes the discovery of the continuous interleaved sampling (CIS) strategy and the first tests with subject SR2. Chapters 5 and 7 describe further studies to evaluate CIS. Chapter 5 presents results from the first seven studied subjects, all of whom were selected for their exceptionally high levels of performance with their clinical "compressed analog" (CA) processors, and Chapter 7 presents those results plus results from tests with four additional subjects specially selected for their low levels of performance with the clinical processor. In addition, Chapter 5 presents a matrix of correlations among test measures, which included high correlations for many of the comparisons and presaged similar results that were reported later by others (e.g., Rabinowitz et al., 1992). Chapter 5 is a superset of our brief publication in *Nature* (Wilson et al., 1991a) and provides much additional information.

The remaining chapters address a variety of topics, including: (1) the designs and evaluations of the "peak picker" and hybrid "peak picker/CIS" strategies (Chapters 4 and 6); (2) design and evaluation of the virtual channel interleaved sampling (VCIS) strategy (Chapters 9 and 11); (3) the psychophysics of virtual channel stimulation (Chapter 10); (4) the dependence of speech reception scores on the overall distance spanned along the length of the cochlea by the activated electrodes and virtual channels (also in Chapter 11); (5) the first use of a "continuous sampling" strategy to greatly improve the speech reception performance of single-channel Auditory Brainstem Implant (ABI) patients (Chapter 8); (6) evaluation of an early design for an inexpensive but nonetheless highly effective CI system, intended primarily for use in China and other low- and mid-income countries (Chapter 12); (7) design and evaluation of the "high rate" n-of-m and other strategies in tests with five subjects implanted with an experimental version of the Nucleus device that included a percutaneous connector (Chapter 13); and (8) the demonstration of an asymptote in speech reception performance with increases in the number of processing channels and associated stimulus sites beyond 4 to 8 (also in Chapter 13)—an outcome that presaged many other observations of this effect.

Many of the reports for the "speech processors" projects at the RTI were on the design and evaluation of novel processing strategies. In addition, many of the reports describe related studies such as the dependence of performance on choices for the values of parameters within a strategy (most often the CIS strategy) and such as changes in speech reception scores over time with accumulated experience in field trials with a particular strategy. A detailed listing of all of these reports is presented under the second major heading in Appendix D.

Chapter 2

COMPARISON OF ANALOG AND PULSATILE CODING STRATEGIES FOR MULTICHANNEL COCHLEAR PROSTHESES*

Blake S. Wilson, Charles C. Finley, and Dewey T. Lawson

In studies conducted in collaboration with investigators at the University of California at San Francisco (UCSF), our team compared a variety of speech processing strategies in tests with patients implanted with the UCSF/Storz electrode array (Wilson et al., 1988a, 1988b, 1988c, 1990b). Some of the largest differences in performance among processing strategies were found in comparisons between the compressed analog (CA) processor of the present UCSF/Storz prosthesis and a type of "interleaved

*From QPR 3:1, May 1, 1989, through July 31, 1989.

pulses" (IP) processor that delivers pulses in sequence to the different channels in the implanted electrode array.

In more recent studies, conducted in collaboration with D. K. Eddington and W. M. Rabinowitz of the Massachusetts Eye and Ear Infirmary and the Massachusetts Institute of Technology, we have extended the comparisons of CA and IP processors to patients implanted with the Symbion electrode array. These later studies are of particular interest inasmuch as the UCSF/Storz and Symbion electrode arrays have fundamentally different designs. (The Symbion array and device are also known as the Ineraid array and device.)

The purpose of the present report is to describe the results obtained with both sets of patients. In particular, results from tests of consonant and vowel identification will be presented, as will results from the open-set tests of the Minimal Auditory Capabilities (MAC) battery (Owens et al., 1985).

PROCESSING STRATEGIES

Four channels of CA stimulation are used in both the UCSF/ Storz and Symbion cochlear prostheses. These stimuli are delivered either to alternate pairs of "radial bipolar" electrodes in the UCSF/Storz device or to the apical four (of six) monopolar electrodes in the Symbion device. The locations of active electrode sites are spaced 4.0 mm apart for both devices, and the depth of electrode array insertion into the scala tympani is similar for the two devices (between 20 and 25 mm for a full insertion). Results from modeling (e.g., Finley et al., 1990) and electrophysiological (e.g., van den Honert & Stypulkowski, 1987a) studies indicate that the spatial selectivity of neural excitation may be much greater for radial bipolar electrodes than for monopolar electrodes, at least for implanted ears in which nerve survival is good.

The basic functions of the CA processor are first to compress the wide dynamic range of input speech signals into the narrow dynamic range available for electrical stimulation and then to filter the compressed signal into individual frequency bands for presentation to each electrode. Typical waveforms of the CA processor are shown in Figure 2–1. The top trace in each panel is the input signal, which in this case is the word "bought." The other waveforms in each panel are the filtered output signals for four channels of intracochlear stimulation. The bottom left panel shows an expanded display of waveforms during the initial part of the vowel in "bought," and the bottom right panel shows an expanded display of waveforms during the final /t/. The lower panels in Figure 2–1 thus exemplify differences in waveforms for voiced and unvoiced intervals of speech.

In the voiced interval the relatively large outputs of channels 1 and 2 reflect the low-frequency formant content of the vowel, and in the unvoiced interval the relatively large outputs

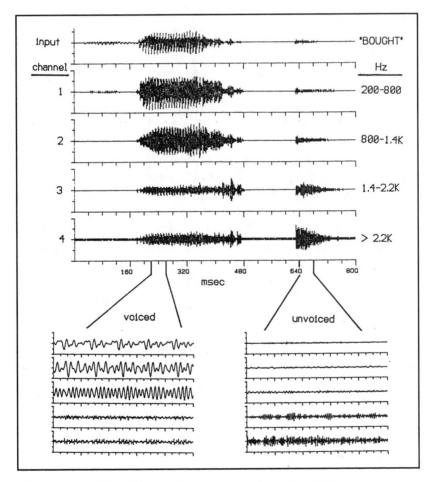

Figure 2-1. Waveforms of a compressed analog (CA) processor.

of channels 3 and 4 reflect the high-frequency noise content of the /t/. In addition, the clear periodicity in the waveforms of channels 1 and 2 reflects the fundamental and first formant frequencies of the vowel during the voiced interval, and the lack of periodicity in the output of any channel reflects the noise-like quality of the /t/ during the unvoiced interval. As has been described elsewhere, this representation of speech features can support high levels of open-set recognition for many (but not all) of the patients implanted either with the UCSF/Storz (Schindler & Kessler, 1987; Schindler et al., 1986, 1987) or the Symbion (Eddington, 1983; Gantz et al., 1988) prosthesis.

A concern associated with the use of multichannel CA processors is that of channel interactions (White et al., 1984). Simultaneous stimulation of two or more channels with continuous waveforms results in summation of the electrical fields from the individual electrodes. This summation can exacerbate interactions among channels, especially for patients who require high stimulation levels. Summation of stimuli from multiple channels also depends on the phase relationships among the waveforms. Because these relationships are not controlled in a multichannel CA processor, the representation of the speech spectrum may be further distorted by continuously changing patterns of channel interaction. A reduction of channel interactions might increase the salience of channel-related cues for implant patients.

The problem of channel interactions is addressed in the IP processor of Figure 2–2 through the use of nonsimultaneous stimuli. There is no temporal overlap between stimulus pulses, so that direct summation of electrical fields produced by different electrode channels is avoided. The energy in each frequency band of the input signal is coded as the amplitude of the pulses delivered to the corresponding stimulus channel. Distinctions between voiced and unvoiced segments of speech are represented by the timing of cycles of stimulation across the electrode array. In this particular IP processor stimulation cycles are timed to occur in synchrony with the detected fundamental frequency for voiced speech sounds and at the maximum rate (with one cycle of stimulation immediately following its predecessor) for unvoiced speech sounds. The timing of stimulation cycles for voiced and unvoiced intervals can be seen in the lower panels of Figure 2–2.

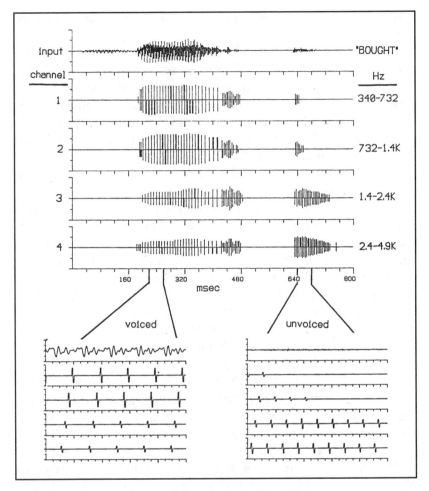

Figure 2-2. Waveforms of an interleaved pulses (IP) processor.

SUBJECTS

Six patients implanted with the UCSF/Storz electrode array (Loeb et al., 1983; Merzenich, 1985) and two patients implanted with the Symbion electrode array (Eddington, 1983) participated as subjects. Tests with the CA processor were conducted with each patient's clinical device, and tests with the IP processor were conducted either with computer simulations (Wilson & Finley,

1985) or with a real-time, microprocessor-based instrument (see QPR 2:7).

Each subject was studied for a one-week period in which: (a) basic psychophysical measures were obtained on thresholds and dynamic ranges for pulsatile stimuli, (b) a variety of IP processors (with different choices of processor parameters) was evaluated with tests of vowel and consonant identification, and (c) the best of these IP processors was further evaluated using a broad spectrum of speech tests.

It is important to note that certain attributes of these subjects favored the CA processor in comparisons of the CA and IP strategies. First, all eight subjects entered the study with substantial experience using the CA processor. The average experience with that processor exceeded one year of daily use. In contrast, experience with the IP processor was limited to that obtained in a 6-day period of testing a variety of processors with each subject. As discussed in detail elsewhere (Dowell et al., 1987; Tyler et al., 1986; Wilson et al., 1988c), such a disparity in experience might strongly favor the CA processor.

An additional factor weighing against the IP processor for the UCSF/Storz subjects was the use of a four-channel transcutaneous transmission system (TTS) for sending stimulus information to the implanted electrodes. The principal limitations of that system for IP processors were: (a) inadequate levels of voltage compliance for stimulation with short-duration pulses, (b) the small number of channels, (c) limited frequency response of each TTS channel (approximately 300 to 7000 Hz), and (d) lack of current control in the stimulus waveforms. Half of the UCSF/Storz subjects were further limited to fewer than four channels due to a mode of TTS failure (Schindler et al., 1986). Because results from preliminary studies with percutaneous cable patients indicate that optimized fittings of IP processors require at least six channels of stimulation and short-duration pulses (Wilson et al., 1988a, 1988b), it seems likely that the present fittings of IP processors were less than ideal for the UCSF/Storz subjects.

The parameters selected for the IP processors used by each of the six UCSF/Storz subjects (subjects 1 through 6) are presented in Table 2–1. The best fulfillments of the fitting criteria for IP processors (Wilson et al., 1988b) were obtained for subjects 2 and 6. Each had the use of all four stimulation channels, and the

Table 2-1. *Parameters of IP Processors for the UCSF/Storz Subjects**

Subject	Channels	Pulse Widths/ Phase (ms)	Pulse Sep. (ms)	Cycle Time (ms)
1	3	0.5	0.5	4.5
2	4	0.5	0.5	6.0
3	3	1.0	0.1	6.3
4	2	0.5	0.1	2.2
5	4	1.0	0.1	6.4
		1.0		
		0.5		
		0.5		
6	4	0.3	0.5	5.2
		0.7		
		0.3		
		0.3		

*All processors used symmetric biphasic pulses with the positive phase leading and with the channels stimulated in base-to-apex order. Stimulation cycles were presented at the fundamental frequency during voiced speech sounds and at the maximum rate (period equal to cycle time) during unvoiced speech sounds.

average pulse width across channels was 0.5 ms/phase or less for these two subjects.

In contrast, relatively poor sets of parameters had to be used for the remaining subjects. Subjects 1 and 3 had only three usable channels for pulsatile stimulation (with phase durations of 1.0 ms or less) and subject 4 only two. In addition, long pulse durations (1.0 ms/phase) had to be used for subjects 3 and 5.

With the exception of subject 4, each of the UCSF/Storz subjects had the same number of usable channels for the CA and IP processors. Subject 4 had the use of his apical-most channel for CA stimulation but not for IP stimulation. Low-frequency analog stimuli presented to that channel produced auditory percepts for subject 4 whereas 1.0 ms/phase pulses did not. The remaining two available channels for subject 4 were used in both the CA and IP processors.

Because the Symbion prosthesis has a percutaneous connector for direct electrical access to the implanted electrodes, implementations of IP processors were not constrained by the limitations of a TTS for the Symbion subjects. Therefore, a greater range of processor variations was used in the studies with those subjects. Processors evaluated in tests with the Symbion subjects (subjects 7 and 8) are described in Table 2–2. The two IP processors evaluated in the tests with subject 7 were identical in all respects except for the polarity of the leading phase of pulses delivered to the active electrodes within the scala tympani. In processor Rb1a the leading phase was negative, and in processor Rb1b the leading phase was positive. This manipulation was made to test the idea that an initially cathodic phase might produce a more localized field of neural excitation around the active electrode than the field produced with an initially anodic phase (see, e.g., Ranck, 1975). A more localized excitation field might in turn lead to an improved representation of frequencies in terms of the site of intracochlear stimulation.

Both IP processors used in the studies with subject 7 had six channels of stimulation and a relatively short stimulation cycle time of 3.0 ms. These favorable values were made possible by the direct percutaneous access to the implanted electrodes.

The choice of processors for the studies with subject 8 was in part guided by the observation with subject 7 that the processor with a positive leading phase of pulses delivered to the active electrodes (Rb1b) produced higher scores on the consonant and vowel identification tests than the processor with negative-leading pulses (Rb1a). Although this result was somewhat surprising, we decided to use positive-leading pulses for all processors evaluated with subject 8. In addition, all processors for subject 8 used 0.1 ms/phase pulses with 0.4 ms separating sequential pulses. These pulse parameters produced stimulation cycle times of 2.4 ms for the four-channel IP processor (4I) and 3.6 ms for the six-channel IP processors (1I, 1A, 1L, and 1B).

Table 2-2. *Parameters of IP Processors for the Symbion Subjects**

Subj	Proc	Chans	dur/ph	Pulses Sep	+/-	v/uv	Update Order v	Update Order uv
7	Rb1a	6	0.1	0.3	-	Y	6,5,4,3,2,1	6,5,4,3,2,1
	Rb1b	6	0.1	0.3	+	Y	6,5,4,3,2,1	6,5,4,3,2,1
8	4I	4	0.1	0.4	+	Y	4,3,2,1	random
	1I	6	0.1	0.4	+	Y	6,5,4,3,2,1	random
	1A	6	0.1	0.4	+	Y	6,5,4,3,2,1	6,5,4,3,2,1
	1L	6	0.1	0.4	+	Y	6,3,5,2,4,1	6,3,5,2,4,1
	1B	6	0.1	0.4	+	N	6,5,4,3,2,1	

*All processors used symmetric biphasic pulses with the indicated phase leading at the "active," intracochlear electrode. Except for processor 1B (the last processor in the list for subject 8), stimulation cycles were presented at the fundamental frequency during voiced speech sounds and at either the maximum rate (period equal to cycle time, processors 4I, 1I, 1A, and 1L) or randomly varied intervals (period between 3.0 and 7.0 ms, processors Rb1a and Rb1b) during unvoiced speech sounds. Stimulation cycles were presented at the maximum rate (278 Hz) during both voiced and unvoiced speech sounds with processor 1B.

35

Manipulations in processor design for the studies with subject 8 included: (a) the number of stimulation channels, (b) the order of channel updates within each stimulation cycle, and (c) the way in which pulses were delivered during voiced and unvoiced speech sounds. The number of stimulation channels was either 4 or 6. Processors 4I and 1I were identical in all respects except for the number of stimulation channels. Thus, comparison of results obtained with those two processors was useful for confirmation of previous findings of increased performance when the number of channels for an IP processor is increased from 4 to 6 (Wilson et al., 1988a, 1988b). In addition, processor 4I (the four-channel IP processor) provided a direct comparison with the four-channel CA processor of the Symbion prosthesis.

The order of channel updates was either from base-to-apex (4,3,2,1 and 6,5,4,3,2,1), as in the previous studies with subjects 1 to 7, or one designed to produce the maximum spatial separation between sequentially stimulated electrodes (6,3,5,2,4,1). The first order mimics the base-to-apex progression of neural excitation imposed by the traveling wave of basilar membrane vibrations in normal hearing, whereas the second order might be expected to provide reductions in channel interactions beyond those already provided with the use of nonsimultaneous stimuli. Processors 1A and 1L were identical in all respects except for the order of channel updates.

The final set of manipulations involved the way in which pulses were delivered during voiced and unvoiced speech sounds. As indicated before, IP processors generally have presented stimulation cycles at the fundamental frequency during voiced speech sounds and at either the maximum rate or randomly varied intervals during unvoiced speech sounds. In addition, the channel update order generally has been the same for stimulation cycles during both types of sounds.

Two variations of this general design were evaluated in the studies with subject 8. In the first variation the order of channel updates was randomized during unvoiced speech sounds. This variation was suggested by recent findings of the Melbourne group (Tong et al., 1989), which indicated that a randomized ordering of channel updates can produce a "scratchy" or "fuzzy" noiselike percept compared with "smoother" percepts produced with fixed orders of channel updates. Inasmuch as unvoiced speech sounds are noise like in character, a randomized update order during those sounds might improve the apparent fidelity of the representation and might also increase the salience of voiced/unvoiced distinctions. Processors 4I and 1I used randomized orders of channel updates during unvoiced speech sounds, and processors 1I and 1A were identical in all respects except that processor 1A used a fixed order of channel updates during unvoiced speech sounds.

The second variation of voiced/unvoiced coding was to eliminate that coding by presenting stimulation cycles at the maximum rate during both voiced and unvoiced speech sounds. This variation increased the "temporal density" of stimulation during voiced speech sounds, and also eliminated the need for the processor to make the voiced/unvoiced decision. Processors 1A and 1B were identical in all respects except that stimulation cycles were presented at the maximum rate (278 Hz) during both voiced and unvoiced speech sounds with processor 1B.

TESTS

Most of the results presented in this report are from tests of consonant and vowel identification. The speech tokens included in these tests are listed in Table 2–3. The first three tests (Iowa videotape test and two RTI tests, see below) were used in the

Table 2-3. Tokens Used in the Tests of Consonant and Vowel Identification

Test	Context	Phonemes
Iowa, videotape	/aCa/	b, d, f, g, dʒ, k, m, n, p, s, ʃ, t, v, z
RTI	/aCa/	d, k, l, n, s, t, ð, z
RTI	/bVt/	i, ɔ, o, u, ɪ
Iowa, videodisc	/aCa/	b, d, f, g, dʒ, k, l, m, n, p, s, ʃ, t, ð, v, z
Iowa, videodisc	/hVd/	i, ɔ, ɛ, u, ɪ, ʊ, ʌ, æ

studies with the UCSF/Storz subjects, and the last two (Iowa videodisc tests) in the studies with the Symbion subjects.

As indicated, two consonant tests were used in the studies with the UCSF/Storz subjects. The first was the one developed at the University of Iowa for measurement of audiovisual consonant perception (Tyler et al., 1983). A videotape of an adult male speaker provided the visual component of each presentation. The audio track of the tape provided an input to the UCSF/Storz processor or the real-time IP processor via direct connection. Each consonant was presented five times in a randomized list of stimulus presentations. After each presentation, the subject responded by pointing to one choice in a table of the 14 response options. No feedback on correct or incorrect responses was provided. Finally, the order of testing for the different conditions was designed to confer any benefits of learning on the CA processor. The order was first to test the IP processor plus vision, then vision alone, and then the CA processor plus vision.

A matrix of stimuli and responses was compiled for each subject and condition. The matrices then were summed across subjects for each of the conditions. These summed matrices provided the inputs to the analyses described in the Results sections of this report.

The second consonant test used in the studies with the UCSF/Storz subjects was one suggested by Earl Schubert (1985). The consonants are those with a nonlabial place of articulation and with high frequencies of occurrence in spoken English. Because consonants with nonlabial places of articulation are difficult or impossible to distinguish with speechreading alone, Schubert reasoned that a pragmatic approach to processor design and evaluation would be to concentrate on these important (but largely invisible) consonants.

The vowel test used for the UCSF/Storz subjects was designed to measure the ability to discriminate relatively large differences in the first and second formant frequencies among the selected vowels.

Single exemplars of the tokens in the last two tests (referred to as the RTI tests) were recorded and digitized from representative utterances of an adult male speaker. The digitized tokens were used as inputs to the UCSF/Storz processor (after appropriate digital-to-analog conversion) or the computer simulation of the IP processor. A single block of trials included three presentations of each of the consonants or five presentations each of the vowels in random order. Multiple repetitions of a token were available at regular intervals during each presentation. At the beginning of each presentation a display of response options was shown on a computer terminal used by the subject. The subject responded by touching a key on the terminal. Usually a response was entered after the first or second repetition. At the end of a block, the subject was given the overall percent correct score and an indication of the principal confusions made during the test. With few exceptions, no feedback was given during a block. In the exceptional cases (12 out of 137 blocks), feedback was provided across conditions so that no processor would receive an advantage over another.

The conditions for both RTI tests included vision only, CA processor plus vision, IP processor plus vision, CA processor only, and IP processor only. For the conditions with a visual component, speechreading information was provided by miming the tokens in synchrony with the stimulus repetitions. The same person (DTL) mimed the tokens for all subjects.

Blocks of trials were repeated as time permitted during the six days of testing with each subject. Because many other tests were being conducted during this same period (Wilson et al., 1988b, 1988c), the total number of trials for the RTI tests was not uniform across subjects and conditions. The actual totals are presented in Table 2–4. For the great majority of subjects and conditions, the number of trials with each token for the consonant test was 6 or more, and the number for the vowel test was 10 or more.

As with the Iowa videotape test, matrices of stimuli and responses were compiled for all subjects and conditions. Each RTI matrix was normalized to show the fraction of responses in each cell, and the normalized matrices were then summed across subjects for each of the conditions. The estimates of matrix responses calculated in this way reflect balanced contributions from all subjects for each condition while still using all of the available data.

As mentioned before, a different set of consonant and vowel tests was used in the studies with the Symbion subjects. The tests with the Symbion subjects were conducted with the newly available laser videodisc materials from the University of Iowa (Tyler

Table 2–4. *Number of Presentations of Each Token in the RTI Tests for the Indicated Subjects*

Test	Subject	Condition* V	CA + V	IP + V	CA	IP
Consonant	1	3	9	15	9	18
	2	6	6	9	3	9
	3	9	9	6	9	6
	4	6	6	9	6	12
	5	3	6	6	9	6
	6	6	3	6	3	6
Vowel	1	10	15	10	15	10
	2	10	10	30	15	15
	3	15	10	5	10	5
	4	10	10	10	10	10
	5	5	10	5	10	5
	6	10	10	10	10	10

*Abbreviations are V for Vision, CA + V for compressed analog plus vision, IP + V for interleaved pulses plus vision, CA for compressed analog only, and IP for interleaved pulses only.

et al., 1987). These materials provided: (a) multiple exemplars of consonant and vowel tokens spoken by both male and female speakers, (b) a larger, more representative set of consonants and vowels than were available in our previously-recorded RTI tests or in the older Iowa videotape test, (c) much better control of visual cues than in the RTI tests, and (d) computer control of videodisc playback, which greatly facilitated randomization of tokens and greatly reduced the time required to complete a block of trials with a given number of tokens. Although we were reluctant to use different sets of tests for the two groups of subjects, we felt that the advantages of the new tests (for the Symbion subjects) outweighed the obvious disadvantage of comparing results from different tests.

A single block of trials for the Iowa videodisc tests included five presentations of each of the 16 consonants or three presentations of each of the 8 vowels. After each presentation, the subject responded by identifying one of the tokens in a video display of response options. No feedback on correct or incorrect responses was provided. Blocks of trials were repeated as time permitted during the six days of testing with each subject. The total number of trials for subjects 7 and 8 are presented in Table 2–5. For all subjects and conditions, the number of trials for the consonant test was 10 or more, and the number for the vowel test was 12 or more. Aggregate matrices of stimuli and responses were compiled and summed for a variety of conditions (see Results) using the procedure outlined above for the RTI matrices.

In addition to the tests of consonant and vowel identification, the CA and IP processors were further evaluated for both the UCSF/Storz and Symbion subjects with an extensive series of speech perception tests. These additional tests included all subtests of the MAC battery (Owens et al., 1985) and connected discourse tracking with and without the prosthesis (De Filippo & Scott, 1978; Owens & Raggio, 1987). The results from the subtests of the MAC battery designed to measure open-set recognition will be discussed in this report.

CONSONANT AND VOWEL IDENTIFICATION, UCSF/STORZ SUBJECTS

To evaluate the patterns of confusions (and correct responses) from the tests of consonant and vowel identification, the combined matrix for the responses of all subjects for each condition was used as an input to the information transmission (IT) analysis of Miller & Nicely (1955). In this analysis the "relative transinformation" is calculated for selected articulatory or acoustic features of the phonemes in the identification tests. The relative transinformation score for each feature, expressed here as percent information transfer, indicates how well that feature was transmitted to the subjects. The consonant features selected for the present study were voicing (voice), nasality (nasal), place of articulation (place), duration (durat), frication (fric), envelope cues (envel), and visual cues (viseme). The vowel features were first formant frequency (F1), second formant frequency (F2), duration (durat), and visual cues (viseme).

Table 2-5. *Number of Presentations of Each Token in the Iowa Laserdisc Tests for the Indicated Subjects*

				Condition*	
Test	Subject	Processor	A	AV	V
Consonant	7	none			10
		CA	25	15	
		Rb1a	20	35	
		Rb1b	20	20	
	8	none			10
		CA	30	20	
		4I	20	10	
		1I	20	10	
		1A	20	15	
		1L	20	15	
		1B	20	10	
Vowel	7	none			12
		CA	24	12	
		Rb1a	24	24	
		Rb1b	12	12	
	8	none			18
		CA	15	12	
		4I	18	15	
		1I	15	15	
		1A	DNT	DNT	
		1L	DNT	DNT	
		1B	12	12	

*Abbreviations are A for Audition only, AV for Audition plus Vision, and V for Vision only.

42

The results from IT analysis of the Iowa videotape matrices (/p, b, m, f, v, ʃ, dʒ, s, z, t, d, n, g, k/, subjects 1 through 6) are presented in Figure 2–3. The open bars show IT scores for the vision-only condition, the bars with diagonal lines show the scores for the CA-processor-plus-vision condition, and the solid bars show the scores for the IP-processor-plus-vision condition. Note that the viseme and place features are transmitted equally well for all three conditions. The high score for place in the vision-only condition is indicative of the high redundancy between assignments for the place and viseme features. That is, a front (bilabial and labiodental) place of articulation usually can be distinguished from other places of articulation through speechreading alone (Owens & Blazek, 1985), and this ability is reflected in the choices for the viseme groupings. Thus, if subjects can distinguish the groups /p, b, m, f, v/, /ʃ, dʒ/, and /d, s, z, t, d, n, g, k/ through speech-reading, then the scores for both viseme and place will be high.

Other features that exhibit some redundancy with the viseme groupings are duration and frication. The relatively high

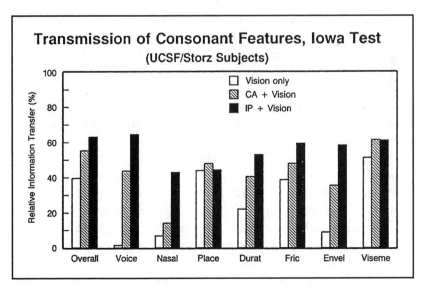

Figure 2–3. Relative information transfer of speech features for the vision-only and vision-plus-processor conditions of the Iowa consonant test (videotape version), UCSF/Storz subjects.

scores for these features with vision alone reflect this overlap. On the other hand, the scores for voicing, nasality, and envelope are all low for the vision-only condition. These features are invisible on the lips and have little or no redundancy with the viseme groupings.

The scores for both processor-plus-vision conditions demonstrate increases over the scores for the vision-only condition. Especially large increases are found for the features of voicing, duration, and envelope. In addition, the scores for overall information transfer are higher for the processor-plus-vision conditions.

Comparison of the scores obtained with the two processors indicates superiority of the IP processor for all features except place and viseme, where the scores are about the same. Scores for the IP processor are much higher for the features of voicing, nasality, and envelope.

The general finding of superior performance with the IP processor also is evident in the results from IT analysis of the RTI consonant matrices (/ð, s, z, t, d, n, k, l/, subjects 1 through 6). Results for the vision-only and processor-plus-vision conditions are presented in Figure 2–4, and results for the processor-only conditions are presented in Figure 2–5. In Figure 2–4 the open, diagonally lined and solid bars again show IT scores for vision only, CA processor plus vision and IP processor plus vision, respectively. In Figure 2–5 the stippled bars show IT scores for the CA processor only, and the vertically lined bars show the scores for the IP processor only.

For the conditions with a visual component (see Figure 2–4), high scores again are obtained for the viseme feature. Because the consonants in the RTI test all have a non-labial place of articulation, however, high scores for the viseme feature merely show that the groups /s, z, t, d, n/, /k, l/, and /ð/ can be distinguished. /ð/ and /l/ usually are visible through tongue protrusion and tongue flap, respectively, even though they have nonlabial places of articulation. Perception of these cues for /ð/ and /l/ can produce relatively high viseme scores for the consonants in the RTI test.

Another effect of the choice of consonants for the RTI test is to hold place of articulation essentially constant. All consonants except /k/ have a middle place of articulation (Singh & Black, 1966). Thus, the only distinction that has to be made to

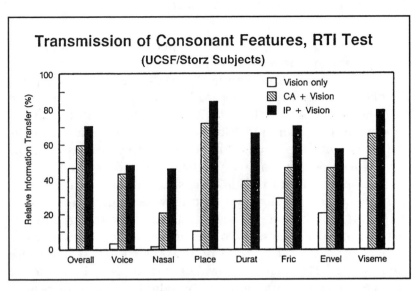

Figure 2–4. Relative information transfer of speech features for the vision-only and vision-plus-processor conditions of the RTI consonant test, UCSF/Storz subjects.

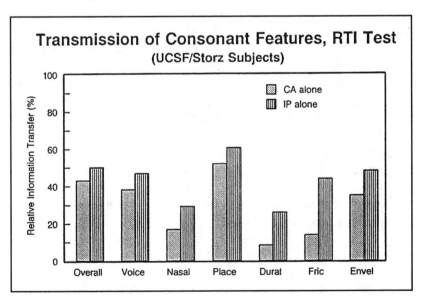

Figure 2–5. Relative information transfer of speech features for the processor-only conditions of the RTI consonant test, UCSF/Storz subjects.

produce high place scores is the one between /k/ (back place of articulation) and the remaining consonants. The low place score for the vision-only condition in Figure 2–4 reflects the fact that the place and viseme features are not redundant for the particular consonants of the RTI test. The scores for all other features (voicing, nasality, duration, frication, and envelope) are generally consistent with the scores for the vision-only condition of the Iowa videotape test (compare Figures 2–3 and 2–4.)

Comparison of results across conditions again shows increases over the vision-only scores when either processor is used with speechreading. The largest increases are found for the features of voicing, nasality, place, and envelope. The increases for voicing and envelope are quite similar to those found for the Iowa test. The increases for nasality and place, however, are not seen (place) or not as large (nasality) in the Iowa results. The difference in the increases for place can be attributed to the particular choice of consonants in the RTI test, as outlined above. The difference in the increases for nasality is one of degree in that increases are found for both tests, but the relative increase for the CA processor plus vision over vision only is not as large for the Iowa test compared with the increase for the RTI test. This difference between tests again might be a consequence of the different choices of consonants: the only nasal in the RTI test is /n/, whereas the Iowa test contains /n/ and /m/.

As with the Iowa test, large increases are found in feature transmission scores when the IP processor is used instead of the CA processor for the vision-plus-processor conditions. The IP processor produces at least some increase in the score for every studied feature, and substantial increases are demonstrated for the features of nasality, duration, and frication. The same pattern of increases is evident in the scores for the Iowa videotape test; however, the relative increases for the voicing and envelope features are greater with the Iowa test, whereas the relative increases for the duration and frication features are greater with the RTI test. These differences probably can be attributed to the differences in the consonant sets and to test variability. In all, the patterns of results from the Iowa and RTI tests are remarkably consistent. Both patterns demonstrate substantial gains over vision alone when either processor is used in conjunction with speechreading, and both patterns show superiority of the IP processor. In addition, the particular differences in feature scores found between conditions for one of the tests usually are found for the other test as well.

The results from the RTI test for the processor-only conditions (see Figure 2–5) mirror those reviewed above for the processor-plus-vision conditions (see Figure 2–4). Specifically, the IP processor again produces an increase in the score for every studied feature, and substantial increases are found for the features of nasality, duration, and frication. Moreover, for all features the ratios of the scores for the CA-processor-plus-vision and IP-processor-plus-vision conditions (see Figure 2–4) closely approximate the ratios for the CA-processor-only and IP-processor-only conditions (see Figure 2–5). These findings suggest that the IP processor provides additional cues which are utilized by the subjects in both the hearing-only and hearing-plus-vision conditions.

In contrast to the results from the Iowa and RTI consonant tests, the IT scores from the RTI vowel test (/i, ɪ, ɔ, o, u/, subjects 1 through 6) indicate superiority of the CA processor. These scores for the vowel test are presented in Figure 2–6, where the coding of the bars for the various conditions is identical to the coding used in Figures 2–3 to 2–5. Comparison of the IT scores between processors shows that the CA processor

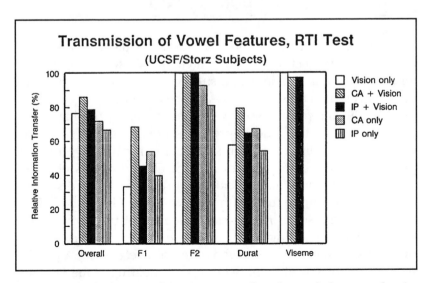

Figure 2–6. Relative information transfer of speech features for the RTI vowel test, UCSF/Storz subjects.

produces higher or equivalent scores for every feature. For the processor-plus-vision conditions higher scores are obtained for overall transmission, F1, and duration; and for the processor-only conditions higher scores are obtained for these features and F2. In the cases where equivalent scores are found (F2 and viseme features, processor-plus-vision conditions), ceiling effects may have masked true differences between the processors. A more difficult test (with, for example, more vowels and less redundancy between assignments for the F2 and viseme features) might provide a more sensitive detector of any difference between processors. In any event, the present results show that the CA processor is superior at least for the transmission of F1 and duration information.

The most general observations from the IT data reviewed above for the UCSF/Storz subjects are that: (a) the IP processor produces higher or essentially equivalent scores for every studied feature of the phonemes in the Iowa and RTI consonant tests and (b) the opposite is found for every studied feature of the phonemes in the RTI vowel test.

CONSONANT AND VOWEL IDENTIFICATION, SYMBION SUBJECTS

Percent correct scores for the processors evaluated in tests with the Symbion subjects (subjects 7 and 8) are shown in Figures 2–7 and 2–8. As in all previous and subsequent figures, the stippled bars represent scores for the CA processor only; the bars with diagonal lines represent scores for the CA processor plus vision; the bars with vertical lines represent scores for the IP processor only; and the solid bars represent scores for the IP processor plus vision. All scores are from the combined results obtained with the male and female speakers of the Iowa videodisc tests.

Results from the tests with subject 7 (see Figure 2–7) show that large increases in identification scores for both vowels and consonants, with and without vision, are obtained when either of the IP processors is used instead of the subject's own CA processor. Scores for vowel identification with hearing alone increase from 55.5% correct with the CA processor to 67 and 85% correct

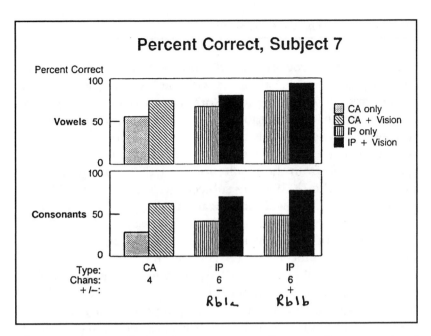

Figure 2–7. Overall percent-correct scores for tests of consonant and vowel identification, subject 7 (Symbion patient RB).

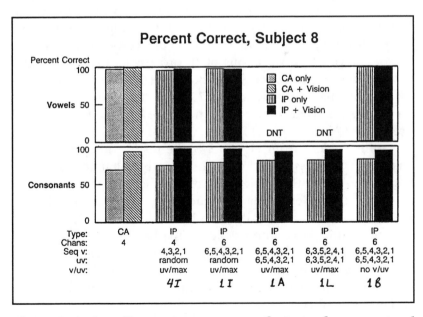

Figure 2–8. Overall percent-correct scores for tests of consonant and vowel identification, subject 8 (Symbion patient MP).

49

with the two IP processors, and scores for consonant identification increase from 28.5% correct with the CA processor to 41 and 48% correct with the IP processors. The increases in the scores for consonant identification are consistent with the increases in those scores found for the UCSF/Storz subjects. The sizable increases in the scores for vowel identification, however, are quite different from the results for the UCSF/Storz subjects. As noted above, the UCSF/Storz subjects generally obtained higher scores on tests of vowel identification with the CA processor.

An additional aspect of the results presented in Figure 2–7 is that the IP processor with the positive-leading pulses (Rb1b, last column) produced higher scores than the IP processor with the negative-leading pulses (Rb1a, middle column). This finding was counter to our expectation (based on Ranck, 1975, for instance) that the use of negative-leading pulses might improve the representation of speech signals via greater spatial specificity of neural excitation around the active electrodes.

Percent correct scores for subject 8 (see Figure 2–8) also demonstrate superior performance of the IP processor for consonant identification. The processors in Figure 2–8 are arranged in an order of increasing scores of consonant identification with hearing alone. Note that all scores are high (ranging from 69.5% correct for the CA processor to 83.5% correct for the last IP processor) and that all variations of IP processors produce higher scores than the CA processor. Among the IP processors, scores for the six-channel processors (79.5, 82, 82.5, and 83.5% correct) are somewhat higher than the scores for the four-channel processor (75.5% correct).

As is evident from Figure 2–8, the tested variations of six-channel IP processors did not produce large changes in performance. However, the subject did report that the processor with an update order designed to produce the maximum spatial separation between sequentially-stimulated channels (1L) sounded "clearer" and "more intelligible" than the otherwise identical processor with a base-to-apex order (1A). In addition, he volunteered that the "maximum rate" processor (1B, no voiced/unvoiced coding) was the most intelligible among all tested variations of IP processors.

The remaining scores in Figure 2–8 all approximate 100% correct. These scores therefore do not indicate superiority of any one processor over another.

Results from IT analyses consonant and vowel matrices from the studies with both Symbion subjects are presented in Figures 2–9 to 2–11. Aggregate matrices submitted to IT analysis were compiled by combining the data obtained from the tests with male and female speakers for each condition. In addition, aggregate matrices for the IP processor were compiled by combining the data obtained from all variations of six-channel IP processors (processors Rb1a, Rb1b, 1I, 1A, 1L, and 1B).

Feature transmission scores for consonant identification with vision only and with vision plus speech processor are presented in Figure 2–9. The pattern of results in Figure 2–9 is almost identical to the pattern shown in Figure 2–3 for the Iowa videotape test with the UCSF/Storz subjects. In particular, the scores for both processor-plus-vision conditions demonstrate large increases over the scores for the vision-only condition, and comparison of the scores for the two processors indicates clear superiority of the IP processor. As before, scores for the IP processor are much higher than those for the CA processor for the features of voicing, nasality, and envelope.

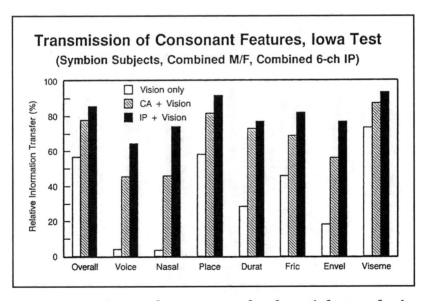

Figure 2–9. Relative information transfer of speech features for the vision-only and vision-plus-processor conditions of the Iowa consonant test (videodisc version), Symbion subjects.

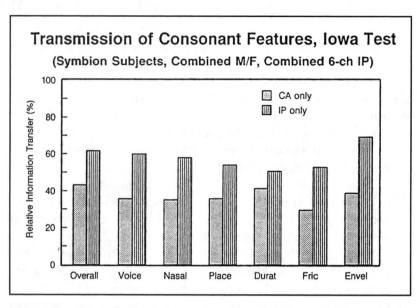

Figure 2-10. Relative information transfer of speech features for the processor-only conditions of the Iowa consonant test (videodisc version), Symbion subjects.

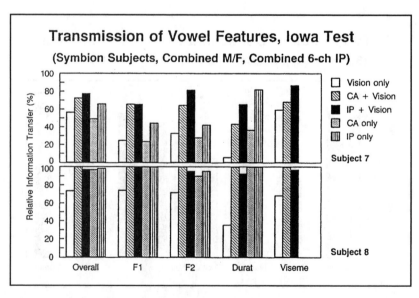

Figure 2-11. Relative information transfer of speech features for the Iowa vowel test, Symbion subjects.

52

Results from IT analyses of consonant matrices from the processor-only conditions are shown in Figure 2–10. As with the previous results from the RTI tests with the UCSF/Storz subjects (see Figure 2–5), increases in transmission scores are demonstrated for every feature when the IP processor is used instead of the CA processor. Here quite large increases are found for the Symbion subjects across all features except duration, where the increase is somewhat smaller. The relatively small increase in the score for duration is consistent with the relatively small increase in that score for the vision-plus-processor conditions shown in Figure 2–9.

Finally, results from IT analyses of the vowel matrices are presented in Figure 2–11. Because subject 8 scored close to 100% correct for all tests of vowel identification, ceiling effects would mask any true differences among processors for this subject. Therefore, the results for subjects 7 and 8 are shown in separate panels of Figure 2–11. As expected, the IT scores for subject 8 approximate 100% for all features when any of the speech processors is used. For subject 7, however, a clear superiority of the IP processor is demonstrated in the IT scores. In particular, substantially higher scores are found for the features of F2 and duration when the IP processor is used in conjunction with speechreading, and substantially higher scores are found for those features and F1 when the IP processor is used without visual cues.

To summarize the IT results for the Symbion subjects, we note that: (a) the IP strategy provides much higher transmission scores than the CA strategy for most consonant features, with and without vision, and (b) the IP strategy provides much higher transmission scores for all vowel features in the hearing-alone condition.

RESULTS FROM TESTS OF OPEN-SET RECOGNITION

The most difficult tests normally administered to assess the performance of patients with cochlear implants are tests of open-set recognition. Performance on these tests probably depends on a host of linguistic and cognitive skills that are not involved in tests of consonant and vowel identification. That is, the open-set tests help to evaluate the integration of segmental identification (consonants and vowels), prosodic cues and contextual information. The open-set tests thus provide complex measures of the representation of speech sounds at the auditory periphery and the interpretation of this representation in the central nervous system.

Results from the open-set tests of the MAC battery for the subjects and processors of this study are presented in Figure 2–12. The tests include those of spondee recognition (Sp), recognition of monosyllabic words from Northwestern Univer-

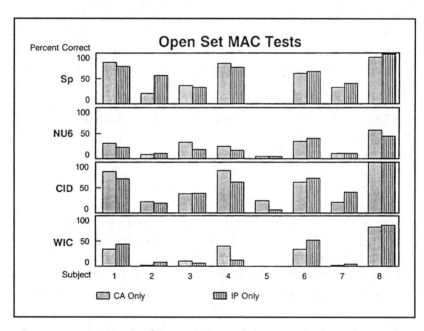

Figure 2–12. Results from subtests of the MAC battery designed to measure open-set recognition of speech. Abbreviations for the subtests are Sp for spondee recognition; NU6 for recognition of monosyllabic words from Northwestern University list 6; CID for recognition of everyday sentences from lists prepared at the Central Institute for the Deaf; and WIC for recognition of words in the context of sentences. Subjects 1 through 6 are the UCSF/Storz subjects, and subjects 7 and 8 are the Symbion subjects.

sity list six (NU6), recognition of everyday sentences from lists prepared at the Central Institute for the Deaf (CID), and recognition of single words in the context of sentences (WIC). Results presented for the IP processors for subjects 7 and 8 are those from processors Rb1a and 1L, respectively (see Table 2–2).

Comparison of the results across subjects for each of the open-set tests demonstrates that there are no significant differences between processors (paired $t < 1.51$ and $p > 0.10$ for all tests). However, substantial differences are found among subjects both in terms of overall performance and in terms of the scores for the two processors. Subjects 1, 4, 6, and 8 have excellent performance with both processors, whereas the remaining subjects have either moderate (subjects 2, 3, and 7) or poor (subject 5) performance with both processors. Between processors, subject 4 has higher scores with the CA processor for all four tests and subject 6 has higher scores with the IP processor for all four tests. Paired t comparisons between processors for these tests show that the CA processor is significantly better for subject 4 (paired $t = 3.25$; $p < 0.05$) and that the IP processor is marginally better for subject 6 (paired $t = 2.90$; $p < 0.10$). No significant differences are found between processors for the remaining subjects (paired $t < 1.67$; $p > 0.10$).

An additional aspect of the open-set results is illustrated in Figure 2–13. In this figure the results are arranged in a rank order of overall scores for each subject. As is obvious from this ordering, subjects who obtained high scores with one processor also did well with the other and vice versa. Thus, patient variables must have played a major role in the measured outcomes for the prostheses and processors of the present studies.

DISCUSSION

In the studies reviewed in this report, the CA and IP processors were compared in tests with six subjects implanted with the UCSF/Storz electrode array and with two subjects implanted with the Symbion electrode array. The tests included those of consonant and vowel identification and of open-set recognition.

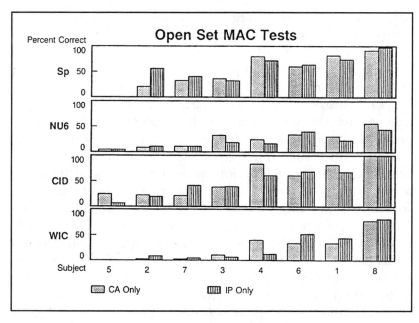

Figure 2-13. Results from the open-set tests (see Figure 2-12) arranged in a rank order of overall scores (average across tests) for each subject.

Large differences between processors were demonstrated in the results from the consonant and vowel tests. The IP processor produced superior results for consonant identification, with and without the addition of visual cues, for both sets of subjects. However, the increases in IT scores for consonant features were generally greater for the Symbion subjects.

In contrast to the consonant results, superiority in tests of vowel identification was split between the two processors for the two sets of subjects. The CA processor produced superior results for the UCSF/Storz subjects, whereas the IP processor produced superior results for Symbion subject 7 (Symbion subject 8 obtained perfect or nearly perfect scores for both processors).

The relatively large gains in performance obtained with the IP processor for the Symbion subjects may have been produced by more optimal fittings of that processor compared to those for the UCSF/Storz subjects. Specifically, the percutaneous connector of the Symbion prosthesis allowed the use of short-duration pulses and up to six channels of intracochlear stimulation. In contrast, limitations of the transcutaneous transmission system for the UCSF/Storz subjects both restricted the number of channels to four or fewer and precluded the use of short-duration pulses.

Although results from the consonant and vowel tests indicated clear differences between the CA and IP processors, results from the open-set tests did not demonstrate an overall superiority of one processor over the other. This latter finding is a little surprising in that consonant identification in particular usually is directly related to speech intelligibility (see, e.g., Denes, 1963; Miller & Nicely, 1955; Minifie, 1973). Thus, in the absence of other factors, one might expect that the IP processor would produce superior scores on the open-set tests. However, other factors may have affected the present results. These factors might include: (a) the huge disparity in the subjects' experience with the two processors and (b) the fact that good performance on the open-set tests probably involves a host of linguistic and cognitive skills that are not tapped in tests of consonant and vowel identification.

The one of these factors that may have favored one processor over the other is the disparity in experience. For the subjects of this study, experience with the CA processor approximated one year of daily use, whereas experience with the IP processor was limited to the tests conducted with that processor (among several) during a one-week period. As mentioned before, many previous studies have demonstrated large learning effects associated with the experience gained from using a prosthesis system. To the extent that such learning is not transferred to a new system (in this case, a new speech processor) (Dowell et al., 1987; Tyler et al., 1986), one might expect the disparity in experience to influence test scores in favor of the CA processor. In any event, equivalent or superior results on the open-set tests are found with the IP processor for seven of the eight subjects in the present study. This finding suggests: (a) that the IP processor could be applied to these seven subjects without any initial deficit and (b) that, with equivalent experience, the IP processor might emerge as the superior processor for most subjects.

CONCLUSIONS

Major conclusions from the results presented in this report include the following:

1. Differences among subjects account for a large proportion of the variance when the CA and IP processing strategies are compared with tests of open-set recognition.
2. However, individual performance can be highly sensitive to the choice of strategy, as measured either with tests of phoneme identification or open-set recognition.
3. The IP strategy generally provides superior identification scores, and may ultimately provide superior open-set scores, for a large majority of implant patients.

Acknowledgments. We thank the subjects of the described studies for their enthusiastic participation and generous contributions of time.

Chapter 3

NEW LEVELS OF SPEECH RECEPTION WITH COCHLEAR IMPLANTS*

Blake S. Wilson, Charles C. Finley, and Dewey T. Lawson

The development and application of cochlear prostheses have improved the lives of many deaf individuals. Nearly all patients enjoy remarkable gains in face-to-face communication when the implant is used as an adjunct to lip-reading, and some patients can recognize words and sentences with hearing alone. However, the ultimate goal of implant research, full restoration of speech perception without visual cues, has remained elusive. In this report we describe a combination of prosthesis elements that produces a close approximation to normal perception for an implant patient.

A cochlear prosthesis consists of: (a) a microphone to sense the acoustic environment, (b) a speech processor to transform the microphone signal into stimuli for direct activation of the auditory nerve, (c) a transcutaneous or percutaneous transmission

---

*From QPR 3:2, August 1, 1989, through October 31, 1989. (The original title for this excerpted section from QPR 3:2 was "New Levels of Speech Perception with Cochlear Implants.")

system for sending stimulus information to implanted electrodes, and (d) the electrodes. The electrodes for a multichannel implant usually are inserted as an array into the scala tympani. This places the electrodes close to residual auditory neurons. In cases of good nerve survival, use of different electrodes can produce shifts in the populations of excited neurons (Hartmann & Klinke, 1990; van den Honert & Stypulkowski, 1987a; Merzenich & White, 1977).

PROCESSORS

The purpose of the present study was to compare strategies for the speech processor in tests with an implant patient who had excellent performance with his standard, clinical device (Symbion subject MP). The strategies included the *compressed analog* (CA) processor used in the clinical device, and the alternative *interleaved pulses* (IP) and *supersampler* (SS) processors. All strategies made use of the tonotopic organization of the auditory nerve by stimulating electrodes near the apex of the cochlea to indicate the presence of low-frequency sounds and by stimulating electrodes near the base of the cochlea to indicate the presence of high-frequency sounds. However, other details of the stimulation patterns were quite different among strategies.

Waveforms of the three processing strategies are shown in Figure 3–1. The CA processor first compresses the wide dynamic range of input speech signals into the narrow dynamic range available for electrical stimulation of the auditory nerve. The compressed signal then is filtered into frequency bands for presentation to each electrode. Filtered output signals for four channels of intracochlear stimulation are illustrated in the figure. The inputs include segments of voiced (/ɔ/) and unvoiced (/t/) speech. During the voiced segment the relatively large outputs of apical channels 1 and 2 reflect the low-frequency formant content (spectral peaks) of the vowel, and the clear periodicity in these waveforms reflects the fundamental and first formant frequencies. During unvoiced speech the stimuli are aperiodic and have greater amplitudes in the higher (more basal) channels.

A concern associated with the use of CA processors is that of channel interactions (White, Merzenich, & Gardi, 1984; Wilson,

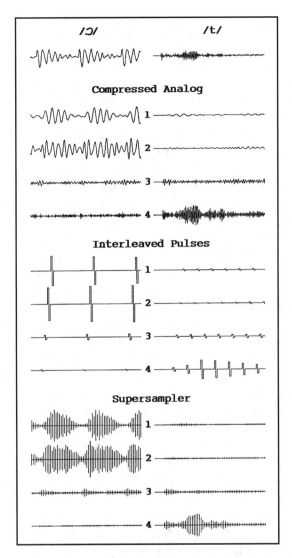

Figure 3-1. Waveforms of three processing strategies. Equalized (6 dB/octave attenuation below 1200 Hz) speech inputs are shown at the top and stimulus waveforms for each of the strategies at the bottom. The left column shows an input and stimulus waveforms for a voiced speech sound and the right column those traces for an unvoiced speech sound. Stimulus waveforms are numbered by channel, with channel 1 delivering its output to the apical-most electrode in the scala tympani. Center frequencies for the bandpass filters associated with channels 1 through 4 are 0.5, 1.0, 2.0, and 4.0 kHz, respectively. The time constants of the integrating filters for bandpass energy detection are 8.0 ms in the IP strategy and 0.4 ms in the SS strategy. The duration of each trace is 25.4 ms.

61

Finley, Lawson, & Wolford, 1988b). Simultaneous stimulation of two or more channels with continuous waveforms results in summation of the electrical fields from the different electrodes. This summation can exacerbate interactions among channels, especially for patients who require high stimulation levels.

The problem of channel interactions is addressed in the IP and SS processors through the use of nonsimultaneous stimuli. There is no temporal overlap between stimulus pulses, so that direct summation of electrical fields is avoided. The energy in each frequency band of the input signal is represented by the amplitudes of the pulses delivered to each electrode. The pulses shown in Figure 3–1 have a one-to-one correspondence with the root-mean-square (RMS) energies in each band. In actual applications of the IP and SS processors, pulse amplitudes are determined with a logarithmic transformation (Wilson et al., 1988a) of RMS energies to compress the dynamic range of those energies into the range of electrically evoked hearing.

Differences between the IP and SS processors are ones of rates of stimulation and of the way in which voiced and unvoiced segments are treated. In the IP processor distinctions between voiced and unvoiced segments are represented by the timing of cycles of stimulation across the electrode array. During voiced segments stimulation cycles are presented at the fundamental frequency of the speech sound, and during unvoiced segments stimulation cycles are presented either at a fixed, high rate or at randomly varied intervals.

In contrast, the SS processor presents stimulation cycles at the maximum rate (with one cycle immediately following its predecessor) during both voiced and unvoiced segments. In addition, the SS processor generally uses the shortest possible durations for pulses and intervals between pulses so that rapid variations in RMS energies can be followed ("sampled") by variations in pulse amplitudes for each channel.

METHODS

The processors of Figure 3–1 were evaluated with a variety of speech perception tests. Because the subject had excellent performance with his CA processor, only the most difficult tests normally administered to implant patients were used. These included identification of 16 consonants (/b, d, f, g, dʒ, k, l, m, n, p, s, ʃ, t, ð, v, z/) in an /a/-consonant-/a/ context (Tyler, Preece, & Lowder, 1987; see QPR 2:14) and the open-set tests of the Minimal Auditory Capabilities battery (Owens, Kessler, Raggio, & Schubert, 1985). In the consonant test multiple exemplars of the /aCa/ tokens were played from laser videodisc recordings of a male speaker and a female speaker. A single block of trials consisted of five randomized presentations of each consonant for one of the speakers. Ten blocks were administered for the CA processor and four blocks each for the IP and SS processors.[1,2]

The open-set tests included recognition of 50 one-syllable words from Northwestern University Auditory Test 6 (NU-6); 25 two-syllable words (spondees); 100 key words in the Central Institute for the Deaf (CID) sentences of everyday speech; and the final word in 50 high-context (WIC) sentences. In these tests single presentations of the words or sentences were played from cassette tape recordings of a male speaker.

In addition to the above, two tests were administered for further evaluation of the CA and SS processors. These were the recognition of key words in the low-context IEEE/Harvard sentences (Rabinowitz, Grant, & Eddington, 1988) and connected discourse tracking (De Filippo & Scott, 1978; Owens & Raggio, 1987). In the IEEE/Harvard test blocks of 10 sentences were played from the audio track of videotape recordings. Each block contained 50 key words, with the utterances made by a male or female speaker. Four blocks were administered for the CA processor and two blocks for the SS processor.[3] New sets of sentences, balanced for difficulty, were used for each block.

All tests were conducted with hearing alone, and all tests except tracking used single presentations of recorded material with no feedback on correct or incorrect responses. In the tracking test the subject's task was to repeat verbatim previously unknown

---

[1]An equal number of blocks was used for the male and female speakers.
[2]The blocks for the CA processor were spread throughout the testing period to evaluate the possibility of learning effects. Results from those blocks were highly repeatable and thus no evidence of such effects was obtained.
[3]An equal number of blocks was used for the male and female speakers.

paragraphs read by a trained speaker (Owens et al., 1987). For items not understood after the first presentation, various strategies such as repetition of phrases or words were used until the items were correctly repeated. The test score was calculated by dividing the number of words in four paragraphs by the time (in minutes) required to complete those paragraphs. Scores for the remaining tests were calculated as the percentage of correct responses. In addition, results for the consonant identification test were expressed as percent information transfer for articulatory and acoustic features that characterize the selected consonants (Miller & Nicely, 1955; Wilson, Finley, & Lawson, 1990b).

As mentioned before, the subject's own clinical device (the Symbion prosthesis) was used for the tests with the CA processor. The implementations of the IP and SS processors were selected by evaluating several variations of each with the consonant identification test. The variations with the best scores then were used for the full battery of remaining tests. Six channels of stimulation were used for the IP and SS processors[4,5] and four channels were used for the CA processor.[6] Detailed information on the clinical CA processor may be found in papers by Eddington (1980; 1983), and additional parameters of the IP and SS processors are presented in Table 3–1.

RESULTS

Results for the consonant identification test are presented in Figure 3–2. The percent correct and feature transmission scores demonstrate a clear picture of relative performance among processors. That is, despite four years of daily experience with the

[4]Results from previous studies with the present subject demonstrated a slight superiority of a 6-channel IP processor over a 4-channel variation of the same processor (see Chapter 2).

[5]Bandpasses for both processors were spaced along a logarithmic scale to span frequencies between 350 and 7000 Hz.

[6]The outputs of the IP and SS processors were delivered via isolated current sources to the six monopolar electrodes of the Symbion implant, and the outputs of the CA processor were delivered to the apical four of those electrodes.

Table 3-1. Parameters of the Interleaved Pulses (IP) and Supersampler (SS) Processors*

Proc	Pulses (μs) dur/ph	Pulses (μs) sep	RMS integrator (ms)	eq (Hz)	Channel sequence	rate (Hz)
IP	100	400	8.0	1200	6-5-4-3-2-1	278
SS	55	0	0.2	600	6-3-5-2-4-1	1515

*The pulse parameters include duration per phase (dur/ph) and separation between pulses (sep), and the remaining parameters include the time constant of the integrating filters for bandpass energy detection (RMS integrator), the frequency below which speech signals are attenuated for input equalization (eq), the sequence of channels for each stimulation cycle (channel sequence; channel 6 is the most basal), and the rate of pulsatile stimulation on each channel (rate). The rate for the IP processor is that used during unvoiced segments.

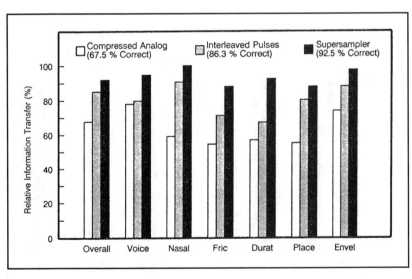

Figure 3-2. Relative information transfer for consonant features. The features include voicing (voice), nasality (nasal), place of articulation (place), duration (durat), frication (fric), and envelope cues (envel).

CA processor, the IP and SS processors immediately produce superior scores. Use of the IP strategy produces gains over the CA strategy for every feature except voicing (where scores are about the same), and use of the SS strategy produces gains over both the IP and CA processors for all features. Especially large increases shared by the IP and SS processors include those for nasality and place of articulation. In addition, substantial increases in the scores for voicing, frication, and duration are obtained when the SS strategy is used instead of the IP strategy.

Because scores for the SS processor approximate the ceilings of perfect performance, the increases shown in Figure 3–2 may in fact underestimate the relative superiority of that processor. In particular, the scores for overall percent correct, overall information transfer, voicing, nasality, duration, and envelope are 92% or higher.

The ranking of processors suggested by the consonant results is affirmed in the results from the remaining tests, presented in Figure 3–3. For the tests with results not at the ceiling of either extremely high (spondee recognition) or perfect (CID sentences)

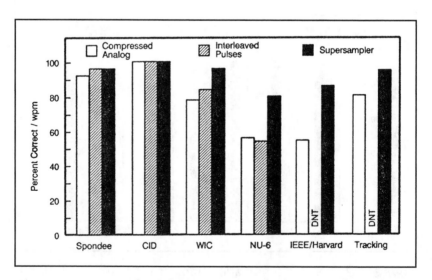

Figure 3–3. Scores from the open-set tests. The scores for the tracking test are given in words per minute, and the scores for the remaining tests are given as the percentage of correct responses.

scores, the IP processor produces scores that are equivalent or superior to those of the CA processor, and the SS processor produces scores that are clearly superior to those of both.

DISCUSSION

To our knowledge, the scores obtained with the SS processor exceed all published results for cochlear implants by wide margins. Also, these scores demonstrate a close approximation to normal speech perception with a cochlear implant.

The performance of the SS processor may be explained in terms of its design. The high rate of stimulation on each channel probably allowed the subject to perceive details in the temporal variations of band energies, whereas the use of nonsimultaneous stimuli eliminated a principal component of channel interactions. Indeed, results from the consonant test are fully consistent with these ideas. Feature transmission scores for nasality and place of articulation, which are largely represented by channel cues (Miller et al., 1955; Wilson et al., 1990b), are improved with the use of either the IP or SS processors. Scores for the remaining consonant features, which are largely or solely represented by temporal variations (Miller et al., 1955; van Tassel, Soli, Kirby, & Widin, 1987) are improved with the SS processor.

Finally, the electrode array and the subject probably played major roles in the outcome of the present tests. Results from psychophysical studies with this subject indicated that he: (a) could rank his electrodes in an appropriate tonotopic order according to pitch percepts produced by stimulation of each electrode, (b) had low levels of measured channel interactions for nonsimultaneous stimuli, and (c) had extremely low thresholds for a variety of stimuli. These results are consistent with a picture of excellent nerve survival (Gardi, 1985; Merzenich, Leake-Jones, Vivion, White, & Silverman, 1978; Merzenich et al., 1977; Pfingst, Glass, Spelman, & Sutton, 1985; Pfingst & Sutton, 1983; Shannon, 1983b). Such survival, in conjunction with the multichannel electrode array, may have been essential to the perception of the temporal and spatial representations provided by the SS processor.

In conclusion, results of this study demonstrate a combination of prosthesis elements that can bring a person from total deafness[7] to nearly normal perception of speech with hearing alone. Our present challenge is to produce similar results across a population of patients with varying degrees of nerve survival.

Acknowledgments. We are pleased to acknowledge the collaboration of R. D. Wolford, D. K. Eddington, and W. M. Rabinowitz in the studies with subject MP. We also are indebted to MP for his precise descriptions of speech percepts and for his enthusiastic participation.

---

[7]Prior to the implant, the subject's hearing levels at octave intervals from 125 Hz to 4000 Hz were 93, 113, 126, 131, 134, and 128 dB, respectively.

Chapter 4

EVALUATION OF ALTERNATIVE IMPLEMENTATIONS OF THE CONTINUOUS INTERLEAVED SAMPLING (CIS), INTERLEAVED PULSES (IP), AND PEAK PICKER (PP) PROCESSING STRATEGIES*

Blake S. Wilson, Charles C. Finley, and Dewey T. Lawson

*From QPR 3:3, November 1, 1989, through January 31, 1990. (The original title for this excerpted section from QPR 3:3 was "Evaluation of Alternative Implementations of the *Continuous Interleaved Sampler, Interleaved Pulses,* and *Peak-Picker* Processing Strategies.")

In an intensive series of studies with subject MP we evaluated four variations of interleaved pulses (IP) processors, four variations of continuous interleaved sampler (CIS) processors, and one variation of a peak picker (PP) processor. As described in Chapter 3, one variation of the IP processor and one variation of the CIS processor (the CIS processor was referred to as the "supersampler" processor in Chapter 3) were compared with each other and with MP's compressed analog (CA) processor using a full battery of speech tests. Results from those comparisons are presented in Chapter 3. The additional processor variations were evaluated with tests of consonant identification (all variations) and vowel identification (some variations). The purpose of this report is to present the phoneme identification results from all tested variations.

PROCESSORS

As mentioned in Chapter 3, results from psychophysical studies with MP indicated that he could rank the six intracochlear electrodes in his Symbion implant in an appropriate tonotopic order. All processors tested with him made use of this ability by stimulating electrodes near the apex of the cochlea to indicate the presence of low-frequency sounds and by stimulating electrodes near the base of the cochlea to indicate the presence of high-frequency sounds. However, other details of the stimulation patterns were quite different among processing strategies and their variations.

Waveforms of the CA, IP and CIS processors are shown in Figure 4–1. Briefly, the CA processor first compresses the wide dynamic range of input speech signals into the narrow dynamic range available for electrical stimulation of the auditory nerve. The compressed signal then is filtered into frequency bands for presentation to each electrode. As can be appreciated from Figure 4–1, CA stimuli contain many temporal details of the input speech signals. In particular, strong periodicities in the apical two channels reflect the fundamental frequency (F0) and first and second formant frequencies (F1 and F2) of the voiced speech sound

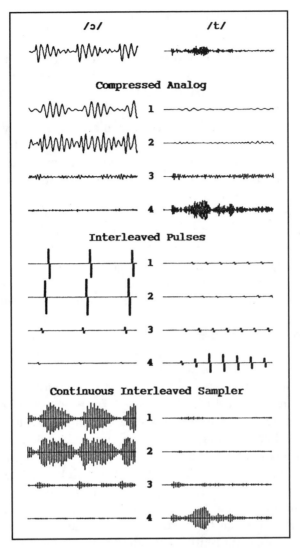

Figure 4-1. Waveforms of three processing strategies. Equalized (6 dB/octave attenuation below 1200 Hz) speech inputs are shown at the top and stimulus waveforms for each of the strategies below. The left column shows input and stimulus waveforms for a voiced speech sound and the right column those for an unvoiced speech sound. Stimulus waveforms are numbered by channel, with channel 1 delivering its output to the apical-most electrode in the scala tympani. Center frequencies for the bandpass filters associated with channels 1–4 are 0.5, 1.0, 2.0, and 4.0 kHz, respectively. The time constants of the integrating filters for bandpass energy detection are 8.0 ms in the IP strategy and 0.4 ms in the CIS strategy. The duration of each trace is 25.4 ms.

71

(left column). In addition, the onset of the unvoiced /t/ burst is represented in the stimuli of the basal channels (right column).

One concern associated with the use of CA processors is that of channel interactions (White et al., 1984; Wilson et al., 1988b). Simultaneous stimulation of two or more channels with continuous waveforms results in summation of the electrical fields from the different electrodes. This summation can exacerbate interactions among channels, and thus may reduce the salience of channel-related cues.

Another concern associated with the use of CA processors is that many of the temporal details present in the stimuli may not be perceived by implant patients. Most patients cannot perceive changes in the frequency of stimulation above a "pitch saturation limit" of about 300 Hz (e.g., Shannon, 1983a). Thus, whereas most patients may be able to perceive changes in F0, only exceptional patients will be able to make use of the F1 information contained in the stimuli for apical channels. It is highly unlikely that any patient would be able to perceive changes in F2 through temporal cues alone.

The problem of channel interactions is addressed in the IP and CIS processors through the use of interleaved nonsimultaneous stimuli. There is no temporal overlap between stimulus pulses, so that direct summation of electrical fields is avoided. The energy in each frequency band of the input signal is represented by the amplitudes of the pulses delivered to the corresponding electrode. The pulses shown in Figure 4–1 have a one-to-one correspondence with the root-mean-square (RMS) energies in each band. In actual applications of the IP and CIS processors, pulse amplitudes are determined with a logarithmic transformation (Wilson et al., 1988a) of RMS energies to compress the dynamic range of those energies into the range of electrically evoked hearing.

Differences between the IP and CIS processors include the rate of stimulation and the way in which voiced and unvoiced segments are treated. In the IP processor distinctions between voiced and unvoiced segments are represented by the timing of cycles of stimulation across the electrode array. During voiced segments stimulation cycles are presented at the fundamental frequency of the speech sound, and during unvoiced segments stimulation cycles are presented either at a fixed, high rate or at randomly varied intervals.

In contrast, the CIS processor presents stimulation cycles at the maximum rate (with one cycle immediately following its predecessor) during both voiced and unvoiced segments. In addition, this processor generally uses the shortest possible durations for pulses and intervals between pulses so that rapid variations in RMS energies can be followed by variations in pulse amplitudes for each channel.

Comparison of the three processors in Figure 4–1 illustrates different tradeoffs between representations of temporal and spatial (channel-related) information. The CA processor provides a high degree of temporal detail, but also may have a high level of channel interactions. The IP processor presents a relatively sparse pattern of stimulation with concomitant loss of temporal detail. However, this loss may not be significant for most implant patients (see above), and, if significant, may be more than compensated for by reduction in channel interactions through the use of nonsimultaneous stimuli. Finally, temporal details are restored in the CIS processor through rapid stimulation rates on each channel. Some patients may be able to make use of this information to perceive changes in F1 and to perceive the rapid temporal variations important for the identification of certain consonants (variations up to about 200 Hz, see Van Tassell et al., 1987).

A fourth tradeoff between representations of temporal and spatial information is embodied in the PP processor. In this processor the position of a peak in either the bandpass output or RMS energy output of a channel is signaled by the presentation of a pulse. Also, as in the IP and CIS processors, the exact timing of the pulses is adjusted so that there is no temporal overlap of stimuli across channels.

The design of the PP processor is illustrated in Figure 4–2. The upper panel shows speech inputs and the middle panel shows bandpass outputs for each of four channels along with the stimulus pulses derived from those outputs. In addition, the positions of the peaks in the bandpass outputs are marked by short vertical lines above each trace. The lower panel shows the stimulus pulses only.

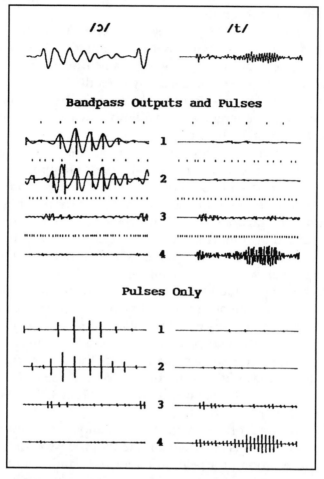

Figure 4–2. Waveforms of the peak picker (PP) processing strategy. Equalized speech inputs are shown at the top and two panels of processor waveforms below. The upper of these two panels shows the bandpass outputs and stimulus pulses for each of four channels. The locations of peaks in the bandpass outputs are marked with short vertical lines above each trace. The lower panel shows the stimulus pulses only. The duration of each trace is 12.25 ms.

In the particular variation of PP processor shown in Figure 4–2, a timer is advanced for each channel in a sequence of stimulation across the electrode array. At each time step a pulse is delivered if a peak occurred in the bandpass output between the previous and present time steps for that channel. The amplitude of the pulse is determined with the same logarithmic transformation used in the IP and CIS processors (i.e., the actual pulse amplitudes would be a logarithmic transformation of the amplitudes shown in Figure 4–2). A fixed time is reserved for each channel in the stimulation sequence whether or not a pulse is delivered. As indicated in Figure 4–2, this variation of the processor produces clusters of pulses at the F0 rate and individual pulses at the F1 rate for voiced speech sounds (left panels). Because the pulses must be presented nonsimultaneously, though, higher frequencies in the bandpass outputs are not followed with pulses at those frequencies. Notice, for instance, that many peaks are missed in channels 3 and 4, and that large offsets between the positions of peaks and subsequent pulses are seen in the waveforms of channel 2.

Alternative implementations of the PP processor are illustrated in Figure 4–3. The uppermost panel beneath the input signals shows the waveforms of the implementation just described ("Bandpass Outputs, Time for Each Channel"); the next panel down shows an implementation in which the time allocated for each channel is *not* used if a pulse is not delivered ("Bandpass Outputs, Channels Skipped"); and the bottom panel shows an implementation in which RMS outputs are used instead of bandpass outputs ("RMS Outputs, Channels Skipped"). As might be expected, the synchronization of pulses to peaks is greatly improved when channels without a pending pulse are skipped in the stimulation sequence.

A summary of waveforms for pulsatile processors is presented in Figure 4–4. All three processors use nonsimultaneous stimuli. Among processors, the CIS processor provides the greatest density of temporal information and the IP processor the least. The PP processor provides an intermediate level of temporal detail, with a representation of F1 in the apical channel(s). In addition, the PP processor presents different rates of stimulation on each channel, which might increase the salience of channel-related cues for some patients.

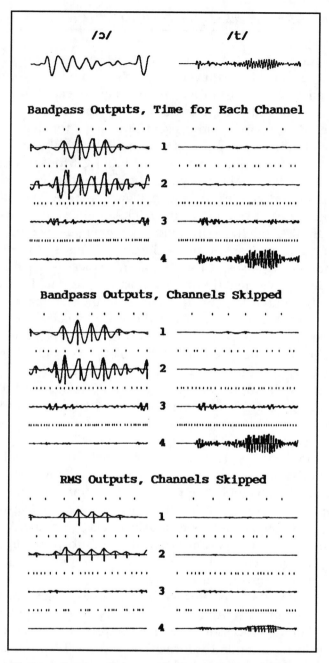

Figure 4–3. Various implementations of the peak picker processor. Equalized speech inputs are shown at the top and waveforms for the processor implementations in the three panels below. The duration of each trace is 12.25 ms.

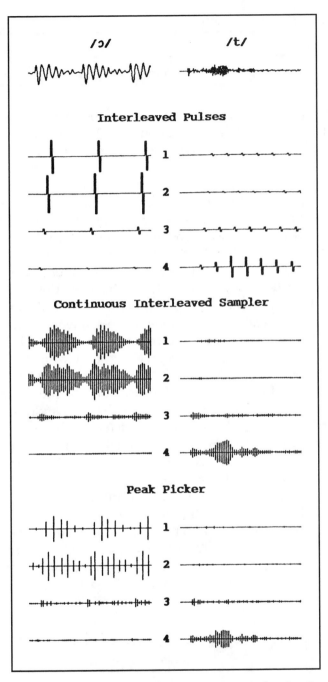

Figure 4-4. Waveforms of three types of pulsatile processors. Equalized speech inputs are shown at the top with stimulus waveforms for each of the strategies below. The duration of each trace is 25.4 ms.

PROCESSOR PARAMETERS

Parameters of all processors used in the tests with MP are presented in Table 4–1. The variations of IP processors included manipulations of the time between sequential pulses and pulse polarity. Processor MP1L presented pulses with the positive phase leading (which produced a stimulus with an initially *cathodic* phase at the intracochlear electrode) and with a separation of 400 μs. Processor MP1LC was identical to MP1L except that the pulse polarity was reversed. Processor MP1L0 was identical to MP1L except that the time between sequential pulses was reduced to zero. Finally, processor MP1LS presented its pulses simultaneously across channels for each stimulation cycle.

All IP processors of the present study used six channels of stimulation, and all delivered stimulation sequences at the fixed rate of 278 Hz during unvoiced intervals. Other variations of IP processors were evaluated in a previous study with MP, and the interested reader is referred to Chapter 2 for the results.

The tested variations of CIS processors included manipulations of the frequency ranges spanned by the bandpass filters, the rectifier used in the RMS energy detector (full wave or half wave), and the update order of sequentially stimulated channels. All CIS processors used six channels of stimulation. The rate of stimulation on each channel was 1515 Hz.

Only one implementation of the PP processor was tested with MP. This implementation used the design outlined in Figure 4–2, that is, with time taken for each channel whether or not a pulse is delivered. The PP processor used six channels of stimulation, with the same update order found to be best in the evaluations of the CIS processors (6-3-5-2-4-1).

TESTS

Tests of consonant and vowel identification were used to evaluate the processors of Table 4–1. These included identification of 16 consonants (/b, d, f, g, dʒ, k, l, m, n, p, s, ʃ, t, ð, v, z/) in an

Table 4–1. Parameters of the Interleaved Pulses (MP1Lx), Continuous Interleaved Sampler (RTSSx), and Peak Picker (RTPP1) Processors*

Proc	Channel update order	Pol	Dur/ ph	Sep	Time between pulse sequences	Round-robin time	Bandpass range	RMS integrator	Rect	eq
MP1L	6-5-4-3-2-1	+	100	400	400	3600	350–6500	25	FW	1200
MP1LS	6-5-4-3-2-1	+	100	**N/A**	**3400**	3600	350–6500	25	FW	1200
MP1LO	N/A	+	100	**0**	**2400**	3600	350–6500	25	FW	1200
MP1LC	6-5-4-3-2-1	**–**	100	400	400	3600	350–6500	25	FW	1200
RTSS2	6-5-4-3-2-1	+	55	0	N/A	660	350–7000	800	FW	600
RTSS3	6-5-4-3-2-1	+	55	0	N/A	660	**350–6000**	800	FW	600
RTSS4	6-5-4-3-2-1	+	55	0	N/A	660	350–6000	800	**HW**	600
RTSS8	**6-3-5-2-4-1**	+	55	0	N/A	660	350–7000	800	FW	600
RTPP1	6-3-5-2-4-1	+	55	0	N/A	N/A	350–7000	N/A	N/A	600

*The pulse parameters include polarity (pol), duration per phase (dur/ph) and separation between pulses (sep), and the remaining parameters include the frequency range spanned by the bandpass filters (bandpass range), the corner frequency of the integrating filters for bandpass energy detection (RMS integrator) and the frequency below which speech signals are attenuated for input equalization (eq). Entries for the last three measures are given in Hertz, and all remaining entries except polarity and channel update order are given in microseconds. Changes in parameters from one processor to the next are highlighted with **boldface type**.

/a/-consonant-/a/ context and identification of 8 vowels (/i, ɔ, ε, u, I, ʊ, ʌ, æ/) in a /h/-vowel-/d/ context. In both the consonant and vowel tests multiple exemplars of the tokens were played from laser videodisc recordings of male and female speakers (Tyler et al., 1987; see QPR 2:14). A single block of trials consisted of five randomized presentations of each consonant or three randomized presentations of each vowel for one of the speakers. The total number of presentations for the processors and tests of this study are presented in Table 4–2.

All tests were conducted with hearing alone, and without feedback as to correct or incorrect responses.

RESULTS

To evaluate the patterns of confusions (and correct responses) from the tests of consonant and vowel identification, matrices of

Table 4–2. Number of Presentations of Each Token in the Tests of Consonant and Vowel Identification

Processor	Consonants		Vowels	
	M	F	M	F
Symbion (CA)	25	25	9	6
MP1L	5			
MP1LS	10	10	9	9
MP1L0	10	10	9	6
MP1LC	5			
RTSS2	5			
RTSS3	5			
RTSS4	5			
RTSS8	10	10	9	9
RTPP1	10	10	6	6

responses for each processor were used as inputs to the information transmission (IT) analysis of Miller and Nicely (1955). In this analysis the "relative transinformation" is calculated for selected articulatory or acoustic features of the phonemes in the identification tests. The relative transinformation score for each feature, expressed here as percent information transfer, indicates how well that feature was transmitted to the subject. The consonant features selected for the present study were voicing (voice), nasality (nasal), frication (fric), duration (dur), place of articulation (place), and envelope cues (envel). The vowel features were first formant frequency (F1), second formant frequency (F2), and duration.

Results for the five processors evaluated with both consonant and vowel tests, and with male and female speakers, are presented in Figures 4–5 and 4–6. The consonant results (Figure 4–5) show clear differences among processors. In particular, comparison of scores for the CA (Symbion), IP (MP1L0) and CIS (RTSS8) processors demonstrate superior performance for the latter two processors despite the subject's four years of daily experience with his Symbion processor. Use of the IP processor produces gains over the CA processor for every feature except voicing (where scores are about the same), and use of the CIS processor produces gains over both the IP and CA processors for all features. In addition, substantial increases in the scores for voicing, frication, and duration are obtained when the CIS processor is used instead of the IP processor.

The remaining scores in Figure 4–5 are those for the "simultaneous pulses" IP processor (MP1LS) and the PP processor (RTPP1). As might be expected from the previous discussion on channel interactions, use of the simultaneous pulses processor produces large decrements in the scores obtained with the otherwise identical IP processor (MP1L0). Especially large decreases are found for overall transmission, nasality, frication, duration, and place of articulation.

In contrast to the simultaneous pulses processor, the PP processor produced high IT scores. Indeed, the overall performance of the PP processor is roughly comparable to that of the CIS processor. Scores for voicing, duration, and envelope are all somewhat higher for the PP processor, and scores for nasality and place of articulation are lower for PP processor.

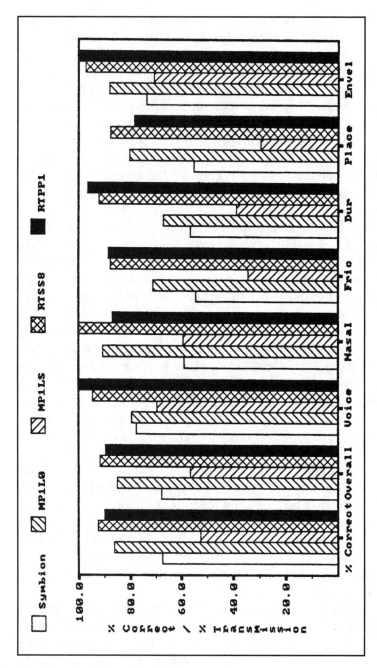

Figure 4–5. Relative information transfer of consonant features for subject MP with various processors, hearing alone, combined male and female speakers. The features include voicing (voice), nasality (nasal), frication (fric), duration (dur), place of articulation (place), and envelope cues (envel).

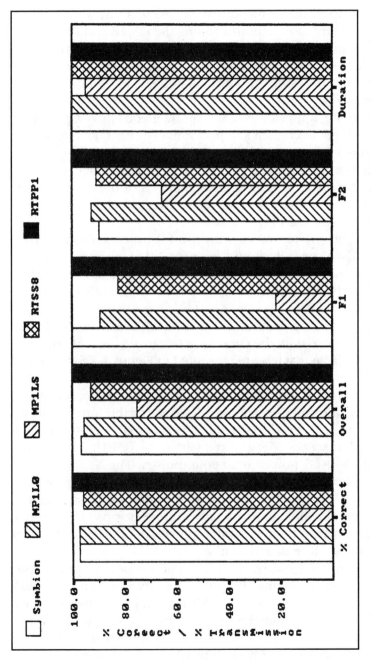

Figure 4–6. Relative information transfer of vowel features for subject MP, for the same processors shown in Figure 4–5, hearing alone, combined male and female speakers. The features include first formant (F1), second formant (F2), and duration.

In comparison to the consonant results, the vowel scores (Figure 4–6) are more uniform among the CA, IP, and CIS processors. The three processors produce identical or nearly-identical scores for percent correct, overall transmission, F2, and duration. The CA processor produces a somewhat higher score for F1, however.

As before, application of the simultaneous pulses processor produces large decrements in performance. Most notable are the reductions in the scores for F1 and F2.

The best performance on the vowel test was obtained with the PP processor. In fact, all presentations of the vowel tokens by both male and female speakers were perfectly identified by MP when using the PP processor.

Although performance with the PP processor was perfect for the vowel test, it should be noted that performance was nearly perfect with the CA, IP, and CIS processors. Thus, ceiling effects might have masked differences that may exist among these processors.

The remaining processors listed in Tables 4–1 and 4–2 were briefly evaluated with the consonant test using the male speaker. The results from that test are presented in Figure 4–7 for all tested variations of IP processors (including MP1L0 and MP1LS) and in Figure 4–8 for all tested variations of CIS processors (including RTSS8). As indicated in Figure 4–7, three of the four variations of IP processors produced similar percent correct and overall transmission scores. These three variations (MP1L, MP1L0, and MP1LC) all used nonsimultaneous pulses. The variation with simultaneous stimulation across channels (MP1LS) produced markedly lower percent correct and overall transmission scores. In addition, the simultaneous pulses processor produced much lower scores than the other three processors for the features of duration and place of articulation.

In examining the results for the three best IP processors, it appears that changing the pulse polarity from positive leading (MP1L) to negative leading (MP1LC) improves the transmission of fricative information, but degrades the transmission of nasality and duration information. In addition, reducing the time between pulses to zero (MP1L0) produces slight increases in the scores for voicing, nasality, and place of articulation.

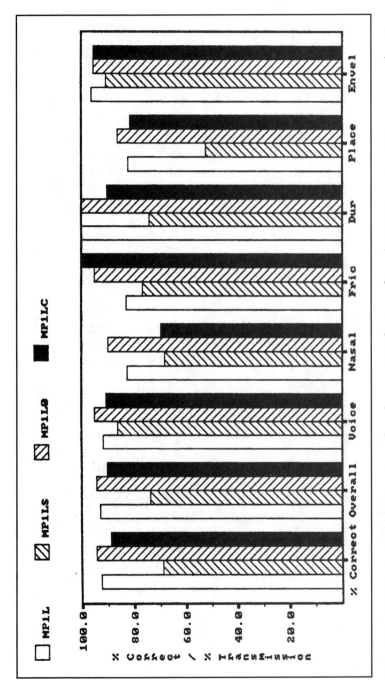

Figure 4–7. Relative information transfer of consonant features for subject MP; various IP processors, hearing alone, male speaker.

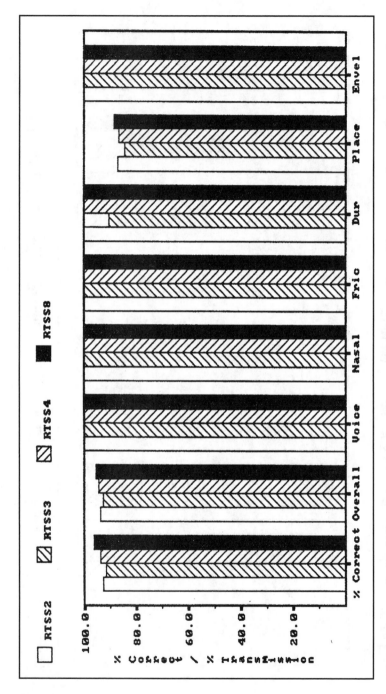

Figure 4–8. Relative information transfer of consonant features for subject MP; various CIS processors, hearing alone, male speaker.

Finally, all tested variations of CIS processors (Figure 4–8) produced similar results. The only clear difference among these processors was a small decrement in the transmission of duration information for the processor with the half-wave rectifier in its RMS energy detectors (RTSS4). All four CIS processors produced perfect transmission scores for voicing, nasality, frication, and envelope cues.

DISCUSSION

Three types of pulsatile processors were compared with each other and with the CA processor of the Symbion device using tests of consonant and vowel identification. With the exception of the "simultaneous pulses" IP processor, all types and variations of the pulsatile processors produced large gains over the CA processor in the transmission of consonant information. In particular, the IP, CIS, and PP processors all produced increases in the IT scores for every consonant feature. Especially large increases shared by all three pulsatile processors included those for nasality and place of articulation. In addition, the CIS and PP processors produced substantially higher scores for voicing, frication, duration, and envelope than did the IP processor.

These results may be understood in terms of processor design. As discussed above, the use of nonsimultaneous stimuli eliminates a principal component of channel interactions. This, in turn, might be expected to increase the salience of channel-related cues and to increase the transmission of consonant features differentiated by those cues. Two such features are nasality and place (Miller & Nicely, 1955; Wilson et al., 1990b), and IT scores for these features are improved by each of the pulsatile processors using nonsimultaneous stimuli.

An additional aspect of processor design is the representation of temporal events. Both the CIS and PP processors present more temporal information than the IP processor, and both produce higher IT scores for the remaining consonant features, which are largely or solely represented by temporal variations in the speech signal (Miller & Nicely, 1955; Van Tassell et al., 1987).

The relatively poor showing of the CA processor in the transmission of temporal information may have been a consequence of severe channel interactions. Because the phase relationships among channels of stimulation are not controlled in the CA processor, a continuously changing (and unpredictable) pattern of channel interaction is produced during ongoing speech. It is highly likely that these changing patterns distort the representation of temporal cues in the neural responses to CA stimuli.

In addition to the problem of continuously varying channel interactions, the CA processor also presents much higher frequencies of stimulation in the basal channels than any of the tested pulsatile processors. Both psychophysical (Shannon, 1983a) and single-unit (Javel, 1990; Moxon, 1971; Parkins, 1986; van den Honert & Stypulkowski, 1987b) studies have demonstrated strong adaptation to high-frequency stimuli. Thus, use of such stimuli in the CA processor could produce temporal distortions in the representation of sustained high-frequency components in speech, a problem that may be avoided with the relatively low frequencies of stimulation used in the pulsatile processors. A faithful representation of sustained high-frequency components would allow discrimination of the long-duration consonants (/ʃ, s, z/) from the remaining consonants in our test. This discrimination would improve the IT score for the duration feature. Also, the IT scores for envelope cues and frication might be enhanced by a representation that maintained perception of sustained high-frequency sounds.

The fact that high frequencies of stimulation can produce adaptation in the nerve suggests a reason for caution in the general application of CIS processors. That is, even though the frequencies used in the CIS processor are substantially lower than the maximum frequencies of the CA processor, the CIS frequencies may be high enough to produce at least some adaptation in some patients. In our experience, patients who exhibit various presumptive signs of poor nerve survival, such as high thresholds, narrow dynamic ranges, and high channel interactions, also exhibit loudness adaptation to sustained high-frequency stimuli. Therefore, these patients might be best served with the IP processor, which presents pulses at rates that do not produce loudness adaptation (e.g., rates below 300 Hz).

An intermediate approach with respect to adaptation would be to use the PP processor. Its rates of stimulation are generally lower than those of the CIS processor and higher than those of the IP processor. Thus, the PP processor may provide temporal details while still not producing loudness adaptation. The findings to date of improvements in the transmission of duration, envelope, and voicing features with the PP processor support this concept.

Finally, improved transmission of vowel features with the PP processor is consistent with an improved temporal representation in the apical channels. In particular, pulses are presented at the rate of F1 in those channels during voiced speech sounds. The large increase in F1 transmission obtained with the PP processor (over that obtained with the IP and CIS processors) may reflect perception of frequency changes in the apical channels.

FUTURE DIRECTIONS

As indicated in the Discussion, different processing strategies may be best for different patients. A major goal of future studies will be to evaluate the CIS and PP processors across a broad population of subjects, and to continue our comparative studies of the CA and IP processors with those same subjects.

Acknowledgments. We are pleased to acknowledge the collaboration of R. D. Wolford, D. K. Eddington, and W. M. Rabinowitz in the studies with subject MP. We also are indebted to MP for his precise descriptions of speech percepts and for his enthusiastic participation.

Chapter 5

COMPARISON OF COMPRESSED ANALOG (CA) AND CONTINUOUS INTERLEAVED SAMPLING (CIS) PROCESSORS IN TESTS WITH SEVEN INERAID SUBJECTS*

Blake S. Wilson, Dewey T. Lawson, and Charles C. Finley

In intensive studies with subject MP (SR2) we evaluated four variations of interleaved pulses (IP) processors, four variations of continuous interleaved sampler (CIS) processors, and one variation of a peak picker (PP) processor. As described in Chapter 3,

---

*From QPR 3:4, February 1, 1990, through April 30, 1990. (The original title for this excerpted section from QPR 3:4 was "Comparison of *Compressed Analog* and *Continuous Interleaved Sampler* Processors in Tests with Symbion Subjects.")

one variation of the IP processor and one variation of the CIS processor (referred to as the "supersampler" processor in Chapter 3) were compared with each other and with MP's compressed analog (CA) processor using a full battery of speech tests. Results from those comparisons indicated superiority of the CIS processor for MP. Indeed, unprecedented levels of speech recognition with a cochlear implant were obtained with that processor and subject.

To evaluate the generality of the results with MP, we initiated a series of studies with seven additional subjects implanted with the Symbion device. (The Symbion device also is known as the Ineraid device.) The purpose of this report is to provide interim results, on comparison of the CA and CIS processors, for the first seven subjects (including MP) in the series.

METHODS

Processors

Waveforms of the CA and CIS processors are shown in Figure 5–1. Briefly, the CA processor first compresses the wide dynamic range of input speech signals into the narrow dynamic range available for electrical stimulation of the auditory nerve. The compressed signal then is filtered into frequency bands for presentation to each electrode. As can be appreciated from Figure 5–1, CA stimuli contain many temporal details of the input speech signals. For example, in the left column strong periodicities in the apical two channels reflect the fundamental frequency (F0) and first and second formant frequencies (F1 and F2) of the voiced speech sound. The onset of an unvoiced /t/ burst is represented in the stimuli of the basal channels, as may be seen in the right column.

One concern associated with the use of CA processors is that of channel interactions (White et al., 1984; Wilson et al., 1988b). Simultaneous stimulation of two or more channels with continuous waveforms results in summation of the electrical fields from the different electrodes. This summation can exacerbate interactions among channels, and thus may reduce the salience of channel-related cues.

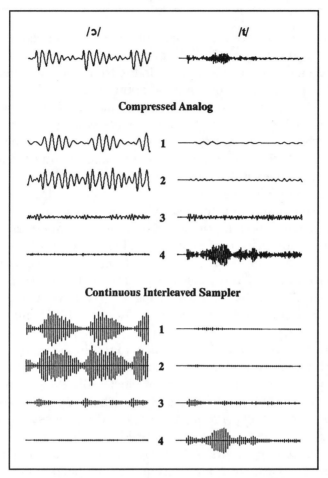

Figure 5-1. Waveforms of the CA and CIS processors. Equalized (6 dB/octave attenuation below 1200 Hz) speech inputs are shown at the top and stimulus waveforms for each of the processors below. The left column shows input and stimulus waveforms for a voiced speech sound and the right column those for an unvoiced speech sound. Stimulus waveforms are numbered by channel, with channel 1 delivering its output to the apical-most electrode in the scala tympani. Center frequencies for the bandpass filters associated with channels 1 through 4 are 0.5, 1.0, 2.0, and 4.0 kHz, respectively. The time constant of the integrating filters for bandpass energy detection in the CIS processor is 0.4 ms. The duration of each trace is 25.4 ms.

Another concern is that many of the temporal details present in CA stimuli may not be perceived by implant patients. Most patients cannot perceive changes in the frequency of stimulation above a "pitch saturation limit" of about 300 Hz (e.g., Shannon, 1983a). Thus, although most patients may be able to perceive changes in F0, only exceptional patients will be able to make use of the F1 information contained in the stimuli for apical channels. It is highly unlikely that any patient would be able to perceive changes in F2 through temporal cues alone.

The problem of channel interactions is addressed in the CIS processor through the use of interleaved nonsimultaneous stimuli. There is no temporal overlap between stimulus pulses, so that direct summation of electrical fields is avoided. The energy in each frequency band of the input signal is represented by the amplitudes of the pulses delivered to the corresponding electrode. The pulses shown in Figure 5–1 have a one-to-one correspondence with the root-mean-square (RMS) energies in each band. In actual applications of the CIS processor, pulse amplitudes are determined with a logarithmic or power-law transformation of RMS energies to compress the dynamic range of those energies into the range of electrically evoked hearing.

In contrast to the IP processor described in previous reports (Wilson et al., 1988a, 1988b, 1990b), the CIS processor presents stimulation cycles at a constant, rapid rate during both voiced and unvoiced segments. In addition, this processor generally uses brief pulses, with one presented immediately after its predecessor, so that rapid variations in RMS energies can be followed by variations in pulse amplitudes for each channel. Some patients may be able to make use of this information to perceive changes in F1 and to perceive the rapid temporal variations important for the identification of certain consonants (variations up to about 200 Hz, see Van Tassell et al., 1987).

Subjects

Subjects for this series were selected on the basis of performance with the Symbion device. In particular, we identified (with the help of others, see Acknowledgments) a population of subjects with levels of performance similar to MP's. As indicated in the Results section, all subjects had scores of 30% or higher on the NU-6 test of monosyllabic word recognition with their CA processors. Such high scores are rare among implant patients.

Each subject was studied for a one-week period in which (a) basic psychophysical measures were obtained on thresholds and dynamic ranges for pulsatile stimuli, (b) a variety of CIS processors (with different choices of processor parameters) were evaluated with tests of consonant and vowel identification, and (c) performance with one or two CIS processors and the clinical CA processor was documented with additional tests.

Tests

The CA and CIS processors were evaluated with a variety of speech perception tests. Because the subjects had excellent performance with both strategies, only results from the most difficult sound-alone tests are reported here. These included identification of 16 consonants (/b, d, f, g, dʒ, k, l, m, n, p, s, ʃ, t, ð, v, z/) in an /a/-consonant-/a/ context; identification of 8 vowels (/i, ɔ, ɛ, u, ɪ, ʊ, ʌ, æ/) in a /h/-vowel-/d/ context; the segmental and open-set tests of the Minimal Auditory Capabilities (MAC) battery (Owens et al., 1985); and connected discourse tracking (De Filippo & Scott, 1978; Owens & Raggio, 1987).

In both the consonant and vowel tests multiple exemplars of the tokens were played from laser videodisc recordings of male and female speakers (Tyler et al., 1987; see QPR 2:14). A single block of trials consisted of five randomized presentations of each consonant or three randomized presentations of each vowel for one of the speakers. At least two blocks were administered for each speaker, processor and subject in the consonant tests, and at least three blocks were administered for each speaker, processor and subject in the vowel tests.

The segmental tests included identification of the word containing the correct vowel, initial consonant (Init Cons), or final consonant (Fnl Cons) among four options for each test item. The vowel test contained 60 items, the initial consonant test 64 items, and the final consonant test 52 items.

The open-set tests included recognition of 50 one-syllable words from Northwestern University Auditory Test 6 (NU-6); 25 two-syllable words (spondees); 100 key words in the Central Institute for the Deaf (CID) sentences of everyday speech; and the final word in 50 sentences from the Speech Perception in Noise (SPIN) test. In both the segmental and open-set tests single presentations of the words or sentences were played from cassette tape recordings of a male speaker.

In the tracking test the subject's task was to repeat verbatim previously unknown paragraphs read by a trained speaker (Owens & Raggio, 1987). For items not understood after the first presentation, various strategies such as repetition of phrases or words were used until the items were correctly repeated.

All tests were conducted with hearing alone, and all tests except tracking used single presentations of recorded material with no feedback as to correct or incorrect responses. The score for the tracking test was calculated by dividing the number of words in four paragraphs by the time taken to complete those paragraphs. Scores for the remaining tests were calculated as the percentage of correct responses. In addition, results for the consonant identification test were expressed as percent information transfer for articulatory and acoustic features that characterize the selected consonants (Miller & Nicely, 1955; Wilson et al., 1990b).

Processor Parameters

Each subject's own clinical device (the Symbion prosthesis) was used for the tests with the CA processor. Four channels of stimulation were used for all subjects. Detailed descriptions of the clinical CA processor may be found in papers by Eddington (1980, 1983).

Selection of parameters for the CIS processors was guided by results from preliminary tests of consonant identification, primarily with the male speaker. The final choices for each subject are presented in Table 5–1. The processors for all subjects used pulses with durations of 102 μs/phase or less, 5 or 6 channels of stimulation, and rates of stimulation above 800 Hz on each channel. In addition, the order of channels in the stimulation cycle was chosen to maximize the spatial separation between sequentially stimulated channels. We expected that this "staggered order" might produce a further reduction in channel interactions.

As indicated in Table 5-1, one CIS processor was evaluated with a full battery of speech tests for subjects SR2-4, SR6 and SR7, and two processors were evaluated for subjects SR5 and SR8. With the exception of the tracking test for subject SR4, all tests were conducted with the first processors listed for each subject. Tests with the second processor for subject SR5 were limited to the segmental and open-set tests of the MAC battery, and tests with the second processor for subject SR8 were limited to those tests and tracking.

Evaluation of Practice and Learning Effects

Because the initial tests with the CA processor preceded those for the CIS processor, we were concerned that practice or learning effects might favor the CIS processor in comparisons of the two strategies. To evaluate this possibility, tests of consonant identification with the CA processor were repeated at the end of the week for each subject. In all cases except one (subject SR3), the retest scores were indistinguishable from the original scores, and data from the second tests were added to those of the first. In the exceptional case, the retest scores were about 10% higher than the original scores for the male speaker and indistinguishable for the female speaker. The retest data for the male speaker, and combined test/retest data for the female speaker, were used in all subsequent analyses for subject SR3.

In addition, the CID sentence and NU-6 word tests were repeated with the CIS processor for five of the subjects (subjects SR3, SR4 and SR6-8) using a different recorded speaker and new lists of words and sentences. Practice or learning effects would be demonstrated by significant differences in the test/retest scores. However, no such differences were found ($p > 0.6$ for paired- t comparisons of the CID scores; $p > 0.2$ for the NU-6 scores), and the scores from the first and second tests were averaged for all subsequent analyses.

Table 5-1 Parameters of CIS Processors*

Subject	RMS			eq (Hz)	Channel sequence	rate (Hz)	mapping
	μs/ph	Rect/	Filters (Hz)				
SR2	55	FW	800	600	6-3-5-2-4-1	1515	logarithmic
SR3	31	FW	400	1200	6-3-5-2-4-1	2688	logarithmic
SR4	63	FW	400	1200	6-3-5-2-4-1	1323	logarithmic
SR5	31	HW	800	1200	2-5-4-6-1[a]	3226	logarithmic
	31	HW	800	1200	2-5-3-1-6-4[b]	2688	logarithmic
SR6	102	FW	400	1200	6-3-5-2-4-1	817	logarithmic
SR7	34	HW	400	1200	5-3-1-4-2[c]	2941	power law ($p = 0.2$)
SR8	100	FW	400	1200	6-3-5-2-4-1	833	logarithmic
	100	FW	400	1200	6-3-5-2-4-1	833	power law ($p = 0.2$)

*The parameters include pulse duration per phase (μs/ph), the type of rectifier (half wave or full wave) used in the circuits for bandpass energy detection (RMS rect), the corner frequency of the integrating filters in those circuits (RMS filters), the frequency below which speech signals are attenuated for input equalization (eq), the sequence of channels for each stimulation cycle (channel sequence; channel 6 is the most basal for all subjects except subject SR5, see footnote a), the rate of pulsatile stimulation on each channel (rate), and the type of transformation used to map pulse amplitudes (mapping). The logarithmic transformation for mapping is of the form $pulse\ amplitude = A \times log(RMS) + k$, and the power-law transformation is of the form $pulse\ amplitude = A \times (RMS)^p + k$, where A and k are set so that pulsatile stimuli derived from processed speech will span the dynamic range from threshold to comfortable loudness on each channel.

aThe electrodes for subject SR5 were inserted into the scala tympani one at a time, instead of as a bundled array. Because of uncertainties in the depths of insertion for the individual electrodes, the electrode positions had to be inferred on the basis of tonotopic ranking. The channel sequence from these inferred positions was 5-3-1-4-2. Electrode 3 was not used in this five-channel processor because stimulation of that electrode produced markedly different pitches at different stimulus levels.

bThe channel sequence from the inferred positions of the electrodes was 6-3-5-2-4-1. (Electrode 3 was used in this processor even though that electrode produced markedly different pitches at different stimulus levels.)

cSubject SR7 used a five-channel processor because stimulation of his sixth channel produced transient sensations of head movements.

RESULTS

Results Across Subjects

Results across subjects are presented in Figure 5–2 and in Tables 5–2 and 5–3. These results were obtained from the tests with the first processors listed in Table 5–1 for each subject. The raw scores from those tests are presented for reference in Appendix Tables A5–1 and A5–2 at the end of this chapter.

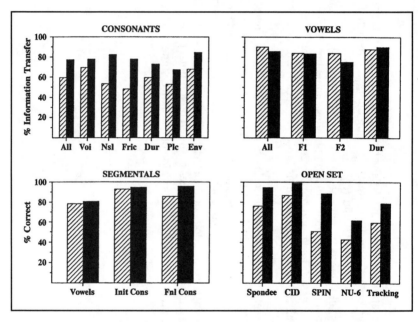

Figure 5–2. Graphs of speech test results for the seven subjects. Scores for the CA processor are indicated by the striped bars, and those for the CIS processor by the solid bars. (**Top**) Relative information transfer of consonant and vowel features. The features include overall transmission (All), voicing (Voi), nasality (Nsl), frication (Fric), duration (Dur), place of articulation (Plc), envelope cues (Env), first formant frequency (F1), and second formant frequency (F2). (**Bottom**) Average scores from the segmental and open-set tests. See text for abbreviations. Note that the scores for the tracking test are given in words per minute; not in percent correct. Thus, full scale corresponds to 100 words per minute for that test.

Table 5–2 and the first halves of Table 5–3 and Figure 5–2 show the results from the tests of consonant and vowel identification. As mentioned before, the patterns of confusions and correct responses were evaluated using information transmission (IT) analysis. In this analysis the "relative transinformation" is calculated for selected articulatory or acoustic features of the phonemes in the identification tests. The relative transinformation score for each feature, expressed here as percent information transfer, indicates how well that feature was transmitted to the subjects. The consonant features selected for the present study were voicing (voice), nasality (nasal), place of articulation (place), duration (dur), frication (fric), and envelope cues (envel). The vowel features were first formant frequency (F1), second formant frequency (F2), and duration (dur). The assignments of these features for the phonemes in the identification tests are presented in Appendix Tables A5–3 and A5–4 at the end of this chapter.

Matrices of stimuli and responses were compiled for each subject and processor by combining the data for the male and female speakers. The combined matrices had a minimum of 20 trials for each of the consonants and 18 trials for each of the vowels.

The overall percent-correct scores and total number of trials for the tests of consonant and vowel identification are presented in Table 5–2. Paired-*t* comparisons of the scores demonstrate superiority of the CIS processor for consonant identification (*p* < .01) and no difference between processors for vowel identification.

Table 5–2. *Results from the Tests of Consonant and Vowel Identification**

Test	Processor	Trials	% Correct	*p*
Consonant	CA	205	66.4	
	CIS	145	81.9	.01
Vowel	CA	132	95.1	
	CIS	126	92.7	NS

*Shown are the number of trials for each token (trials), the mean percent-correct scores (% correct), and the significance levels from paired-*t* comparisons (*p*).

Table 5-3. Results of Speech Tests for the Seven Subjects*

	CA		CIS			Wil-coxon
	Mean	SD	Mean	SD	Paired-*t*	
Consonants						
Overall	67.8	9.8	83.1	11.1	.01	.05
Voice	70.6	10.4	80.4	17.4		
Nasal	60.4	26.0	86.4	18.1	.01	.02
Fric	51.5	19.3	81.2	16.8	.01	.05
Dur	60.5	9.1	76.1	19.8	.05	
Place	55.7	8.5	72.9	19.3	.02	.05
Envel	71.7	14.6	86.8	12.1	.05	.05
Vowels						
Overall	93.0	8.0	88.9	5.9	.05	
F1	88.3	16.6	85.4	13.6		
F2	88.1	16.9	78.8	10.6		
Dur	90.6	13.4	91.5	6.2		
Segmental						
Vowel	78.3	6.2	80.3	7.8		
Init Cons	92.7	5.5	94.6	3.5		
Fnl Cons	85.7	6.7	95.6	3.3	.02	.05
Open Set						
Spondee	76	16.2	94.3	8.6	.05	.05
CID	86.9	13.8	98.8	1.8		.05
SPIN	50.3	29.3	88.6	11.9	.01	.02
NU-6	42.9	14.6	61.4	13.8	.01	.05
Tracking	59.2	14.6	78.8	14.2	.01	.05

*Means and standard deviations (SD) are shown for the CA and CIS processors. Levels of significance from paired-*t* tests and Wilcoxon signed ranks (nonparametric) tests are indicated in the right columns.

Although percent correct scores provide a rough indication of processor performance, IT analyses can demonstrate specific strengths and weaknesses of a given strategy. Means of the scores from those analyses are presented in Table 5–3, along with the results from paired-t and Wilcoxon (nonparametric) comparisons of the scores for the two processors. IT scores for all consonant features except voicing are significantly higher with CIS processor, with especially large differences found for overall transmission, nasality, frication, and place of articulation. The IT scores for the vowel features are indistinguishable except for overall transmission, where the scores for overall transmission are higher for the CA processor ($p < .05$).

In addition to the IT analyses of matrices for each of the subjects, analyses were performed using aggregate matrices across subjects. These were compiled for each processor by combining the subject matrices, and are presented for reference in Appendix Tables A5–5 and A5–6 at the end of this chapter.

Results from IT analyses of the aggregate matrices are shown in Figure 5–2. Large gains in the consonant features of overall transmission, nasality, frication, and place of articulation again are seen when the CIS processor is used instead of the CA processor. In addition, substantial increases are found for consonant duration and envelope cues. Finally, notice that the absolute scores for most features approximate the ceiling of perfect performance when the CIS processor is used. The scores for nasality and envelope each exceed 80%, and the scores for all remaining features except place (67.3%) exceed 70%. The greatest strengths of the CIS processor are in the transmission of nasality, frication, and envelope information, whereas the greatest strengths of the CA processor are in the transmission of voicing, duration, and envelope information. A relative weakness shared by both processors is in the transmission of place information. Further weaknesses of the CA processor lie in the transmission of nasality and frication information.

Scores from IT analyses of the aggregate matrices for vowels approximate the ceilings of perfect performance for both processors and all features. Transmission scores are nearly identical for F1 and duration, and somewhat higher with the CA processor for overall transmission and F2.

The remaining results presented in Figure 5–2 and Table 5–3 are those for the segmental and open-set tests of the MAC battery, and for connected discourse tracking. The means of scores from the seven subjects are shown for all tests except tracking, where the means for six subjects are shown.

Results from the segmental tests all approximate perfect performance and mirror, to some extent, the results from the tests of vowel and consonant identification. In particular, the scores for the vowel test are indistinguishable, whereas the scores for the final consonant test demonstrate superiority of the CIS processor ($p < .02$). The scores for the initial consonant test do not favor either processor. However, ceiling effects may have masked a true difference between processors for that test (absolute scores are greater than 90% for both processors).

Finally, the open-set and tracking results demonstrate clear superiority of the CIS processor. Remarkable gains are found for all tests not subject to ceiling effects. The mean score for the SPIN test increases from 50.3 to 88.6% ($p < .01$); the mean score for the NU-6 test increases from 42.9 to 61.4% ($p < .01$); and the mean score for the tracking test increases from 59.2 to 78.8 words per minute ($p < .01$).

Individual Scores

An additional aspect of the open-set and tracking results is the pattern of increases for each subject. The individual scores for the CA and CIS processors are presented in Table 5–4. The scores for the CIS processor are those from the best tested variation of that processor. This variation was processor 1 for subjects SR2-4, SR6 and SR7, and processor 2 for subjects SR5 and SR8.

As indicated in Table 5–4, every subject obtained a higher score, or repeated a score of 100% correct, for every test when the CIS processor was used instead of the CA processor. The increases across subjects are significant for spondee recognition ($p < .05$) and highly significant for recognition of the last word in the SPIN sentences ($p < .01$), recognition of the NU-6 words ($p < .002$), and the rate of speech tracking ($p < .02$). The increase for recognition of key words in the CID sentences is not significant,

Table 5–4. Individual Results from the Open-Set Tests

Subjects	Spondee		CID		SPIN		NU-6		Tracking	
	CA	CIS	CA	CIS	CA	CIS	CA	CIS	CA	CIS
SR2	92	96	100	100	78	96	56	80	81	94
SR3	52	96	66	98	14	92	34	58	51	89
SR4	68	76	93	95	28	70	34	40	--	--
SR5	100	100	97	100	94	100	70	80	--	--
SR6	72	92	73	99	36	74	30	49	43	56
SR7	80	100	99	100	66	98	38	71	51	68
SR8	68	100	80	100	36	94	38	66	56	94

in part because the performance of several subjects is perfect or nearly so with both processors.

The overall pattern of scores in Table 5–4 was evaluated further with a two-way analysis of the variance (ANOVA), using the five tests and two processors as the factors. This analysis demonstrated highly significant differences among tests ($F(4,56) = 13.5$; $p < .0001$) and between processors ($F(1,56) = 34.1$; $p < .0001$), with no interaction between factors ($F(4,56) = 1.4$; $p > .2$).

Correlation Analyses

A final aspect of the results is shown in Table 5–5, a matrix of correlations among test scores for all subjects and both processors. The CIS processors are the ones listed first for each subject in Table 5–1.

As might be expected from the redundancy in assignments for consonant features (see Table A5–3 and Wang & Bilger, 1973), high correlations are found among the transmission scores for those features. Also, overall transmission is highly correlated with all six consonant features ($r = .86$ or higher; $p < .001$), with especially high correlations observed for the features of nasality, frication, place, and envelope ($r = .94$ or higher).

Similarly, high correlations are found among transmission scores for the vowel features. In particular, a strong relationship is demonstrated between the scores for F1 and F2 ($r = .83$; $p < .001$). As with the consonant features, all vowel features are strongly correlated with overall transmission ($r = .80$ or higher; $p < .001$). Among these, F1 and F2 have higher correlations ($r = .88$ and .93, respectively) than duration ($r = .80$).

Correlations among scores for the segmental tests are either insignificant or barely significant (scores for the vowel and initial consonant test are weakly correlated: $r = .64$; $p < .02$). This suggests that these tests are relatively independent.

In contrast, correlations among the open-set tests generally are quite high. With the exception of the correlation for the NU-6 and CID tests ($r = .67$; $p < .01$), all correlations are .84 or higher ($p < .001$). This suggests that the open-set tests are not independent of each other and further that one or more of these tests might be omitted in future studies without any significant loss in information.

Table 5–5. Correlations Among Test Results for All Seven Subjects and Both Processors*

	1	2	3	4	5	6	7	8	9	10	11	12	13	14	15	16	17
Consonants																	
1. Overall																	
2. Voice	.84																
3. Nasal	.96	.73															
4. Fric	.94	.84	.89														
5. Dur	.86	.65	.80	.74													
6. Place	.94	.78	.87	.85	.90												
7. Envel	.95	.89	.93	.92	.74	.83											
Vowels																	
8. Overall	.42	.38	.55	.27	.38	.40	.50										
9. F1	.52	.50	.58	.44	.37	.46	.61	.88									
10. F2	.35	.33	.45	.18	.33	.27	.46	.93	.83								
11. Dur	.56	.50	.69	.46	.47	.51	.64	.80	.62	.62							

continues

107

Table 5–5. *continued*

	1	2	3	4	5	6	7	8	9	10	11	12	13	14	15	16	17
Segmentals																	
12. Vowel	.61	.64	.54	.40	.62	.66	.60	.54	.49	.46	.64						
13. Init Cons	.66	.59	.65	.48	.70	.55	.70	.55	.51	.62	.55	.64					
14. Fnl Cons	**.80**	.65	**.80**	**.81**	.52	.60	**.82**	.13	.20	.09	.47	.32	.55				
Open Set																	
15. Spondee	**.86**	.68	**.86**	**.84**	.69	.76	**.82**	.32	.42	.22	.53	.51	.63	**.85**			
16. CID	.70	.53	.70	.71	.52	.57	.69	.27	.37	.28	.37	.38	.52	.69	**.84**		
17. SPIN	**.83**	.60	**.84**	**.82**	.66	.73	.77	.27	.31	.15	.56	.44	.54	**.87**	**.97**	**.84**	
18. NU-6	**.79**	.60	.75	.71	**.79**	**.81**	.66	.24	.19	.12	.49	.59	.61	.69	**.87**	.67	**.89**

*Correlation coefficients of .53, .61, .66, .70, .75, and .78 are significant at $p < .05$, .02, .01, .005, .002, and .001, respectively. Correlation coefficients that are significant at $p < .001$ are highlighted with **boldface type**.

108

Examination of correlations among classes of tests demonstrates strong relationships between feature transmission scores from tests of consonant identification and scores from the tests of open-set recognition. With the exception of the CID sentence test, significant correlations are found for every consonant feature, with relatively high correlations for overall transmission ($r = .83$ or higher; $p < .001$), nasality ($r = .75$ or higher; $p < .002$), frication ($r = .71$ or higher; $p < .005$), and place ($r = .73$ or higher; $p < .005$). The lack of high correlations for the CID test may be a result of the very high scores obtained for that test across processors and subjects (see Tables A5–1 and A5–2).

In addition to the high correlations between consonant features and open-set scores, high correlations are found between consonant features and the scores from the final consonant test of the MAC battery. Somewhat surprisingly, similar correlations are not found for the initial consonant test. As with the relative lack of correlations with the CID scores, though, this might be attributable to the uniformity of scores across subjects and processors for the initial consonant test.

As might be expected from the strong relationship between consonant features and scores from the final consonant test, the latter scores also are predictive of outcomes on the open-set tests. The correlations are .69 or higher ($p < .01$), with especially high correlations found for the spondee and SPIN tests ($r = .85$ and .87, respectively; $p < .001$).

Unlike the high correlations found for consonant features and scores from the open-set tests, only weak or insignificant correlations are observed for vowel features and those scores. Similarly, scores for the vowel test of the MAC battery are not generally predictive of the open-set scores. The only exception is a weak correlation between scores for the vowel and NU-6 tests ($r = .59$; $p < .05$).

In summary, the correlation results appear to reflect the average scores presented in Figure 5–2 and Table 5–3. Large differences in scores between processors are found for most consonant features, most open-set tests, and the final consonant test of the MAC battery. The correlation results show that these differences between processors co-vary across subjects. The remaining tests produce similar scores for the two processors (vowel features, vowel and initial consonant tests of the MAC battery, and, to some extent, the CID sentence test), and therefore those scores are not predictive of each other or of scores from the majority of open-set tests.

DISCUSSION

The CA and CIS processing strategies were compared in tests with seven subjects implanted with the Symbion electrode array. Every subject obtained a higher score, or repeated a score of 100% correct, for all five open-set tests when the CIS processor was used instead of the CA processor. In addition, significant gains in the transmission of consonant information were demonstrated for the CIS processor. Performances on tests of vowel identification, and on the vowel and initial consonant tests of the MAC battery, were similar for the two processors. Finally, scores for the open-set tests were highly correlated (across subjects and processors) with transmission scores for consonant features.

The absolute levels of performance obtained with the CIS processor exceed by wide margins the previous levels reported in the open literature for any cochlear implant patient, using any type of device. The highest previously reported score for the NU-6 test, for example, was 60% correct (Dorman et al., 1989). Four of the seven subjects in the present series exceeded this previous record, and two of the subjects had scores of 80% correct. This latter score is in the range of scores obtained by people with mild-to-moderate hearing losses when taking the same test (Bess & Townsend, 1977; Goetzinger, 1978). Also, most scores for the remaining tests are near the respective upper scale limits: four subjects had scores of 96% or higher for the spondee test; all seven subjects had scores of 95% or higher for the CID test; five subjects had scores of 92% or higher for the SPIN test; and three of five tested subjects had tracking rates of 89 wpm or higher. Indeed, scores of 100% correct were not uncommon for the spondee and CID tests, and two subjects had tracking scores of 94 wpm. These scores are indistinguishable from those obtained by control subjects with normal hearing (e.g., four subjects with normal hearing took the same tracking test and got scores of 94, 94, 96, and 97 wpm; see Owens & Raggio, 1987).

The overall pattern of increases in open-set performance is even more compelling when one considers the large disparity in experience the subjects had with the two processors. Each subject had multiple years of daily experience with the CA processor at the time of our tests, but had only 15 minutes of experience (with informal conversation) before formal evaluation of the CIS processor. In previous studies using within-subject controls, such differences in experience have strongly favored the processor with the greatest duration of use (Dowell et al., 1987; Tyler et al., 1986).

Collectively the present findings show that close approximations to normal levels of speech recognition are possible with multichannel cochlear implants. In addition, they demonstrate clear superiority of the CIS processor for identification of consonants and for open-set recognition of words and sentences. The unprecedented performance obtained with the CIS processor offers new hope for implant recipients.

Acknowledgments. We are pleased to acknowledge the collaboration of Bob Wolford in the studies with all seven subjects, and of Don Eddington and Bill Rabinowitz in the studies with subject SR2. We also are indebted to Michael Dorman, Richard Tyler, Mary Lowder, and Korine Dankowski for their help in identifying the subjects for this series. Finally, we are most grateful for the time and interest contributed by each of the subjects.

Appendix

Table A5–1. Scores from Tests with the CA Processor

	Subject						
	SR2	SR3	SR4	SR5	SR6	SR7	SR8
Consonants							
1. Overall	67.7	50.1	63.3	80.1	68.9	77.2	67.0
2. Voice	77.9	53.7	67.1	83.0	75.9	75.8	61.1
3. Nasal	59.0	18.8	38.2	92.2	61.3	89.0	64.1
4. Fric	54.4	28.5	40.2	74.8	57.6	74.8	30.5
5. Dur	56.8	50.4	56.3	78.5	55.6	64.7	60.9
6. Place	55.0	45.4	48.8	67.2	51.7	67.2	54.4
7. Envel	73.8	43.2	64.9	86.2	78.1	84.5	71.3
Vowels							
8. Overall	96.7	77.4	87.0	97.4	95.2	100.0	97.4
9. F1	100.0	53.3	84.3	89.4	100.0	100.0	90.8
10. F2	89.7	50.8	90.1	86.4	93.4	100.0	96.4
11. Dur	100.0	74.4	69.3	100.0	90.8	100.0	100.0
Segmentals							
12. Vowel	88.3	70.0	75.0	76.7	76.7	76.7	85.0
13. Init Cons	93.8	82.8	93.8	100.0	92.2	89.1	96.9
14. Fnl Cons	86.5	75.0	80.8	96.2	88.5	88.5	84.6
Open Set							
15. Spondee	92.0	52.0	68.0	100.0	72.0	80.0	68.0
16. CID	100.0	66.0	93.0	97.0	73.0	99.0	80.0
17. SPIN	78.0	14.0	28.0	94.0	36.0	66.0	36.0
18. NU-6	56.0	34.0	34.0	70.0	30.0	38.0	38.0
19. Tracking	81.0	51.0	53.0	73.0	43.0	51.0	56.0

Table A5-2. Scores from Tests with the CIS Processor

	Subject						
	SR2	SR3	SR4	SR5	SR6	SR7	SR8
Consonants							
1. Overall	91.9	74.5	63.2	95.0	83.0	83.8	90.0
2. Voice	94.7	69.2	57.2	100.0	87.8	61.6	92.6
3. Nasal	100.0	68.8	54.7	100.0	85.5	96.1	100.0
4. Fric	87.9	63.9	56.0	100.0	88.9	74.8	97.2
5. Dur	92.4	55.1	46.7	96.7	81.4	92.2	68.2
6. Place	87.8	58.4	39.4	94.5	66.7	79.5	84.1
7. Envel	97.5	75.7	69.3	100.0	91.3	78.5	95.3
Vowels							
8. Overall	93.1	79.9	84.7	95.3	84.4	93.9	91.0
9. F1	82.2	63.6	75.3	100.0	82.2	94.7	100.0
10. F2	90.7	59.8	74.3	87.2	74.4	86.6	78.5
11. Dur	100.0	84.3	87.4	100.0	87.4	90.8	90.8
Segmentals							
12. Vowel	91.7	76.7	66.7	86.7	80.0	80.0	80.0
13. Init Cons	98.4	90.6	90.6	98.4	96.9	95.3	92.2
14. Fnl Cons	98.1	100.0	92.3	96.2	96.2	90.4	96.2
Open Set							
15. Spondee	96.0	96.0	76.0	100.0	92.0	100.0	100.0
16. CID	100.0	98.0	95.0	100.0	99.0	100.0	99.5
17. SPIN	96.0	92.0	70.0	100.0	74.0	98.0	90.0
18. NU-6	80.0	58.0	40.0	70.0	49.0	71.0	62.0
19. Tracking	94.0	89.0	—	81.0	56.0	68.0	85.0

Table A5–3. Assignment of Consonant Features

Consonant	Voicing	Nasality	Frication	Duration	Place	Envelope
m	2	2	1	1	1	4
n	2	2	1	1	2	4
f	1	1	2	1	1	3
v	2	1	2	1	1	2
s	1	1	2	2	2	3
z	2	1	2	2	2	2
ʃ	1	1	2	2	3	3
ð	2	1	2	1	1	2
p	1	1	1	1	1	1
b	2	1	1	1	1	2
t	1	1	1	1	2	1
d	2	1	1	1	2	2
g	2	1	1	1	4	2
k	1	1	1	1	4	1
dʒ	2	1	2	1	3	2
l	2	1	1	1	2	4

Table A5–4. Assignment of Vowel Features

Vowel	F1	F2	Duration
i	1	1	1
ɔ	2	2	1
ɛ	2	1	2
u	1	2	1
ɪ	1	1	2
ʊ	1	2	2
ʌ	2	3	2
æ	2	1	1

Table A5–5. Consonant Matrix for the CA Processor

Stimulus	Response															
	m	n	f	v	s	z	ʃ	ð	p	b	t	d	g	k	dʒ	l
m	122	45	1	4				6		5		4	1			20
n	3	189		1	1	1		3		1	1	6			1	2
f	1	119	13	4	1		29	14	11		4	7	2		1	
v	13	3	8	60	2	5		37	2	58		3	2	1		15
s	1	3	11	2	138	17	8	5	4	2	1	3				
z	2	7		23	5	123	1	18		1		4	9			
ʃ					2		202	1								
ð	13	9	2	45	1	16		67		25		10	8			10
p	1	3	6	2	2	1		5	136	1	41			12		
b	9	3	3	17	1			7	3	156	1	3	6			6
t		1	2					1	15		138	1		46		
d	1	4		5	1	3	1	6		4	1	139	43	1	1	
g	1	14	3	9		2		8		2		21	142	3		3
k		2	2						33		40	2		128		
dʒ												2			203	1
l	16	43		3				4		1		4		1		137

Table A5–6. Consonant Matrix for the CIS Processor

Stimulus								Response								
	m	n	f	v	s	z	ʃ	ð	p	b	t	d	g	k	dʒ	l
m	116	25						1								3
n	10	130														4
f			116	13	3	2	1	10		12		2				
v	7	3	8	80	1	9	9	29	2	1		2				4
s			15	1	108	5		5								
z			4	9		114	1	16								
ʃ					11	1	133									
ð	2	1	3	41		2		88	1	1		1	1		3	
p								1	105		25			5	9	
b			1	3				5		131		5				
t					3		1			4	122	113		7	12	
d											5	4	25		2	
g													141			
k									7		2			131	1	
dʒ		7													143	
l	11											1				127

117

Table A5-7. Vowel Matrix for the CA Processor

Stimulus	i	ɔ	ɛ	u	ɪ	ʊ	ʌ	æ
i	132							
ɔ		131						1
ɛ			125	7				
u				127	5			
ɪ	2	1			128	1		
ʊ			6	1	10	116		
ʌ		1	1			9	120	2
æ			1			1	3	127

Table A5-8. Vowel Matrix for the CIS Processor

Stimulus	i	ɔ	ɛ	u	ɪ	ʊ	ʌ	æ
i	123			2	1			
ɔ		106					6	14
ɛ			116	4			6	
u	1			123	1	1		
ɪ		9			116	1		
ʊ			1	2		119	4	
ʌ			8	1	2	4	111	
æ		4	2					120

118

Chapter 6

EVALUATION OF OTHER PROMISING STRATEGIES*

Blake S. Wilson, Dewey T. Lawson, Charles C. Finley, and Mariangeli Zerbi

Although very high levels of speech recognition have been obtained with the *continuous interleaved sampling* (CIS) strategy, other strategies may well be better, at least for certain classes of patients. One possibility is the *peak picker* (PP) strategy first described in Chapter 4. In studies with one of our Ineraid patients, this strategy produced transmission scores for several consonant features that were higher than the scores obtained with the CIS strategy. Overall transmission of consonant information was approximately the same for the PP and CIS strategies. Transmission of vowel features to this patient by the PP strategy was perfect for our eight vowel test (compared with high, but not perfect, scores for the CIS strategy). The PP strategy obviously has promise and should be investigated further with additional tests and subjects.

A possible advantage of the PP strategy is that it uses generally lower rates of stimulation than the CIS strategy. This may

---

*From QPR 3:10, August 1, 1991, through October 31, 1991.

allow useful implementations of the PP strategy for patients implanted with the Nucleus device, whose transcutaneous transmission system (TTS) does not permit the rapid sequencing of pulses required by typical implementations of the CIS strategy.

In addition to the PP strategy, we have conducted preliminary studies to evaluate a hybrid PP/CIS strategy. In this strategy PP stimuli are delivered to the apical-most electrodes (usually the two most apical electrodes in an array of six), and CIS stimuli are delivered to the remaining electrodes. This hybrid strategy attempts to combine attributes of the PP and CIS approaches.

In this section we summarize results reported in Chapter 4 for the PP strategy, and we describe preliminary studies with the new PP/CIS strategy.

PEAK PICKER (PP) PROCESSOR

The design of the PP processor is illustrated in Figure 6–1. In this processor the position of a peak in either the bandpass or envelope detector output is signaled by the presentation of a pulse. Also, as in the *interleaved pulses* (IP) and CIS processors, the exact timing of the pulses is adjusted so that there is no temporal overlap of stimuli across channels.

In Figure 6–1 the middle panel shows bandpass outputs for each of four channels along with the stimulus pulses derived from those outputs. In addition, the positions of the peaks in the bandpass outputs are marked by short vertical lines above each trace. The lower panel shows the stimulus pulses only.

In this particular implementation of the PP strategy, a timer is advanced for each channel in a sequence of stimulation across the electrode array. At each time step a pulse is delivered if a peak occurred in the bandpass output between the previous and present time steps for that channel. The amplitude of the pulse is determined with the same logarithmic transformation used in the IP and some CIS processors (i.e., the actual pulse amplitudes would be computed using a logarithmic transformation of the amplitudes shown in the figure). A fixed time is reserved for each channel in the stimulation sequence whether

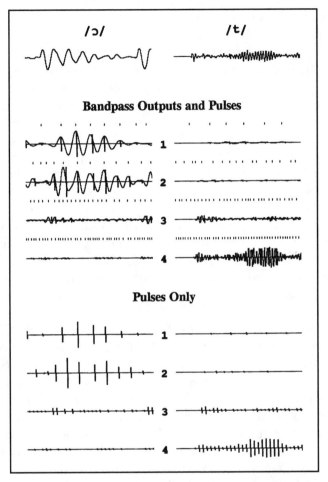

Figure 6–1. Waveforms of the peak picker (PP) processing strategy. Equalized speech inputs are shown at the top and processor waveforms are shown in the middle and bottom panels. The middle panel shows the bandpass outputs and stimulus pulses for each of four channels. The location of peaks in the bandpass outputs are marked with short vertical lines above each trace. The bottom panel shows the stimulus pulses only. The duration of each trace is 12.25 ms.

or not a pulse is delivered. As indicated in Figure 6–1, this variation of the processor produces clusters of pulses at the F0 rate and individual pulses at the F1 rate for voiced speech sounds (left panels). Because the pulses must be presented nonsimultaneously, higher frequencies in the bandpass outputs are not followed with pulses at those frequencies. Notice, for instance, that many peaks are missed in channels 3 and 4, and that large offsets between the positions of peaks and subsequent pulses are seen in the waveforms of channel 2.

Alternative implementations of the PP processor are illustrated in Figure 6–2. The uppermost panel beneath the input signals shows the waveforms of the implementation just described ("Bandpass Outputs, Time for Each Channel"); the next panel down shows an implementation in which the time allocated for each channel is *not* used if a pulse is not delivered ("Bandpass Outputs, Channels Skipped"); and the bottom panel shows an implementation in which the outputs of the envelope detectors are used instead of the bandpass outputs ("Envelope Detector Outputs, Channels Skipped").

A summary of waveforms for various types of pulsatile processors is presented in Figure 6–3. All three types of processors use nonsimultaneous stimuli. Among these, the CIS processor delivers the greatest number of pulses per unit time, and the IP processor the least. The PP processor provides an intermediate level of temporal detail, with a representation of F1 in the apical channel(s). In addition, the PP processor presents different rates of stimulation on each channel, which might increase the salience of channel-related cues for some patients (i.e., channel cues might be represented both by place of stimulation and by rate of stimulation).

One implementation of a PP processor was evaluated in preliminary tests with Ineraid subject SR2. The design illustrated in Figure 6–1 was used, with time taken for each channel whether or not a pulse is delivered. The PP processor used six channels, with the staggered update order found to be best in (contemporaneous) evaluations of CIS processors (6-3-5-2-4-1).

The tests included identification of 16 consonants and 8 vowels, for male and female speakers (see Chapter 4 for a complete description of the tests and related procedures).

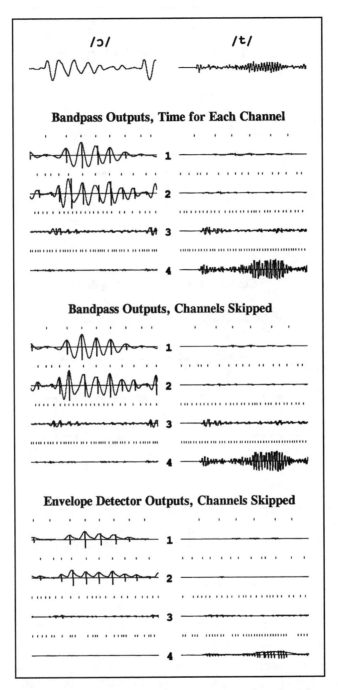

Figure 6–2. Various implementations of peak picker (PP) processors. See text for details.

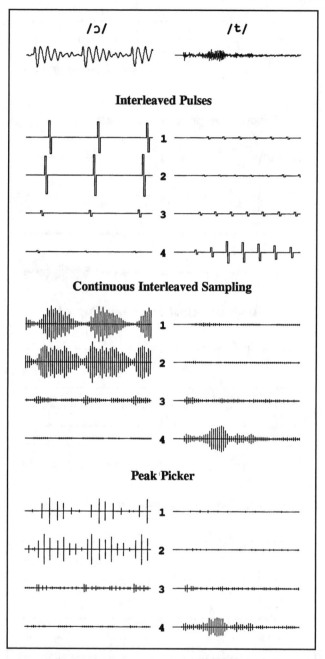

Figure 6-3. Waveforms of three types of pulsatile processors. The duration of each trace is 25.4 ms. Note that the prolonged stimulation in the interleaved pulses (IP) processor for the /t/ burst is a consequence of the long time constant of the lowpass filters in the envelope detectors (25 Hz cutoff versus 400 Hz cutoff for the other processors).

Results for a contemporaneous implementation of the CIS strategy (processor RTSS8) and the PP strategy (processor RTPP1) are presented in Figure 6–4. As noted above, both processors used a staggered update order. In addition, both used pulse durations of 55 μs/phase, no time delay between sequential pulses, and a 600 Hz corner frequency for the input equalization filter (present versions of CIS processors generally use shorter pulses and a 1200 Hz corner frequency for the equalization filter). Finally, the envelope detectors in the CIS processor used half-wave rectifiers and 800 Hz low-pass filters (present CIS processors generally use lower cutoff frequencies for the lowpass filter).

Comparison of the scores for the two processors shows a similarity in feature transmission for consonants. Overall transmission

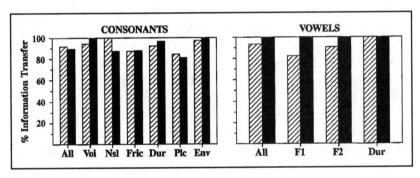

Figure 6–4. Comparison of speech test scores for an early implementation of a continuous interleaved sampling (CIS) processor (*striped bars*) and a peak picker (PP) processor (*solid bars*) evaluated at the same time. Twenty presentations of each of 16 consonants were used in the consonant identification test for both processors. The presentations were equally divided between the male and female speakers. For the vowel identification tests, 18 presentations were used for evaluation of the CIS processor (*striped bars*) and 12 were used for the PP processor (*solid bars*). The presentations were equally divided between the male and female speakers. Overall information transfer (IT) scores are presented for the consonant and vowel tests. In addition, IT scores are presented for the consonant features of voicing (Voi), nasality (Nsl), frication (Fric), duration (Dur), place of articulation (Plc), and envelope cues (Env), and for the vowel features of the first formant frequency (F1), the second formant frequency (F2), and duration (Dur).

approximates 90% for both strategies. The PP strategy produces somewhat higher scores for the temporal features of voicing, duration, and envelope cues, and the CIS strategy produces somewhat higher scores for the features of nasality and place of articulation. Scores for frication are quite similar for the two processors.

In contrast to the overall picture for consonants, transmission of vowel information appears to be better with the PP processor. In fact, the 8 vowels of our vowel identification test were perfectly identified for both the male and female speakers when the PP processor was used.

The large gain in the transmission of vowel feature information found for F1 is consistent with the explicit representation of F1 in the apical channels with the PP processor.

With the exception of this one feature, and possibly nasality for the consonant test, no obvious differences are found in the results for the two processors. We note, however, that many of the scores approach or encounter the 100% ceiling for these particular tests. More difficult tests will be needed to detect additional differences between the processors, if indeed such differences exist.

SR2 remarked that percepts produced with the PP processor were more "pitch appropriate" than percepts produced with the contemporaneous versions of the CIS processor, particularly for low frequency sounds such as the fundamental frequency of voiced speech. Although the PP processor sounded a bit more natural to SR2, both processors were judged by him to be highly intelligible, with no clear difference between processors for recognizing connected speech. (SR2 has scored substantially higher with subsequently developed CIS versions.)

HYBRID PP/CIS PROCESSOR

In much more recent studies we have evaluated a hybrid of the PP and CIS strategies. In this PP/CIS processor, PP stimuli were delivered to the apical two electrodes in the Ineraid array and CIS stimuli were delivered to the remaining four electrodes. The speech processor was programmed to examine the signals from the envelope detectors in the apical-most two channels just before the scheduled delivery of a CIS pulse on one of the more basal channels. If the processor detected a peak in one or both of the apical channels, then the CIS pulse would be delayed to allow the delivery of a (nonsimultaneous) PP pulse for each channel with a detected peak. This process was repeated for each CIS pulse.

Results from an initial evaluation of this hybrid PP/CIS processor are presented in Figure 6–5. In addition, results from a CIS

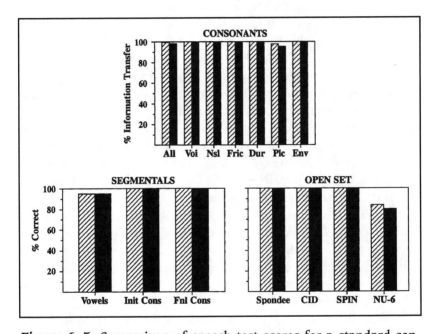

Figure 6–5. Comparison of speech test scores for a standard continuous interleaved sampling (CIS) processor (*striped bars*) and a hybrid peak picker/CIS (PP/CIS) processor (*solid bars*). Five presentations of each of 24 consonants by the male speaker were used in the consonant identification tests for both processors. The results from the consonant tests are given as percent information transmission scores, as in Figure 6–4. Abbreviations in the present figure for the consonant results are the same as those used in Figure 6–4. Additional abbreviations used in the present figure include: Init Cons for Initial Consonant, Fnl Cons for Final Consonant, Spondee for Spondee words, CID for the Central Institute for the Deaf sentences, SPIN for the Speech in Noise Test sentences (presented in quiet in the present tests), and NU-6 for the Northwestern University Auditory Test 6 for the recognition of monosyllabic words.

processor with parameters similar or identical to those of the CIS channels in the PP/CIS processor are shown. The consonant test used for these evaluations included 24 consonants. Tests were conducted with the male speaker only. The CID, SPIN and NU-6 tests were conducted using novel lists of recorded sentences and words (with a different male speaker). (The full names of these latter tests are presented in the figure caption.)

Clearly, both processors support high levels of speech recognition. All scores except those for the NU-6 test approach or hit the 100% ceiling. The NU-6 scores are 84 and 80% correct for the CIS and PP/CIS strategies, respectively.

Anecdotally, the PP/CIS processor sounded quite natural, especially for music. Indeed, SR2, who was a musician before he lost his hearing, indicated that percepts produced with the PP/CIS processor had greater "pitch appropriateness" and musical clarity than percepts produced with his clinical CA processor or with the CIS processor (this observation was made while listening to small ensemble jazz recordings, which were familiar to the subject only through use of his clinical CA processor). Because the sound was so enjoyable to SR2 ("music is wonderful through this [PP/CIS] processor, like nothing I've even dreamed of ever hearing again with my implant"), we took some time off from testing so that he could listen to tapes of music he remembered from years ago (rock band material, which was familiar to the subject before loss of his normal hearing). Again, SR2 heard nuances in the material that could not be perceived with the other processors.

These high levels of performance for the PP/CIS strategy are encouraging. We plan further studies, with additional subjects and tests, to evaluate further the PP and PP/CIS strategies. The preliminary results, along with anecdotal comments, suggest that use of PP stimuli, at least for the apical channels, may provide an improved representation of frequencies in the F0 and F1 ranges, at least for some of the better subjects.

Acknowledgments. We thank subject SR2 for his enthusiastic participation and generous contribution of time.

Chapter 7

COMPLETION OF "POOR PERFORMANCE" SERIES*

Blake S. Wilson, Dewey T. Lawson, Mariangeli Zerbi, and Charles C. Finley

Recent studies in our laboratory have focused on comparisons of *compressed analog* (CA) and *continuous interleaved sampling* (CIS) processors (see Chapter 5; Lawson et al., 1993; Wilson et al., 1991a). Both use multiple channels of intracochlear electrical stimulation, and both represent waveforms or envelopes of speech input signals. No specific features of the input, such as the fundamental or formant frequencies, are extracted or explicitly represented. CA processors use continuous analog signals as stimuli, whereas CIS processors use nonsimultaneous pulses. The CA approach is used in the widely applied Ineraid device (Eddington, 1980, 1983) and in the now discontinued UCSF/Storz device (with some differences in details of processor implementation; see Merzenich et al., 1984). Wearable devices capable of supporting the CIS approach are just becoming available for use in clinical settings.

We have completed a study of eleven subjects, seven selected for their high levels of speech recognition with the Ineraid CA

---

*From QPR 3:12, February 1, 1992, through April 30, 1992.

processor and four selected for their relatively poor performances with that processor. The "high performance" subjects were representative of the best patients, in terms of their speech recognition scores, using any commercially available implant system (Wilson et al., 1991a). The purpose of this report is to provide a summary of results for both sets of subjects.

PROCESSING STRATEGIES

Distinctions between CA and CIS processors are illustrated in Figures 7–1 and 7–2. In CA processors a microphone input signal varying over a wide dynamic range is compressed or restricted to the narrow dynamic range of electrically evoked hearing (Pfingst, 1984; Shannon, 1983a) using an automatic gain control. The resulting signal then is filtered into four contiguous frequency bands for presentation to each of four electrodes. As shown in Figure 7–1, information about speech sounds is contained in the relative stimulus amplitudes among the four electrode channels and in the temporal details of the waveforms for each channel.

A concern associated with this method of presenting information is that substantial parts of it may not be perceived by implant patients (Wilson et al., 1990b). For example, most patients cannot perceive frequency changes in stimulus waveforms above about 300 Hz (see, e.g., Shannon, 1993). Thus, many of the temporal details present in CA stimuli are not likely to be accessible to the typical user.

In addition, the simultaneous presentation of stimuli may produce significant interactions among channels through vector summation of the electric fields from each electrode (e.g., White et al., 1984). The resulting degradation of channel independence would be expected to reduce the salience of channel-related cues. That is, the neural response to stimuli from one electrode may be significantly distorted, or even counteracted, by coincident stimuli from other electrodes.

The CIS approach addresses the problem of such channel interactions through the use of interleaved nonsimultaneous stimuli (see Figure 7–2). Trains of balanced biphasic pulses are

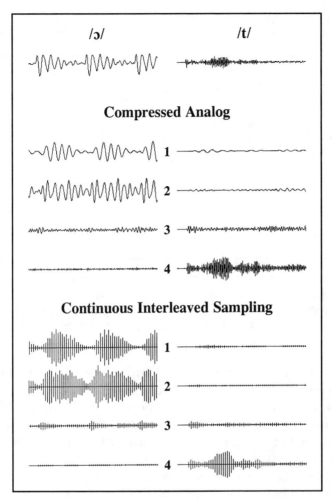

Figure 7–1. Waveforms produced by simplified implementations of CA and CIS strategies. The top panel shows pre-emphasized (6 dB/octave attenuation below 1.2 kHz) speech inputs. Inputs corresponding to a voiced speech sound ("aw") and an unvoiced speech sound ("t") are shown in the left and right columns, respectively. The duration of each trace is 25.4 ms. The remaining panels show stimulus waveforms for CA and CIS processors. The waveforms are numbered by channel, with channel 1 delivering its output to the apical-most electrode. To facilitate comparisons between strategies, only four channels of CIS stimulation are illustrated here. In general, five or six channels have been used for that strategy. The pulse amplitudes reflect the envelope of the bandpass output for each channel. In actual implementations the range of pulse amplitudes is compressed using a logarithmic or power-law transformation of the envelope signal.

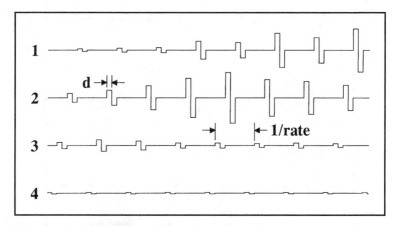

Figure 7–2. Expanded display of CIS waveforms. Pulse duration per phase ("d") and the period between pulses on each channel ("1/rate") are indicated. The sequence of stimulated channels is 4-3-2-1. The total duration of each trace is 3.3 ms.

delivered to each electrode with temporal offsets that eliminate any overlap across channels. The amplitudes of the pulses are derived from the envelopes of bandpass filter outputs. In contrast to the four-channel clinical CA processors, five or six bandpass filters (and channels of stimulation) generally have been used in CIS systems to take advantage of additional implanted electrodes and reduced interactions among channels. The envelopes of the bandpass outputs are formed by rectification and lowpass filtering. Finally, the amplitude of each stimulus pulse is determined by a logarithmic or power-law transformation of the corresponding channel's envelope signal at that time. This transformation compresses each signal into the dynamic range appropriate for its channel.

A key feature of the CIS approach is its relatively high rate of stimulation on each channel. Other pulsatile strategies present sequences of interleaved pulses across electrodes at a rate equal to the estimated fundamental frequency during voiced speech and at a jittered or fixed (often higher) rate during unvoiced speech (Clark, 1987; Wilson, 1993; Wilson et al., 1991b). Rates of stimulation on any one channel rarely have exceeded 300 pulses per second (pps). In contrast, CIS processors generally use brief pulses and minimal delays, so that rapid variations in speech can be tracked by pulse amplitude variations. The rate of stimulation on each channel usually exceeds 500 pps and is constant during both voiced and unvoiced intervals. A constant high rate allows relatively high cutoff frequencies for the lowpass filters in the envelope detectors. With a stimulus rate of 800 pps, for instance, lowpass cutoffs can approach (but not exceed) 400 Hz without introducing aliasing errors in the sampling of the envelope signals at the time of each pulse (see Rabiner and Shafer [1978] for a complete discussion of aliasing and its consequences).

METHODS

Each subject has been studied for a one-week period during which: (a) basic psychophysical measures were obtained on thresholds and dynamic ranges for pulsatile stimuli, (b) a variety of CIS processors (with different choices of processor parameters) were evaluated with preliminary tests of consonant identification, and (c) performance with the best of the CIS processors and the clinical CA processor was documented with a broad spectrum of speech tests. Experience with the clinical processor exceeded one year of daily use for all subjects. In contrast, experience with the CIS processors was limited to no more than several hours before formal testing. All comparisons within this 11-subject study are on the basis of a single week of CIS optimization. In subsequent visits by some of the same subjects a potential for significant further optimization has been demonstrated.

Tests

The comparison tests included open-set recognition of 50 one-syllable words from Northwestern University Auditory Test 6 (NU-6), 25 two-syllable words (spondees), 100 key words in the Central Institute for the Deaf (CID) sentences of everyday speech, and the final word in each of 50 sentences from the Speech Perception in Noise (SPIN) test (presented in our studies without noise). All tests were conducted with hearing alone, using single presentations of recorded material, and without feedback as to correct or incorrect responses.

Processor Parameters

Each subject's own clinical device was used for the tests with the CA processor. As mentioned above, selection of parameters for the CIS processor was guided by preliminary tests of consonant identification. The standard four channels of stimulation were used for the clinical CA processors (Eddington, 1980, 1983), whereas five or six channels were used for the CIS processors. Additional parameters of the CIS processors are presented in Table 7–1. As indicated there, all CIS processors for the "high per-

Table 7–1. Parameters of CIS Processors*

Subject	Channels	Pulse Duration (µs/phase)	Rate (pps)	Integrating Filter Cutoff (Hz)
SR2	6	55	1515	800
SR3	6	31	2688	400
SR4	6	63	1323	400
SR5	6	31	2688	800
SR6	6	102	817	400
SR7	5	34	2941	400
SR8	6	100	833	400
SR1	5	34	833	400
SR10	6	167	500	200
SR9	5	167	500	200
SR11	6	167	500	200

*The parameters include number of channels, pulse duration, the rate of stimulation on each channel (Rate), and the cutoff frequency of the low-pass integrating filters for envelope detection (Integrating Filter Cutoff). The subjects are listed in the chronological order of their participation in the present studies. SR2 through SR8 are the "high performance" subjects, whereas SR1 and SR9-11 belong to the "low performance" group.

formance" subjects, SR2-8, had pulse durations of 102 µs/phase or less, zero delay between the sequential pulses on different channels, pulse rates of 817 pps or higher on each channel, and a cutoff frequency for the lowpass filters of 400 Hz or higher. The best processor for subject SR1 also fit this description, except that a delay of 172 µs was interposed between sequential pulses. The best processors for subjects SR9-11 used long-duration pulses (167 µs/phase), paired with a relatively low rate of stimulation on each channel (500 pps) and a relatively low cutoff frequency for the lowpass filters (200 Hz).

Evaluation of Practice and Learning Effects

Because the tests with the CA processor preceded those with the selected CIS processor for each subject, we were concerned that practice or learning effects might favor the latter in comparisons of the two strategies. To evaluate this possibility, the CID and NU-6 tests were repeated with the CIS processor for five of the "high performance" subjects (subjects SR3, SR4 and SR6-8), using a different recorded speaker and new lists of words and sentences. Practice or learning effects would be demonstrated by significant differences in the test/retest scores. However, no such differences were found ($p > 0.6$ for paired-t comparisons of the CID scores; $p > 0.2$ for the NU-6 scores), and the scores from the first and second tests were averaged for all subsequent analyses.

RESULTS

The results from one-week studies with each of the eleven subjects are presented in Table 7–2 and Figure 7–3. CA and CIS scores for each of the "high performance" subjects are connected by the light lines near the top of each panel in Figure 7–3, and scores for the four "low performance" subjects are connected by the dark lines closer to the bottom of each panel. We note that low-performance subject SR1 had participated in an earlier study not involving CIS processors (Wilson et al., 1991b). Results from his first week of testing with CIS processors are presented

Table 7–2. *Individual Results from the Open-Set Tests*

Subjects	Spondee CA	Spondee CIS	CID CA	CID CIS	SPIN CA	SPIN CIS	NU-6 CA	NU-6 CIS
SR2	92	96	100	100	78	96	56	80
SR3	52	96	66	98	14	92	34	58
SR4	68	76	93	95	28	70	34	40
SR5	100	100	97	100	94	100	70	80
SR6	72	92	73	99	36	74	30	49
SR7	80	100	99	100	66	98	38	71
SR8	68	100	80	100	36	94	38	66
SR1	40	60	25	70	2	30	6	32
SR10	0	56	1	55	0	26	0	14
SR9	8	34	9	34	2	2	2	4
SR11	46	66	40	71	12	30	18	22

here. This is also true of high-performance subject SR2, who has returned to the laboratory for many additional studies with various implementations of CIS processors (see, e.g., Lawson et al., 1993). In those subsequent tests SR2 has achieved even higher scores using a variety of six-channel CIS processors, with NU-6 percent-correct scores ranging from the high 80s to the low 90s.

As is evident from the figure, scores for all eleven subjects are improved with the use of a CIS processor. The average scores across subjects increased from 57 to 80% correct on the spondee test ($p < 0.002$), from 62 to 84% correct on the CID test ($p < 0.005$), from 34 to 65% correct on the SPIN test ($p < 0.001$), and from 30 to 47% correct on the NU-6 test ($p < 0.0005$). Note that the range of difficulty among the four tests provides sensitivity to performance differences across the rather wide range of absolute performance represented in this 11-subject study.

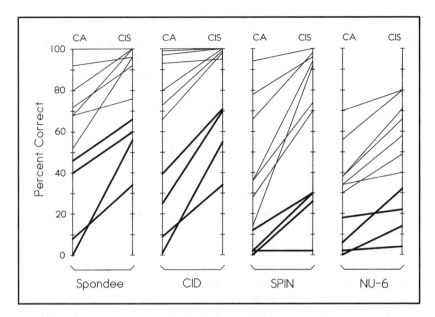

Figure 7-3. Speech recognition scores for CA and CIS processors. A line connects the CA and CIS scores for each subject. Light lines correspond to the seven subjects selected for their excellent performance with the clinical CA processor, whereas the heavier lines correspond to the four subjects selected for relatively poor performance.

Perhaps the most encouraging of these results are the improvements for the four low-performance subjects. SR1, for instance, achieved scores with the CIS processor that would have qualified him for membership in the high performance group (with the clinical CA processor). Similarly, SR10 achieved relatively high scores with the CIS processor. The score on the spondee test increased from 0 to 56% correct, on the CID test from 1 to 55% correct, on the SPIN test from 0 to 26% correct, and on the NU-6 test from 0 to 14% correct. These increases were obtained with no more than several hours of aggregated experience with CIS processors, compared to more than a year of daily experience with the clinical CA processor.

Note that although these gains for SR10 are large, they are not atypical of results for the other subjects. His improvements follow the pattern of the other subjects, that is, generally large gains in the scores of tests that are not limited by ceiling effects. The distinctive aspect of SR10's results is that he enjoys such gains even though he started at or near zero on all four tests. Thus, the relative improvements for SR10 are larger than those for any other subject in the series.

DISCUSSION

The findings presented above demonstrate that use of CIS processors can produce large and immediate gains in speech recognition for a wide range of implant patients. Indeed, the sensitivity of some of the administered tests has been limited by ceiling (or saturation) effects: five of the seven "high performance" subjects scored 96% or higher for the spondee test using CIS processors; all seven scored 95% or higher for the CID test; and five scored 92% or higher for the SPIN test. Scores for the NU-6 test, although not approaching the ceiling, still were quite high. The 80% score achieved by two of the subjects corresponds to the middle of the range of scores obtained by people with mild-to-moderate hearing losses when taking the same test (Bess & Townsend, 1977; Dubno & Dirks, 1982).

The improvements are even more striking when one considers the large disparity in experience with the two processors. At the time of our tests each subject had 1 to 5 years of daily experience with the CA processor, but only several hours over a few days with CIS. In previous studies involving within-subjects comparisons, such differences in experience have strongly favored the processor with the greatest duration of use (Dowell et al., 1987; Dowell et al., 1990; Tyler et al., 1986).

Factors contributing to the performance of CIS processors might include (a) reduction in channel interactions through the use of nonsimultaneous stimuli, (b) use of five or six channels instead of four, (c) representation of rapid envelope variations through the use relatively high pulse rates, (d) preservation of amplitude cues with channel-by-channel compression, and (e) the shape of the compression function.

An interesting aspect of the studies with low-performance subjects is that the best CIS processors seem to involve parameters distinct from those of the best processors for subjects in the high-performance group. The best processor for SR1 used short-duration pulses (34 μs/phase) presented at a relatively low rate (833 pps), and the best processors for SR9-11 used long-duration pulses (167 μs/phase) presented at an even lower rate (500 pps). The subjects in the high-performance group, however, often obtained their best scores with processors tending to minimize pulse widths and maximize pulse rates (e.g., 31 μs/phase pulses presented at 2688 pps).

The use of such shorter pulses and higher rates allows representation of higher frequencies in the modulation waveform for each channel, that is, the cutoff frequency of the lowpass filter in the envelope detectors for each channel may be raised to 1/2 the pulse rate without introducing aliasing effects. In addition, the dynamic range (DR) of electrical stimulation—from threshold to most comfortable loudness—typically is a strong function of pulse rate and a weaker function of pulse duration (see QPR 3:9 and Shannon, 1993). Large increases in DR generally are found with increases in pulse rates from about 400 pps to 2500 pps. Smaller increases often (but not always) are observed with increases in pulse duration (at a fixed rate of stimulation) from roughly 50 μs/phase to higher values (e.g., out to 200 μs/phase for practical CIS designs).

For some patients, though, these advantages may be outweighed by other factors. For several subjects in our Ineraid series, for instance, we have observed that the salience of channel ranking can decline with decreases in pulse widths below 100 μs/phase. A favorable tradeoff for such subjects might involve the use of long-duration pulses (e.g., 100 μs/phase or greater) to preserve channel cues, while foregoing any additional DR obtainable with shorter pulses and higher rates of stimulation.

Another possible advantage of relatively low rates of stimulation is further reduction of channel interactions. Providing time between pulses on sequential channels can reduce the "temporal integration" component of channel interactions (a component produced by the accumulation of charge at neural membranes from sequential stimuli, see, e.g., White et al., 1984). Thus, use of time delays between short-duration pulses in the stimulation sequence across electrodes may reduce interactions. Alternatively, use of long-duration pulses with no time delay also might reduce temporal interactions in that a relatively long period still is realized between the excitatory phases of successive pulses.

Collectively, the present results indicate that: (a) the performance of at least some patients with poor clinical outcomes can be improved substantially with the use of a CIS processor, (b) use of long-duration pulses produced large gains in speech test scores for three such subjects, (c) use of short-duration pulses presented at a relatively low rate produced similar improvements in another such subject, and (d) the optimal tradeoffs among pulse duration, pulse rate, interval between sequential pulses, and cutoff frequency of the lowpass filters appear to vary from patient to patient.

Acknowledgments. We thank the subjects of the described studies for their enthusiastic participation and generous contributions of time. We also are pleased to acknowledge the important scientific contributions of Michael F. Dorman, Donald K. Eddington, William M. Rabinowitz, and Robert V. Shannon. This report is an updated version of a paper that has been submitted for publication in the *Journal of Rehabilitation Research and Development*, "Design and Evaluation of a Continuous Interleaved Sampling (CIS) Processing Strategy for Multichannel Cochlear Implants."

Chapter 8

AUDITORY BRAINSTEM IMPLANT (ABI) STUDIES*

Blake S. Wilson, Dewey T. Lawson, Mariangeli Zerbi, and Charles C. Finley

The Auditory Brainstem Implant (ABI) has been used to restore some hearing for people with bilateral loss of the cochlear nerve. To date, approximately 20 people have been implanted with the ABI device, following the removal of acoustic tumors resulting from neurofibromatosis II.

We have studied two of these patients, in collaboration with Robert V. Shannon and others at the House Ear Institute (HEI). The studies were conducted in our laboratory at the Duke University Medical Center, beginning in the fall of 1989.

The ABI was placed in the first patient immediately after removal of his second acoustic tumor. In contrast, the device was placed in the second patient immediately after removal of her first tumor. This second patient still had normal hearing in her second ear at the time of our tests and no experience with prosthetic stimulation of her implant. The first patient was totally deaf without his prosthesis, and had approximately five months of experience with his ABI at the time of our tests. Both subjects

---

*From QPR 3:12, February 1, 1992, through April 30, 1992. (The original title for this excerpted section from QPR 3:12 was "Auditory Brainstem Implant.")

had percutaneous access to their implanted electrodes, and in both cases only one of the two implanted electrodes offered the possibility of stimulating purely auditory percepts.

Results for the first subject are shown in Figure 8–1. A single-channel *continuous sampling* (CS) processor was compared with the subject's clinical HEI processor (identical in most respects to the 3M/House processor). The stimuli presented by the CS processor, a single-channel variation of *continuous interleaved sampling* (CIS) processors, consisted of a train of short duration pulses whose amplitudes were modulated (via a logarithmic mapping function) with the envelope of the broadband speech signal. The tests included identification of 16 consonants, using male and female speakers; identification of 8 vowels, using male and female speakers; the segmental tests of the Minimal Auditory Capabilities (MAC) battery (Owens et al., 1985); and all open-set tests of the MAC battery except for the SPIN test, which was omitted for this subject. All tests were conducted with hearing alone, with no feedback as to correct or incorrect responses.

As is obvious from the figure, use of the CS processor produced large gains in the transmission of consonant information. In particular, scores for the temporal features of voicing, frication, duration, and envelope cues are much higher with the CS processor. In addition, the score for place of articulation is more than doubled with the application of the CS processor. The only score not improved with the CS processor is the one for nasality, which is about the same for the two processors.

Transmission of vowel features is about the same for the two processors, except for the transmission of F1 information, which is approximately doubled with the use of the CS processor. In addition, the scores for the vowel test in the MAC battery are essentially equivalent for the two processors.

In contrast to the vowel scores, remarkable gains in the initial- and final-consonant tests, and in open-set recognition, are produced with the use of the CS processor. For the open-set tests, for example, the score for spondee recognition is increased from 2 to 40% correct, for CID sentences from 11 to 25% correct, and for NU-6 words from 2 to 12% correct.

These increases, particularly for open-set recognition, are all the more remarkable when one considers the disparity in experience with the two processors. This subject had 5 months of

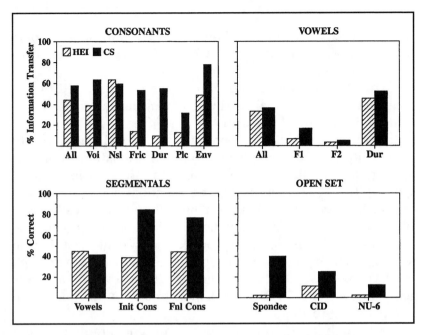

Figure 8–1. Comparison of speech test scores for the first ABI patient studied in the laboratory at Duke. Scores for the HEI processor are indicated by the striped bars, and those for the CS processor by the solid bars. The top panels show relative information transfer for articulatory and acoustic features of consonants and vowels (see Miller & Nicely, 1955). The features for consonants include overall transmission (All), voicing (Voi), nasality (Nsl), frication (Fric), duration (Dur), place of articulation (Plc), and envelope cues (Env). The features for vowels include overall transmission (All), first formant frequency (F1), second formant frequency (F2), and duration (Dur). Twenty presentations of each of 16 consonants were used in the consonant identification tests for both processors, and eighteen presentations of each of 8 vowels were used in the vowel identification tests for both processors. Presentations for both the consonant and vowel tests were equally divided between male and female speakers. The bottom panels show scores from the segmental and open-set tests of the Minimal Auditory Capabilities (MAC) battery. Those tests include vowels (Vowels), initial consonants (Init Cons), and final consonants (Fnl Cons) for the segmentals, and spondee words (Spondee), the Central Institute for the Deaf sentences (CID), and the Northwestern University Auditory Test 6 monosyllabic words (NU-6). The CS processor (processor SS2B) used 110 µs/phase pulses, presented at the rate of 1818 pulses/s. The cutoff frequency of the lowpass filter in the envelope detector was 400 Hz.

143

daily experience with his HEI processor, but only several hours of (aggregated) experience with CS processors before these tests were conducted.

Studies with the second subject were complicated by the facts that she had normal hearing, and that she lacked any experience with electrical stimulation.

Most studies with her were directed at acclimating her to electrically evoked percepts and to initial evaluations of the CS strategy as an adjunct to lip-reading. As indicated in detail in QPR 3:6 (in the section "Parametric Variations and the Fitting of Speech Processors for Single-Channel Brainstem Prostheses"), use of the CS strategy in conjunction with lipreading (from the Iowa laser videodisc images) produced consonant identification scores in the high 90s. Such scores are compatible with high levels of open-set speech recognition. Thus, even in a totally naive listener, the CS strategy demonstrated its potential as an adjunct to lip-reading.

Although these findings are most encouraging, recent results from studies with CIS processors suggest that substantial improvements in speech recognition might be obtained with additional channels. In particular, consonant identification increased almost linearly with increases in channel number from 1 to 6 for a subject using a scala tympani implant (Lawson et al., 1993). Effective use of such additional channels for the ABI device would of course depend on the number of perceptually distinct sites of stimulation.

The present HEI implant has two large electrode surfaces that overlie the dorsal cochlear nucleus. In most cases, only one of these electrodes is useful, in that (monopolar) stimulation of the other produces various nonauditory percepts such as dizziness. In the few cases in which both electrodes produce auditory sensations, the percepts have been described as identical (Robert V. Shannon, personal communication to Wilson, 1992).

Although distinct auditory percepts have not been demonstrated in ABI patients, studies of Frederickson and Gerken (1977) indicate that penetrating electrodes, properly positioned (in the ventral cochlear nucleus), can produce tonotopically restricted patterns of activation in the central auditory system. Use of such electrodes may allow the effective application of multichannel CIS processors.

Electrodes under development include the penetrating electrodes at the University of Michigan and at the HEI in collaboration with the Huntington Medical Research Institutes. In addition, Cochlear Corporation has developed an array of surface electrodes (including 8 electrodes) in a separate cooperative effort with the HEI. We plan to continue our collaborative studies with Bob Shannon and others at the HEI to: (a) study additional patients with the present electrode system and (b) study patients who might be implanted in the future with one of the new electrode systems.

Acknowledgments. We thank the subjects of the described studies for their enthusiastic participation and generous contributions of time. This work was conducted in collaboration with investigators at the HEI, including Bob Shannon, John Wygonski, and Albert Maltan.

Chapter 9

VIRTUAL CHANNEL INTERLEAVED SAMPLING (VCIS) PROCESSORS: INITIAL STUDIES WITH SUBJECT SR2[*]

Blake S. Wilson, Dewey T. Lawson, Mariangeli Zerbi, and Charles C. Finley

Recent studies in our laboratory have focused on development of *continuous interleaved sampling* (CIS) processors (e.g., see Wilson et al., 1991a). A block diagram and waveforms for CIS processors are presented for reference in Figures 9–1 and 9–2, respectively. Each channel includes a bandpass filter and an envelope detector. The amplitudes of stimulus pulses are determined with a logarithmic or power-law transformation of the envelope signal.

[*]From QPR 4:1, August 1, 1992, through October 31, 1992. (The original title for this excerpted section from QPR 4:1 was "Virtual Channel Interleaved Sampling (VCIS) Processors.")

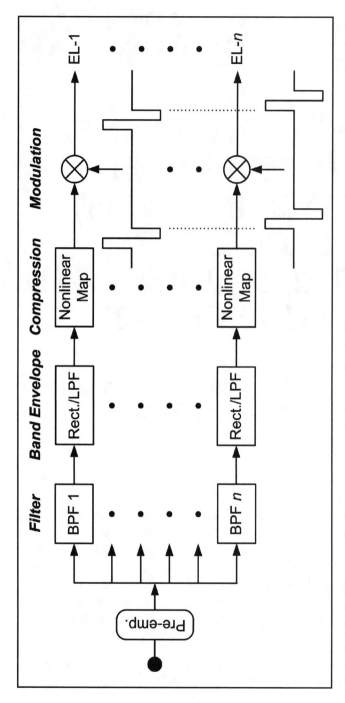

Figure 9–1. Block diagram of a CIS processor. A pre-emphasis filter (Preemp.) is used to attenuate strong low frequency components in speech that otherwise might mask important high frequency components. The pre-emphasis filter is followed by n channels of processing. Each channel includes stages of bandpass filtering (BPF), envelope detection, compression, and modulation. The envelope detector consists of a rectifier (Rect.) followed by a lowpass filter (LPF). Carrier waveforms for two of the modulators are shown immediately below the two corresponding multiplier blocks.

148

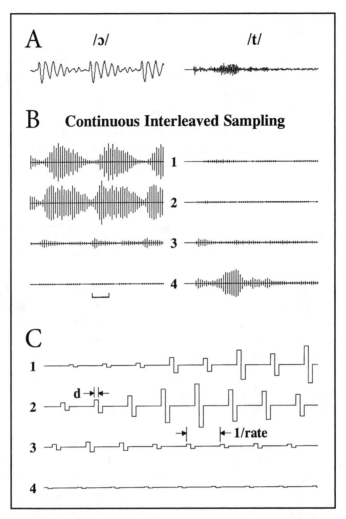

Figure 9–2. Waveforms of a four-channel CIS processor. **A.** Pre-emphasized (6 dB/octave attenuation below 1.2 kHz) speech inputs. Inputs corresponding to a voiced speech sound (/ɔ/) and an unvoiced speech sound (/t/) are shown in the left and right columns, respectively. The duration of each trace is 25.4 ms. **B.** Stimulus waveforms. The waveforms are numbered by channel, with channel 1 delivering its output to the apical-most electrode. The pulse amplitudes in the illustration reflect the envelope of the bandpass output for each channel. In actual implementations the range of pulse amplitudes is compressed using a logarithmic or power-law transformation of the envelope signal. **C.** Expanded display of CIS waveforms (from the bracketed interval in **B**). Pulse duration per phase (**d**) and the period between pulses on each channel (1/rate) are indicated. The sequence of stimulated channels is 4-3-2-1. The duration of each trace is 3.3 ms.

The corner (or cutoff) frequencies of the bandpass filters span the frequency range from 350 to 5500 Hz, evenly spaced along a logarithmic scale. In typical implementations five or six channels are used, with 400 Hz lowpass smoothing filters in the envelope detectors. The information represented by the implant thus consists of envelope variations, below 400 Hz, in each of five or six frequency bands of speech.

DESIGN OF VCIS PROCESSORS

A possible refinement and extension of the CIS approach is illustrated in Figure 9–3. Here adjacent electrodes may be stimulated simultaneously to shift the perceived pitch in any direction with respect to the corresponding single-electrode percepts. Studies with implant subject SR2 indicate that perceived pitch can be manipulated through various choices of simultaneous and nonsimultaneous conditions. If, for instance, the apical-most electrode of his Ineraid electrode array (electrode 1) is stimulated alone, a low pitch is reported. If the next electrode in the array (electrode 2) is stimulated alone, a higher pitch is reported. An intermediate pitch can be produced by stimulating the two electrodes together with identical, in-phase pulses. Finally, by reversing the phase of one of the simultaneous pulses pitch percepts outside the interval represented by the single-electrode percepts can be obtained. The availability of pitches other than those elicited with stimulation of single electrodes may provide additional channels of stimulation. We call these additional channels "virtual channels," and processors that use them *virtual channel interleaved sampling* (VCIS) processors.

An important feature shared by CIS and VCIS processors is interleaving of stimulus pulses. Pulses, or simultaneous combinations of pulses, are presented for each channel in a nonoverlapping sequence, such as the one shown for a CIS processor in the bottom panel C in Figure 9–2. Without interleaving, electric fields from other electrodes would interact (i.e., sum) with the fields produced by the stimuli for any given channel, thereby reducing the independence among channels.

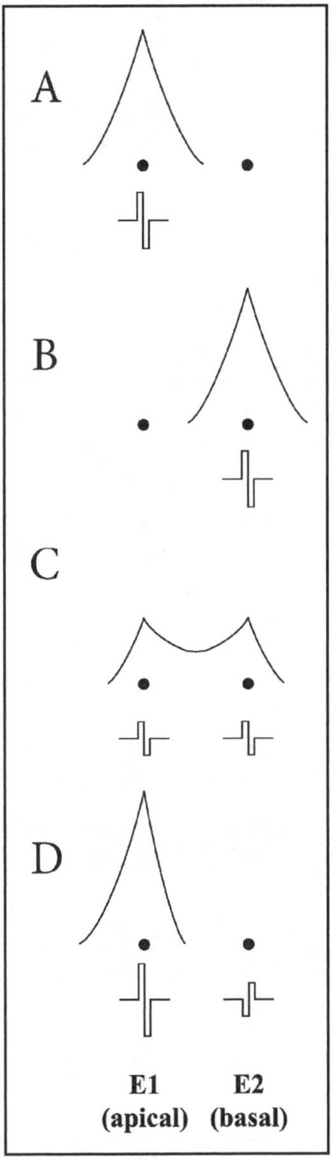

Figure 9–3. Schematic illustrations of neural responses for various conditions of stimulation. The top curve in each panel sketches a hypothetical profile of the number of neurons responding to the pulse or pulses at the bottom of the panel. The positions of two adjacent electrodes are indicated by the dots in each panel. Profiles for stimulation of either electrode alone are presented in **A** and **B**, and profiles for paired stimulation in **C** and **D**. Implant subject SR2, listening to these different stimuli, can rank them according to their distinct pitches. Otherwise the percepts are similar, in that percepts arising from paired pulse conditions and those arising from single pulse conditions seem to differ only in pitch. For the tested subject (using the Ineraid electrode array), stimulation of electrode 1 alone (**A**) produced a low pitch, whereas stimulation of electrode 2 alone (**B**) produced a higher pitch. Simultaneous stimulation of both electrodes, with identical pulses having approximately half the amplitude of the single pulse conditions (**C**), produced an intermediate pitch at an equally loud sensation level. Pairing stimulation of electrode 1 with a reversed-polarity pulse on electrode 2 (**D**) produced the lowest pitch among the illustrated conditions. Various lower pitches could be produced by manipulating the ratio of the pulse 2 to pulse 1 amplitudes over the range of 0.2 to 0.8. A ratio of 1.0 produced a pitch higher than that elicited by stimulation of electrode 1 alone. Similarly, pitches higher than that elicited by stimulation of electrode 6 alone (the basal-most electrode) could be produced by presenting a reversed-phase pulse (of lower amplitude) on electrode 5. Additional discriminable pitches between electrodes also might be produced by manipulating the amplitude ratio of in-phase pulses, but this possibility was not tested. The pulse width used for the listening tests was 33 µs/phase.

151

SUBJECT AND TESTS

Ineraid subject SR2 has participated in an extensive series of studies to evaluate effects of parametric changes in CIS processors and more recently to evaluate several implementations of VCIS processors. Results from his first tests with CIS processors are presented in earlier reports from our group (see Chapter 5 and Wilson et al., 1991a) and are summarized here in Table 9–1 for reference. The tests included open-set recognition of 25 two-syllable words (spondees), 100 key words in the Central Institute for the Deaf (CID) sentences of everyday speech, the final word in each of 50 "high predictability" sentences in the Speech Perception in Noise (SPIN) test (presented without noise in our

Table 9–1. *Percent-Correct Scores from Speech Tests with 6-Electrode Processors, Subject SR2. The processors included a 6-channel CIS processor, a refined 6-channel CIS processor, and an 11-channel VCIS processor.*

Test	CIS	Refined CIS	VCIS[a]
Spondees	96	100	100
CID	100	100	100
SPIN	96	100	100
NU-6	80	90, 94[b]	98
Consonants	*	98.1 ± 0.7[c]	97.1 ± 0.8

[a]VCIS and refined CIS processors both used 12th-order bandpass filters, full-wave rectifiers, 400 Hz lowpass filters (1st order), and 33 µs/phase pulses. The rate of stimulation for each channel was 1365 pulses/s for the VCIS processor and 2500 pulses/s for the refined CIS processor.

[b]Scores from two separate administrations of the NU-6 test; total phoneme score was 287/300.

[c]SEM of percent-correct scores for the blocks in the administered consonant tests.

*The 24 consonant test was not conducted during this initial fitting and evaluation of a CIS processor.

studies), and 50 one-syllable words from Northwestern University Auditory Test 6 (NU-6). All tests were conducted with hearing alone and the test items were presented from standard recordings without feedback or repetition.

RESULTS

These tests and others have been used to evaluate the subsequent implementations of CIS and VCIS processors. Results from a refined implementation of a CIS processor, using parameters somewhat different from those of the original implementation, are presented in the second column of numeric entries in Table 9–1. Results for a VCIS processor are presented in column 3. This processor used in-phase pulses to produce pitches between each pair of electrodes. Thus, six channels corresponded to conditions involving stimulation of one electrode alone, while five additional channels corresponded to conditions involving in-phase paired stimulation. As a precaution against possible learning or familiarization effects, different lists of words and sentences were used in each of the CID, SPIN and NU-6 tests for the different processors. Also, the NU-6 test was repeated for the "refined CIS" processor using another new list of words. The additional test listed in Table 9–1 involved identification of 24 consonants (/b, d, f, g, dʒ, h, j, k, l, m, n, ŋ, p, r, s, ʃ, t, tʃ, ð, θ, v, w, z, ʒ/) in an /a/-consonant-/a/ context, with each of the 24 played in block-randomized order 10 times for a male speaker and 10 times for a female speaker.

Multiple exemplars of each token were drawn from laser videodisc recordings under computer control (Lawson et al., 1993). As with the other tests, the medial consonant tokens were presented in a sound-alone condition, with no feedback as to correct or incorrect responses.

Scores for all three processors are quite high. Indeed, most of the scores are at or near the upper scale limits for each of the tests. The only exception is the NU-6 test, for the two implementations of CIS processors. The NU-6 scores indicate an improvement in performance with the refined CIS processor over the original implementation. The refined processor used a somewhat higher rate of stimulation on each channel (2500 versus 1515 pulse/s), shorter pulses (33 versus 55 μs/phase), a higher corner frequency for the input equalization filter (1200 versus 600 Hz), sharper bandpass filters (12th versus 6th order), and a lower cutoff frequency for the lowpass filters in the envelope detectors (400 versus 800 Hz). Also, the refined processor was evaluated in the 10th week of testing various CIS and other processors with this subject, spread over a 3-year period. Learning effects associated with this additional experience also may have contributed to his improved scores (Dorman et al., 1990; Dowell et al., 1987; Tyler et al., 1986).

With the 11-channel VCIS processor SR2 achieved a score of 98% correct on the NU-6 test, making only one phoneme error (149/150 phonemes). He obtained scores of 100% correct on all remaining open-set tests, and a score of 97% correct on the consonant test. The few errors on the consonant test included five /v/-/ð/ confusions; two /f/-/θ/ confusions; and single confusions between /n/-/m/, /f/-/s/, /s/-/θ/, /ð/-/z/, /ð/-/b/, /b/-/d/, and /g/-/d/.

DISCUSSION

These results indicate quite high levels of speech recognition. The NU-6 score of 80% correct falls in the middle of the range of scores obtained by listeners with mild-to-moderate hearing losses (Bess & Townsend, 1977; Dubno & Dirks, 1982); the score of 92% correct falls in the range of scores obtained by listeners with mild hearing losses (Dubno et al., 1984); and it is not unusual for a subject with normal hearing to score 98% correct (e.g., Davis & Silverman, 1978; Frank & Craig, 1984).

The attainment of such scores with a cochlear implant is noteworthy. The sensitivities of standard audiometric tests of open-set speech recognition are inadequate for this subject with the best of these processors. Obviously, tests of even greater difficulty (e.g., tests involving presentation of low context sentences in noise) will be required in the future to discriminate differences in speech reception under such circumstances.

Although it seems unlikely that many patients will be able to enjoy the high levels of performance obtained by SR2 (e.g., see Wilson et al., 1993), the present results demonstrate what is possible with electrical stimulation of the auditory system, using only six monopolar electrodes. In fact, the scores reported here are highly consistent with scores reported in the early literature on analysis/synthesis systems (sometimes called "vocoder" systems) for the reduced bandwidth transmission of speech. In those experiments speech test scores for listeners with normal hearing began to asymptote at high levels when 6 to 10 bandpass channels were used in an acoustic representation of envelope signals (Flanagan, 1972). The present results suggest that most or all of the information contained in such envelope signals can be transmitted across the electrode-nerve interface of a cochlear implant, and that quite high levels of speech reception can be supported with 6 or 11 channels.

Although the indications from preliminary implementations of VCIS processors are encouraging, much work remains to evaluate fully the potential of the VCIS approach. For example, only one combination of virtual channels was involved in the processor described here. As suggested in Figure 9–3, this combination, using identical in-phase pulses on adjacent electrodes, might produce substantial overlaps in neural excitation fields across single-electrode and two-electrode channels (compare the hypothetical fields sketched for conditions A, B, and C in Figure 9–3). Other combinations may reduce such overlaps. Also, conditions utilizing reversed-phase pulses (e.g., condition D in Figure 9–3) may prove useful in VCIS processors, as may simultaneous pulsatile stimulation of more than two electrodes.

Acknowledgments. We thank subject SR2 for his enthusiastic participation and generous contribution of time. We also note that modeling studies, conducted under the auspices of Project IV in NIH Program Project Grant P01-DC00036, have played an important role in the formulation of VCIS processors. We expect that continued modeling studies may offer further insights into the fine control of the shapes and extents of neural excitation fields in the electrically stimulated cochlea.

Chapter 10

IDENTIFICATION OF VIRTUAL CHANNELS ON THE BASIS OF PITCH*

Blake S. Wilson, Mariangeli Zerbi, and Dewey T. Lawson

The concept of virtual channels was introduced in Chapter 9. Briefly, virtual channels involve simultaneous stimulation of two or more electrodes and may be used in *virtual channel interleaved sampling* (VCIS) processors to provide pitch percepts that are different from those elicited by stimulation of single electrodes. VCIS processors thereby offer the possibility of increasing the number of effective channels beyond the number of available electrodes.

The construction of various types of virtual channels is illustrated in Figure 10–1. The top curve in each panel is a hypothetical sketch of the number of neural responses, as a function of position along the cochlea, for a given condition of stimulation. The condition of stimulation is indicated by the pulse waveform(s) below each dot, which represent the positions of three adjacent electrodes. Conditions involving stimulation of

---

*From QPR 4:3, February 1, 1993 through April 30, 1993. (The original title for this excerpted section from QPR 4:3 was "Identification of Virtual Channel Conditions on the Basis of Pitch.")

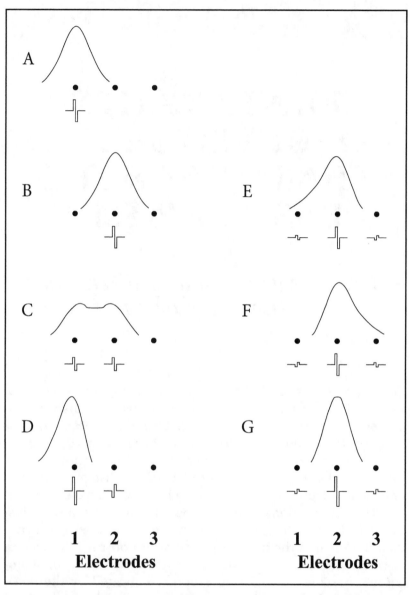

Figure 10–1. Conditions of single-electrode and multiple-electrode (virtual channel) stimulation. See text for a description of the different types of information presented in each panel.

one electrode only are shown in panels A and B, and conditions involving simultaneous stimulation of more than one electrode are shown in panels C through G.

As indicated in Chapter 9, Ineraid subject SR2 previously reported that many of these conditions can be ranked according to their distinct pitches. In informal listening tests stimulation of apical-most electrode 1 alone (A) produced a low pitch, whereas stimulation of electrode 2 alone (B) produced a higher pitch. Simultaneous stimulation of both electrodes, with identical pulses having approximately half the amplitude of the single-pulse conditions (C), produced an intermediate pitch. Pairing stimulation of electrode 1 with a reversed-polarity pulse on electrode 2 (D) produced the lowest pitch among the illustrated conditions. Various lower pitches could be produced by manipulating the ratio of the pulse 2 to pulse 1 amplitudes over the range of 0.2 to 0.8. A ratio of 1.0 produced a pitch higher than that elicited by stimulation of electrode 1 alone. Similarly, pitches higher than that elicited by stimulation of electrode 6 alone (the basal-most electrode in the Ineraid array) could be produced by presenting a reversed-phase pulse (of lower amplitude) on electrode 5. Additional pitches could be produced by constructing triads of pulses, as illustrated in E and F.

Condition G in Figure 10–1 suggests a way in which the width of a neural excitation field might be reduced without altering the centroid or peak of the field, by supplying reversed-phase pulses on either side of a primary pulse. Subject SR2 reported that the pitch percept of this condition was indistinguishable from that of condition B.

Stimuli used for the informal listening tests consisted of 50 ms bursts of 33 μs/phase pulses, presented at 1364 pulses per second. The duration and rate of the pulses are typical of those used in VCIS processors. The stimuli were presented at current amplitudes corresponding to most comfortable loudness (MCL) for each condition.

Although the informal listening tests indicated apparent differences in pitch percepts across conditions, we wanted to evaluate the anecdotal reports in a formal test. In this way we could rank the conditions in an order of ascending pitch and estimate the magnitude and reliability of pitch differences between conditions producing adjacent pitches.

METHODS

An identification experiment was conducted, with each of the seven stimulus conditions in Figure 10–1 presented 30 times in a randomized order. The subject was asked to nominate a pitch from 1 to 7 following each trail, with a nomination of 1 corresponding to the lowest pitch among the conditions and a nomination of 7 corresponding to the highest pitch among conditions. Condition D was presented prior to the formal test as an example of a low pitch among conditions, and condition F was presented prior to the formal test as an example of a high pitch among conditions. No feedback was provided during the formal test. As before, all conditions were presented at MCL, with at least an approximate balance of loudness across conditions (MCL judgments are highly repeatable for this subject). The amplitude ratio of pulses for condition D was 0.5 and the amplitude ratio of flanking pulses to the central pulse for conditions E through G was 0.2. Identical amplitudes were used for the two pulses of condition C.

RESULTS

The results are presented in Figure 10–2, which shows the ranking of conditions in the leftmost column and histograms of pitch nominations in the adjacent column. The mean and standard deviation of the pitch nominations for each condition are shown in the remaining columns.

Note that the overall ranking of conditions is consistent with SR2's anecdotal reports. In particular, the mean of pitch nominations is lowest for condition D; the mean for condition C lies between the means for conditions A and B; the means for conditions E and F are lower than and higher than the mean for condition B, respectively; and the mean of condition G is adjacent to the mean of condition B. Note also that the variance of pitch nominations is not reduced with the use of reversed-phase flanking pulses on either side of a principal pulse (compare standard deviations for conditions G and B).

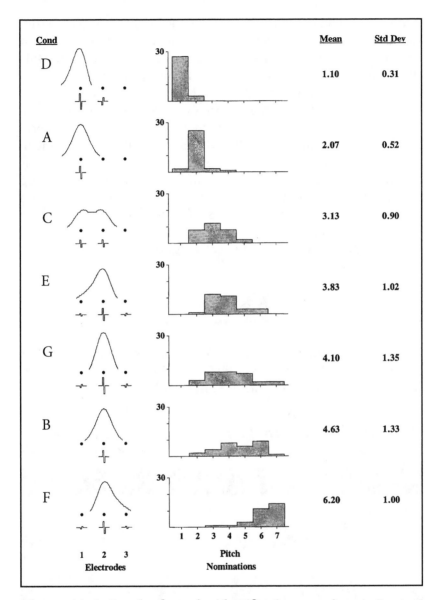

Figure 10–2. Results from the identification experiment. See text for details.

To evaluate the significance of differences among conditions, a one-way analysis of the variance (ANOVA) was conducted using the pitch nomination data. The result indicated that at least some of the means were different from each other ($F[6,203] = 87.5$; $p < .00000001$). Following the ANOVA, a post hoc analysis was conducted with Tukey's HSD statistic. The HSD (the "honestly significant difference" between any pair of means) for the $p = .05$ level was 0.78, and the HSD for the $p = .01$ level was 0.91. Table 10–1 shows a matrix of the differences in means among the tested conditions. Note that half of the adjacent conditions (D and A, A and C, and B and F) are statistically different, at $p = .01$, according to this (conservative) analysis. All of the means separated by one position in the ranking are different (compare conditions C and G, E and B, and G and F). A final observation from Table 10–1 is that the means of conditions C and E, E and G, and G and B are similar, that is, the differences in means for these conditions are not statistically significant.

DISCUSSION

These results indicate that percepts elicited by virtual channels may be separable from those elicited by single-electrode stimulation at adjacent positions in the pitch ranking order. Consistent

Table 10–1. Differences in Means of Pitch Nominations Among Single-Channel and Virtual-Channel Conditions (see Figure 10–2)*

	D	A	C	E	G	B
A	0.97					
C	2.03	1.06				
E	2.73	1.76	0.70			
G	3.00	2.03	0.97	0.27		
B	3.53	2.56	1.50	0.80	0.53	
F	5.10	4.13	3.07	2.37	2.10	1.57

*Differences greater than or equal to 0.78 are significant at the $p = .05$ level, and differences greater than or equal to 0.91 are significant at the $p = .01$ level.

with SR2's anecdotal reports, percepts elicited by conditions A, C, and B form a continuum, with distinct increases in pitch for the order A, C, B. The difference in means between A and C was 1.06, and the difference in means between C and B was 1.50.

Similarly, pitch may be shifted with triads of pulses. Condition E produces a significantly lower pitch than condition B, and condition F produces a significantly higher pitch than condition B. The difference in means between E and B was 0.80, and the difference between B and F was 1.57.

As noted above, conditions G and B produced similar pitches, again consistent with SR2's anecdotal reports. However, use of reversed-phase flanking pulses in condition G did not appear to reduce the variance of pitch judgments, as might have been expected from a sharpening of the neural excitation field.

In general, the present results demonstrate the feasibility of the VCIS approach at a basic psychophysical level. A challenge for future work is to examine possibilities for constructing virtual channels that will: (a) have a greater degree of perceptual independence from adjacent channels and (b) produce equal steps in pitch across channels in a VCIS processor. Use of conditions with a small variance in pitch judgments, for instance, may allow the addition of independent channels. Also, fine adjustment of flanking pulse amplitudes may be helpful in shifting pitches so that equal steps across channels can be approximated. We plan to evaluate several such possibilities in the next quarter, using identification measures like those presented in this report, along with measures of d' and cumulated d' (see, e.g., Braida & Durlach, 1972; Tong & Clark, 1985) to map perceptual distances across conditions.

Acknowledgment. We thank subject SR2 for his enthusiastic participation and generous contribution of time.

Chapter 11

FURTHER EVALUATION OF VCIS PROCESSORS*

Blake S. Wilson, Dewey T. Lawson, and Mariangeli Zerbi

Initial studies with *virtual channel interleaved sampling* (VCIS) processors have been described in Chapters 9 and 10. The concept of virtual channels was introduced in Chapter 9. Results from speech reception tests with one subject also were presented in that chapter. Results from psychophysical studies of virtual channel stimuli were presented in Chapter 10. In the present report we summarize these prior results and present new results from evaluation of VCIS processors with reduced numbers of electrodes and from comparisons of *continuous interleaved sampling* (CIS) and VCIS processors in tests with additional subjects.

PERCEPTS ELICITED BY VCIS STIMULI

Virtual channels involve simultaneous stimulation of two or more electrodes and may be used in VCIS processors to provide pitch percepts that are different from those elicited by stimulation of single electrodes. VCIS processors thereby offer the possibility of

---

*From QPR 4:6, November 1, 1993, through January 31, 1994. (The original title for this excerpted section was "Evaluation of VCIS Processors.")

increasing the number of effective channels beyond the number of available electrodes.

The construction of various types of virtual channels is illustrated in Figure 11–1. The top curve in each panel is a hypothetical sketch of the number of neural responses, as a function of position along the cochlea, for a given condition of stimulation. The condition of stimulation is indicated by the pulse waveform(s) below each dot, with the dots representing the positions of three adjacent electrodes. Conditions involving stimulation of one electrode only are shown in panels A and B, and conditions involving simultaneous stimulation of more than one electrode are shown in panels C through G.

As indicated in Chapters 9 and 10, Ineraid subject SR2 can rank conditions A through F according to their distinct pitches. Stimulation of the apical-most electrode 1 alone (condition A) produces a low pitch, whereas stimulation of electrode 2 alone (condition B) produces a higher pitch. Simultaneous stimulation of both electrodes, with identical pulses having approximately half the amplitude of the single-pulse conditions (condition C), produces an intermediate pitch. Pairing stimulation of electrode 1 with a reversed-polarity pulse on electrode 2 (condition D) produces the lowest pitch among the illustrated conditions. Similarly, pitches higher than that elicited with stimulation of electrode 6 alone (the basal-most electrode in the Ineraid array) can be produced by presenting a reversed-phase pulse (of lower amplitude) on electrode 5. Additional pitches between electrodes can be produced by constructing triads of pulses, as illustrated in panels E and F. The pitch produced with the stimulus of condition E is lower than that elicited with stimulation of electrode 2 alone (condition B), whereas the pitch produced with the stimulus of condition F is higher than that elicited with stimulation of electrode 2 alone.

Condition G in Figure 11–1 suggests a way in which the width of a neural excitation field might be reduced without altering the centroid or peak of the field, by supplying reversed-polarity pulses on either side of a principal pulse. Subject SR2 reports that the pitch percept of this condition is indistinguishable from that of condition B. We note that this general type of "sharpened field" stimulation also has been described by Townshend and coworkers (1987) and by Jolly, Spelman, and Pfingst (1994).

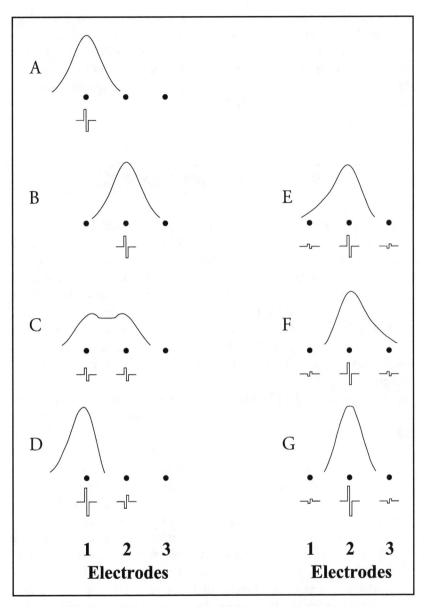

Figure 11–1. Conditions of single-electrode and multiple-electrode (virtual channel) stimulation. See text for a description of the different types of information presented in each panel.

Ineraid subjects SRl0 and SR13 also have participated in psychophysical studies to evaluate perceptual differences among virtual channel and single-electrode stimuli. Subject SR10 was tested with conditions A through C and subject SR13 with conditions A through D. The results were the same qualitatively as those indicated above for SR2.

INITIAL CIS/VCIS COMPARISON

One implementation of a VCIS processor is illustrated in Figure 11–2. The virtual channels use identical in-phase pulses presented simultaneously on adjacent electrodes. These channels are combined with six single-electrode channels to form an 11-channel processor. As in standard CIS processors, the stimulus for each of the channels is presented in a nonoverlapping sequence. Without such interleaving of stimuli, electric fields from other electrodes would interact (i.e., sum) with the fields produced by the stimulus for any given channel, thereby reducing the independence among channels.

An 11-channel VCIS processor of the type illustrated in Figure 11–2 has been compared with 6-channel CIS processors in initial tests with subject SR2 (Chapter 9; Wilson et al., 1994). This subject has participated in an extensive series of studies to evaluate effects of parametric changes in CIS processors and more recently to evaluate implementations of VCIS processors. Results from his first tests with CIS processors are presented in earlier reports from our group (e.g., Wilson et al., 1991a) and are summarized here in Table 11–1 for reference. The tests included open-set recognition of 25 two-syllable words (spondees), 100 key words in the Central Institute for the Deaf (CID) sentences of everyday speech, the final word in each of 50 "high predictability" sentences in the Speech Perception in Noise (SPIN) test (presented without noise in our studies), and 50 one-syllable words from Northwestern University Auditory Test 6 (NU-6). All tests were conducted with hearing alone and the test items were presented from standard recordings without feedback or repetition.

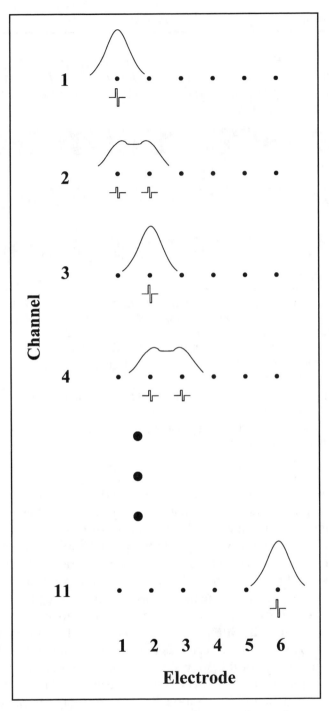

Figure 11-2. Construction of an 11-channel VCIS processor.

Table 11–1. *Percent-Correct Scores from Speech Tests with 6-Electrode Processors, Subject SR2. The processors included a 6-channel CIS processor, a refined 6-channel CIS processor, and an 11-channel VCIS processor.*

Test	CIS	Refined CIS	VCIS[a]
Spondees	96	100	100
CID	100	100	100
SPIN	96	100	100
NU-6	80	90, 94[b]	98
Consonants	*	98.1 ± 0.7[c]	97.1 ± 0.8

[a]VCIS and refined CIS processors both used 12th-order bandpass filters, full-wave rectifiers, 400 Hz lowpass filters (1st order), and 33 μs/phase pulses. The rate of stimulation for each channel was 1365 pulses/s for the VCIS processor and 2500 pulses/s for the refined CIS processor.

[b]Scores from two separate administrations of the NU-6 test; total phoneme score was 287/300.

[c]SEM of percent-correct scores for the blocks in the administered consonant tests.

*The 24 consonant test was not conducted during this initial fitting and evaluation of a CIS processor.

These tests and others have been used to evaluate the subsequent implementations of CIS and VCIS processors. Results from a refined implementation of a CIS processor, using parameters somewhat different from those of the original implementation, are presented in the second column of numeric entries in Table 11–1. Results for the 11-channel VCIS processor are presented in column 3. As a precaution against possible learning or familiarization effects, different lists of words and sentences were used in each of the CID, SPIN, and NU-6 tests for the different processors. Also, the NU-6 test was repeated for the "refined CIS" processor using another new list of words. The additional test listed in Table 11–1 involved identification of 24 consonants in an /a/-consonant-/a/ context. Each of the 24 was presented in block-randomized order 10 times for a male speaker and

10 times for a female speaker. As with the other tests, the medial consonant tokens were presented in a sound-alone condition, with no feedback as to correct or incorrect responses.

Scores for all three processors are quite high. Indeed, most of the scores are at or near the upper scale limits for each of the tests. The only exception is the NU-6 test, for the two implementations of CIS processors. The NU-6 scores indicate an improvement in performance with the refined CIS processor over the original implementation. The refined processor used a somewhat higher rate of stimulation on each channel (2500 versus 1515 pulses/s), shorter pulses (33 versus 55 µs/phase), a higher corner frequency for the input equalization filter (1200 versus 600 Hz), sharper bandpass filters (12th versus 6th order), and a lower cutoff frequency for the lowpass filters in the envelope detectors (400 versus 800 Hz). Also, the refined processor was evaluated in the 10th week of testing various CIS and other processors with this subject, spread over a 3-year period. Learning or practice effects associated with this additional experience also may have contributed to his improved scores (Dorman et al., 1990; Dowell et al., 1987; Tyler et al., 1986).

With the 11-channel VCIS processor SR2 achieved a score of 98% correct on the NU-6 test, making only one phoneme error (149/150 phonemes). He obtained scores of 100% correct on all remaining open-set tests, and a score of 97% correct on the consonant test.

EVALUATION OF VCIS PROCESSORS WITH REDUCED NUMBERS OF ELECTRODES

Following the initial comparison of CIS and VCIS processors, we decided to evaluate a variety of CIS and VCIS processors with reduced numbers of electrodes. The principal motivation for these additional studies was to reduce test scores to a range where differences among processors might be clearly demonstrated. In addition, we were interested in evaluating the potential benefit of virtual channels for patients with a limited number of usable electrodes.

The conditions and results of the additional studies, again with subject SR2, are presented in Figure 11–3. The horizontal lines indicate the positions of six physical electrodes. An open circle on one of the lines indicates a channel of stimulation with a single electrode. An open circle between lines indicates a virtual channel formed by stimulation of adjacent electrodes with identical in-phase pulses (corresponding to condition C in Figure 11–1). A closed circle indicates a virtual channel formed by presentation of a principal pulse at one electrode paired with simultaneous presentation of a reversed-polarity, half-amplitude pulse on an adjacent electrode (corresponding to condition D in Figure 11–1). As an example, the leftmost condition in Figure 11–3 is that of a 3-channel processor using two single-electrode channels and one virtual channel. Electrodes 2 and 3 are used for the single-electrode channels, and electrodes 2 and 3 are stimulated together with identical in-phase pulses for the virtual channel. The next condition in Figure 11–3 also has three channels, but in this case each of the channels is a virtual channel formed with identical in-phase pulses. The next condition uses the three channels of the first condition along with two additional virtual channels formed with reversed-polarity pulses. The apical-most virtual channel is produced by simultaneous stimulation of electrode 2 with a principal pulse and electrode 3 with a reversed-polarity pulse at half the amplitude of the principal pulse. Similarly, the basal-most virtual channel is produced with a principal pulse on electrode 3 and a reversed-polarity pulse on electrode 2. Note that in this condition five channels of information are presented with only two electrodes.

The processors for each of the conditions in Figure 11–3 were evaluated with the consonant test. Each of 24 consonants was presented at least 10 times with the male speaker for each of the conditions. The results are presented in terms of overall information transfer (Cons. IT Overall) and the information transfer score for the place of articulation feature (Cons. IT Place). The results and conditions are arranged in order of increasing scores for overall information transfer.

The ranking of conditions from left to right seems to indicate improvements in scores with increases in the total distance along the cochlea spanned by the channels. The addition of virtual

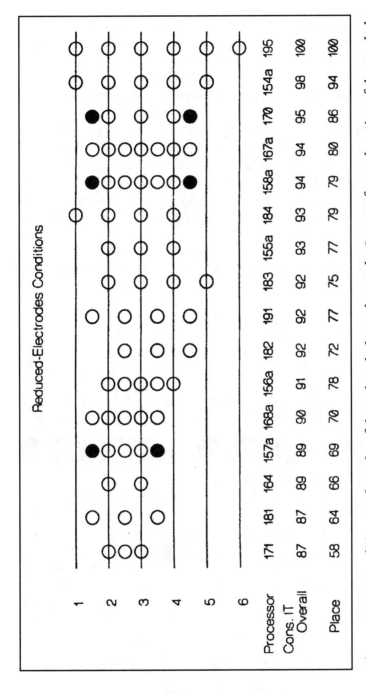

Figure 11–3. Conditions and results of the reduced-electrodes study. See text for explanation of the symbols denoting conditions at the top of the figure. Results from tests of consonant identification are presented at the bottom, and include overall information transfer (Cons. IT Overall) and information transfer for the place of articulation feature (Cons. IT Place).

channels per se does not appear to improve scores, even with an increase the number of channels. Improvements in scores can be produced by increasing cochlear distance either with single-electrode channels or with virtual channels.

To evaluate these impressions, we conducted stepwise linear regression analyses of the data, where the dependent variable was either overall information transfer or information transfer for the place of articulation feature. The independent variables for both analyses included the variables listed in Table 11–2.

The regression analyses indicated that the single variable of cochlear distance accounted for 83.3% of the variance in the overall IT scores ($p < .000002$) and for 84.1% of the variance in the place IT scores ($p < .000002$). No other variable accounted for a significant portion of the variance for either dependent variable once cochlear distance was factored out. The regression equations were:

$$\text{Overall IT} = 3.1 \times \text{dist} + 84.2$$
$$\text{Place IT} = 9.6 \times \text{dist} + 51.8$$

Table 11–2. Independent Variables Used in the Stepwise Linear Regression Analyses of Results from the Reduced-Electrodes Study

Variable	Description
nchans	number of channels
Pivc	fraction interior virtual channels
eacr	exterior virtual channels, reversed phase
eacin	exterior virtual channels, in phase
dist	total cochlear distance spanned by the channels
center	center of cochlear distance
space	average spacing between channels
ratio	number of channels/number of electrodes
vc	presence of virtual channels

The addition of interior virtual channels does not figure in the regression analyses. It may be that much of the information on intermediate pitches already is available with CIS processors, using single-electrode channels. That is, even though stimuli are presented nonsimultaneously, intermediate pitches might be produced between adjacent electrodes. A critical question relates to the time over which the central auditory system integrates inputs to make inferences about pitch. Recent studies by Colette McKay and Hugh McDermott of the Melbourne team (personal communication to Wilson, 1993) suggest that this interval is at least 400 μs, which is much longer than the time between sequential pulses in typical implementations of CIS processors.

CIS/VCIS COMPARISONS WITH ADDITIONAL SUBJECTS

In parallel with the reduced-electrodes study, we also evaluated full VCIS processors with additional subjects. The results are presented in Figure 11–4. The initial findings for SR2 are repeated in the top panel. Scores for subjects SR10 and SR13 are shown in the middle and bottom panels, respectively. The consonant tests for SR2 included 24 consonants with both male and female speakers, whereas the tests for SRl0 and SR13 included 16 consonants. Tests with both male and female speakers were used for SR10, whereas only the male speaker was used for SR13.

The processors implemented for SR13 used the five apical electrodes only, because stimulation of basal-most electrode 6 elicited a somatic sensation at levels just above auditory threshold. Each subject was fitted with an 11-channel VCIS processor. The 11-channel processors for SR2 and SR10 used interior virtual channels, as illustrated in Figure 11–2. The processor for SR13 used four interior virtual channels (corresponding to the positions between the five available electrodes) and two exterior virtual channels, formed with a principal pulse on the apical-most or basal-most electrode paired with a half-amplitude, reversed-polarity pulse on the adjacent electrode (i.e., on electrode 2 for a principal pulse on apical-most electrode 1, or on electrode 4 for a principal pulse on basal-most electrode 5).

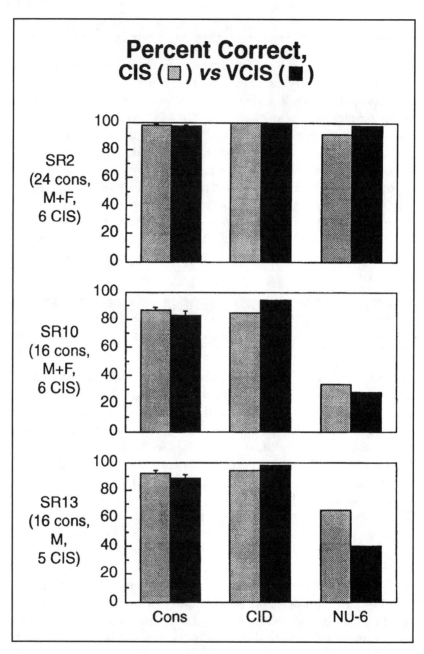

Figure 11–4. Comparisons of CIS and VCIS processors for three subjects. Tests included identification of consonants in an /a/-consonant-
/a/ context (Cons), recognition of key words in the Central Institute
for the Deaf sentences of everyday speech (CID), and recognition of
monosyllabic words from Northwestern University Auditory Test 6
(NU-6).

In general, the results do not demonstrate an advantage of VCIS processors. Scores from the consonant tests are not statistically different for any of the subjects. Results from the open-set tests are mixed, with somewhat better scores for VCIS in some cases (e.g., the NU-6 test for SR2 and the CID test for SR10) and for CIS in others (e.g., the NU-6 test for SR10). The only large difference between processors is in the NU-6 scores for SR13, where the score for the CIS processor is clearly better than the score for the VCIS processor.

Although the speech reception scores for the two types of processors were similar, each of the subjects expressed a strong preference for the VCIS processor. Each of them said that the VCIS processor sounded more natural and seemed more intelligible than the CIS processor. SR2 and SR13 also compared the two processors for listening to music, and both said the VCIS processor produced a richer and more natural sound than the CIS processor.

DISCUSSION

Present implementations of VCIS processors offer no obvious advantage over CIS despite some very encouraging initial results, and despite the strong preference for VCIS expressed by all three subjects. It is possible that we have not selected the best tests to demonstrate a difference between processors, as suggested by the anecdotal remarks of the subjects. For example, a difficult test of vowel identification might demonstrate a difference between processors with sparse *versus* dense spatial representations (e.g., CIS versus VCIS, where each of the processors use the same number of electrodes). In initial tests of vowel identification, involving 12 different synthesized vowels of equal durations, SR2 obtained a higher score with a VCIS processor than with a CIS processor (percent correct identification was 82% with VCIS versus 72% with CIS; Michael F. Dorman, personal communication to Wilson, 1992). Also, tests of music perception may demonstrate differences between processors. Studies of complex tone perception, as described in QPR 4:4, are underway with subject SR2 using both VCIS and CIS processors.

We are not quite ready to discontinue our studies with VCIS processors. Evaluation of VCIS with different tests seems warranted. Also, we note that alternative implementations of VCIS processors may be superior to the present implementations. For example, selective use of single-electrode and multiple-electrode channels may allow implementation of a processor with a relatively large number of channels (e.g., 7 or 8) with a high degree of perceptual distinctness among channels. We are exploring the potential of such alternative implementations with psychophysical studies of channel scaling and channel identification. As indicated in QPR 4:5, we also are assessing the spatial patterns of neural excitation produced with single-electrode and multiple-electrode stimulation using a forward masking technique. Results from those studies should indicate whether additional information can be provided with the selective use of virtual channels or with types of virtual channels different from those used in the present implementations of VCIS processors.

Acknowledgments. We thank the three subjects of the studies described in this report for their enthusiastic participation and generous contributions of time. We also are grateful to M. F. Dorman and C. C. Finley, who helped us in various scientific aspects of the work.

Chapter 12

DESIGN FOR AN INEXPENSIVE BUT NONETHELESS HIGHLY EFFECTIVE COCHLEAR IMPLANT SYSTEM*

Blake S. Wilson, Dewey T. Lawson, Mariangeli Zerbi, and Charles C. Finley

The 1993 Zhengzhou International Conference on Cochlear Implants and Linguistics was held in Zhengzhou, China, October 23–26, 1993. The Conference was organized by Min-Sheng Dong, MD, Professor and Chief Surgeon of the Henan Medical University in Zhengzhou, and by Fan-Gang Zeng, PhD, Research Scientist at the House Ear Institute in Los Angeles, California. Approximately 130 physicians, scientists, and engineers attended the Conference, including representatives from most centers in China involved with the development or clinical application of implant systems. A panel of five experts from the United States and Canada was invited to provide information on recent developments in implant design and performance. The panel also

---

*From FR 4, August 1, 1992, through July 31, 1995. (The original title for this excerpted section from FR 4 was "Design for an Inexpensive But Effective Cochlear Implant System.")

was invited to offer recommendations for the design of an inexpensive but effective implant system that might be suitable for widespread use in China. The panelists included Gerald Loeb, Stephen Rebscher, Robert Shannon, Blake Wilson, and Fan-Gang Zeng. Blake Wilson's participation in the conference was supported by the Commission of Science and Technology of Henan Province. Support for the subsequent evaluation of a prototype system, as described below, was provided by this project. Dewey Lawson and Mariangeli Zerbi conducted the evaluation studies.

The system recommended by the panel includes a speech processor, four pairs of transmitting and receiving coils, and an electrode array with four monopolar electrodes. All implanted components are passive, reducing to a minimum the complexity of manufacture and allowing high reliability. A transcutaneous link is used to minimize the possibility of infection, which in turn should minimize medical costs in maintaining device function. The electrode array has a mechanical memory to position the electrodes in close proximity to the inner modiolar wall of the scala tympani. A reference electrode is implanted in the temporalis muscle. A four-channel CIS strategy is used for the speech processor. The speech processor and transcutaneous link have been evaluated in preliminary tests with a patient implanted with the Ineraid electrode array and percutaneous connector. A prototype of the link, consisting of four pairs of transmitting and external receiving coils, was used, with the outputs of the receiving coils routed to the apical four electrodes of the Ineraid array via the percutaneous connector. The tests included identification of 24 consonants in an /a/-consonant-/a/ context. The subject scored 89 ± 2% correct with a standard laboratory implementation of the four-channel CIS processor using current-controlled stimuli and 92 ± 1% correct with the prototype system. These scores show that use of the coils does not degrade performance. Results from other studies indicate that many patients can achieve high levels of speech recognition with CIS processors and monopolar electrodes. The system recommended here includes those components along with: (a) an electrode array that may improve placement of the intracochlear contacts, and (b) a simple transcutaneous link that does not degrade performance.

The excellent performance obtained with the prototype system supports development of a commercial system that can be easily manufactured at low cost. Such a system may be especially appropriate for widespread use in countries like China, with large numbers of people with profound hearing loss and highly limited resources for procurement of medical devices.

Acknowledgments. We thank research subject SR2 for his enthusiastic participation and generous contribution of time.

Chapter 13

22-ELECTRODE PERCUTANEOUS STUDY: RESULTS FOR THE FIRST FIVE SUBJECTS*

Dewey T. Lawson, Blake S. Wilson,
Mariangeli Zerbi, and Charles C. Finley

With NIH support, our group is participating with Duke University Medical Center (DUMC) and Cochlear Corporation in a study of patients implanted with a percutaneous research version of the standard Nucleus 22 electrode array. Five patients (NP1 through NP5) have been selected thus far and implanted by DUMC surgeon Debara Tucci. It has been agreed that a total of seven patients will be included in the study. Each subject agrees to participate in three 2-week research visits to our laboratory.

During the percutaneous phase of the studies each patient's everyday processor is a monopolar variation of the standard clinical *spectral peak* (SPEAK) strategy. That processor is fitted and maintained by DUMC audiologist Patricia Roush and evaluated by our group along with various *continuous interleaved*

---

*From QPR 5:3, February 1, 1996, through April 30, 1996.

sampling (CIS) and other research designs. The subjects also participate in our intracochlear evoked potential studies.

A core protocol of processor comparisons is carried out with each of these subjects. As outlined in QPR 5:1, the contents of the protocol evolved significantly in the course of the early patient visits, as initial results were obtained. In this report we will review the final design of the protocol and present its results for each of the first five subjects.

The sixteen core protocol processors to be compared are outlined in Table 13–1. All processors use 33 µs/phase pulses, full-wave rectification, 12th-order bandpass filters, 4th-order smoothing filters, and our normal pre-emphasis filter and logarithmic mapping functions. All stimulate chosen intracochlear electrodes with respect to a reference electrode in the temporalis muscle ipsilateral to the implanted cochlea. In addition, there are reference settings that are departed from only in processors designed to assess the variation of a single parameter. These reference settings include: positive phase leading at the intracochlear electrodes in balanced biphasic pulses, a pulse rate on each channel of 833 pulses/s, a staggered order of stimulation within each cycle (e.g., 6, 3, 5, 2, 4, 1 for a 6-channel processor), a 200 Hz cutoff frequency for the smoothing filters in the envelope (or energy) detectors, and a 350 to 5500 Hz overall bandpass range allocated to the channels in contiguous bands of logarithmically equal widths.

Five of the sixteen protocol processors use the reference settings to implement different numbers of CIS channels. These five processors are labeled as **21**, **11**, **8**, **6ref**, and **4**, corresponding to 21, 11, 8, 6, and 4 channels of stimulation, respectively. (Note that the reference pulse rate for the 21-channel processor is necessarily 721 rather than 833 pulses/s, given 33 µs/phase pulse widths.) Seven additional processors represent single parameter variations with respect to **6ref**. These variations include **6els** (differing only in that it utilizes a different set of six electrodes), **6ord** (using an apex-to-base rather than staggered order of stimulation), **6sth** (using a 400 Hz rather than a 200 Hz smoothing filter cutoff frequency), **6pol** (using balanced biphasic pulses that begin with the negative rather than the positive phase to the intracochlear electrode), **6rng** (with frequency bands covering the range of 350 to 9500 Hz rather than 350 to 5500 Hz),

Table 13–1. 22-Electrode Percutaneous Study Protocol Processors*

Type	Label	Chans	Pulse Polarity	Stimul. Rate	Stimul. Order	Smoother Cutoff	Freq. Range	Selected Electds.
n chan	21	21	+/–	721	stag	200 Hz	5500 Hz	
	11	11	+/–	833	stag	200	5500	
	8	8	+/–	833	stag	200	5500	
	4	4	+/–	833	stag	200	5500	
6 chan	ref	6	+/–	833	stag	200	5500	ref
	ord	6	+/–	833	a-b	200	5500	ref
	sth	6	+/–	833	stag	400	5500	ref
	pol	6	–/+	833	stag	200	5500	ref
	rng	6	+/–	833	stag	200	9500	ref
	slo	6	+/–	250	stag	200	5500	ref
	fst	6	+/–	2525	stag	200	5500	ref
	els	6	+/–	833	stag	200	5500	alt

continues

Table 13-1. continued

Type	Label	Chans	Pulse Polarity	Stimul. Rate	Stimul. Order	Smoother Cutoff	Freq. Range	Selected Electds.
n-of-m	slo	6/18	+/−	250	a-b	200	5500	
	fst	6/18	+/−	833	a-b	200	5500	
	rngslo	6/18	+/−	250	a-b	200	**9500**	
	rngfst	6/18	+/−	833	a-b	200	**9500**	

*Abbreviations: Chans for Channels; Stimul. for Stimulation; Freq. for Frequency; Electds. for Electrodes; n chan for processors in which the number of channels is manipulated; stag for staggered; ref for reference; ord for an alternative stimulation order; a-b for apex-to-base; sth for an alternative smoother cutoff frequency; pol for the alternative polarity; rng for the upper end of the frequency range represented by an implant processor set to 9500 Hz; slo for a relatively slow rate of stimulation for each channel; fst for a relatively fast rate of stimulation for each channel; els for an alternative selection of electrodes; alt for the same alternative selection of electrodes; rngslo for the features of rng plus slo in the same processor; and rngfst for the features of rng plus fst in the same processor.

186

6slo (with a pulse rate on each channel of 250 rather than 833 pulses/s), and **6fst** (with a pulse rate of 2525 rather than 833 pulses/s). The remaining four processors are what we call *n*-of-*m* designs, in which a total of *m* frequency bands are analyzed and only the *n* electrodes corresponding to the *n* highest energy bands are stimulated on a given processing cycle. In the protocol, *n* is set to 6, whereas *m* may vary somewhat depending on each subject's number of available electrodes. For the first five subjects, *m* has been held constant at 18. For all subjects, four variations of *n*-of-*m* processors will be or have been tested. These variations include processors using the standard frequency range and relatively fast (**nmfst**) or slow (**nmslo**) rates of stimulation at the 6 electrodes selected for each update cycle across electrodes, and processors using the extended frequency range and the fast (**nmrngfst**) or slow (**nmrngslo**) rates. The faster rate for the *n*-of-*m* processors is 833 pulses/s/selected electrode, and the slower rate is 250 pulses/s/selected electrode. A summary of all processor variations and their labels is presented in Table 13–2.

This set of protocol processors has been chosen to support a wide array of comparisons. The effects of varying the number of CIS channels are explored through comparisons among **21**, **11**, **8**, **6ref**, and **4**. The sensitivity of performance to choices among available electrodes may be probed by comparing **6ref** and **6els**. The effects of various single parameter variations are studied in comparisons of performance between **6ref** and, in turn, **6ord**, **6sth**, **6pol**, **6rng**, **6fst**, and **6slo**. The **nmrngslo** processor is designed to be equivalent in some respects to the clinical SPEAK processor, which also analyzes an extended frequency range, selects a subset of the analyzed bands for stimulation on each processing cycle, and stimulates the corresponding electrodes at a variable rate that averages approximately 250 pulses/s. Comparisons are available with a basic 6-channel CIS processor at the same rate (**6slo**), an *n*-of-*m* processor at the same rate but without the extended frequency range (**nmslo**), and *n*-of-*m* processors running at a rate substantially higher than is possible for the present SPEAK strategy (**nmfst**, **nmrngfst**). The latter processors also may be compared with a CIS processor running at the same rate (**6ref**). Depending on performance test results with individual subjects, various features of the protocol designs can be combined in additional processors for further evaluations.

Table 13-2. Key to Processor Labels

Processor Label(s)*	Description
21, 11, 8, 4, 6ref	21, 11, 8, 4, and 6 channels, reference parameters
6els	6 channel, alternative selection of electrodes
6ord	6 channel, apex-to-base stimulation order
6sth	6 channel, 400 Hz smoothing cutoff
6pol	6 channel, reversed polarity
6rng	6 channel, extended frequency range
6fst	6 channel, fast rate (2525 pulse/s)
6slo	6 channel, slow rate (250 pulse/s)
nmfst	*n*-of-*m* (*6*-of-*18*) strategy, fast rate (833 pulses/s)
nmslo	*n*-of-*m* (*6*-of-*18*) strategy, slow rate (250 pulses/s)
nmrngfst	*n*-of-*m* (*6*-of-*18*) strategy, extended frequency range, fast rate
nmrngslo	*n*-of-*m* (*6*-of-*18*) strategy, extended frequency range, slow rate

*When 6-channel and *n*-of-*m* processors are grouped separately and no confusion will result, the "6" and "*nm*" label prefixes may be omitted.

The performance of the monopolar clinical SPEAK processor is tested during each of the three visits to our laboratory, to assess possible learning effects. A bipolar SPEAK processor is fitted during the last of the three research visits and its performance is tested after extended use outside of the laboratory.

After completion of these visits to the laboratory, it is anticipated that each subject will undergo a second surgery to receive a standard clinical transcutaneous device. Only subject NP1 has undergone that second surgery to date; she is doing well with her clinical bipolar SPEAK processor.

Tables 13–3 through 13–7 summarize contemporaneous 24 or 16 consonant identification data from subjects NP1 through NP5 for the 16 protocol processors and the monopolar version of the clinical SPEAK processor that each subject had used daily for approximately one and a half years. (Not all of the subjects have high enough levels of performance to justify use of the 24-consonant tests; 16-consonant tests have been used with three of the first five subjects: NP3, NP4, and NP5.) Results for tests using male and female talkers are listed separately, in descending order of overall information transmission (overall % IT) in each case. For subject NP1 these results (in Table 13–3) are the same as in Table 4 of QPR 5:1, except that results for corrected versions of two of the processors, **nmfst** and **nmslo**, were obtained after submission of QPR 5:1 and those updated results are included in the present Table 13–3.

To facilitate comparisons, Tables 13–3 through 13–7 have separate columns for: (1) single parameter variations among 6 channel CIS processors, (2) speed and frequency range variations among *n*-of-*m* processors, (3) comparisons among otherwise similar processors differing in the number of CIS channels, and (4) the monopolar variation of the clinical SPEAK processor. Experience with all tested processors except the clinical SPEAK processor was limited to a brief period of informal conversation and loudness adjustment prior to testing. The SPEAK processor was used by each of the subjects in their everyday lives and for at least a year and a half prior to the tests with any other processor.

Appendix 1 in QPR 5:3 (the QPR from which this chapter is drawn) presents both the overall % IT and percent-correct scores with standard deviations of the means for each subject and each protocol processor. (The complete QPR, including the appendices, can be viewed by visiting http://www.rti.org/capr/caprqprs. html, scrolling down to Project N01-DC-5-2103, and then clicking on the "pdf" or "hmtl" link for QPR 3.) Each percent-correct or IT value is based on presentation of a minimum of 10 randomized blocks of the 16 or 24 consonant tokens, sound alone, from videodisc recordings. Multiple exemplars of each token were used, and there was no feedback as to correct or incorrect responses.

Table 13–3. Protocol Processor Rankings, Subject NP1*

Overall % IT	24 Consonants Male				24 Consonants Female			
	6 chan	*n*-of-*m*	n chan	clin	6 chan	*n*-of-*m*	n chan	clin
84	rng				rng			
83		fst,slo	11, 21					
82						fst	11, 21	
81					els		6'	
80		rngfst	4			rngfst	8	
79	ord, els		6', 8			slo		
78	pol				ord			
77	ref		6		pol	rngslo		
76	fst							
75				SPEAK	ref		6	
74	sth	rngslo			fst			
73					sth, slo		4	SPEAK
72								
71	slo							

*All abbreviations are the same as those used in Table 13–1, except for the 6' abbreviation used in the "n chan" columns of the present figure. The 6' abbreviation is a further abbreviation of 6els.

190

Table 13–4. Protocol Processor Rankings, Subject NP2*

Overall % IT	24 Consonants Male				24 Consonants Female			
	6 chan	*n-of-m*	n chan	clin	6 chan	*n-of-m*	n chan	clin
93	sth							
92	rng							
91	ref		6					
90								
89	ord, pol	rngfst						
88	fst		11	SPEAK				
87	els	fst	6', 8					SPEAK
86			4			rngfst		
85	slo				rng			
84					ref		6	
83					sth			

continues

Table 13–4. continued

Overall % IT	24 Consonants Male				24 Consonants Female			
	6 chan	n-of-m	n chan	clin	6 chan	n-of-m	n chan	clin
82					fst	fst		
81		slo			slo,ord		11	
80								
79								
78					pol	slo		
77								
76							8	
75							4	
74								
73					els		6'	

*All abbreviations are the same as those used in Table 13–1, except for the 6' abbreviation used in the "n chan" columns of the present figure. The 6' abbreviation is a further abbreviation of 6els.

*Table 13–5. Protocol Processor Rankings, Subject NP3**

Overall % IT	16 Consonants Male				16 Consonants Female			
	6 chan	*n*-of-*m*	n chan	clin	6 chan	*n*-of-*m*	n chan	clin
87						rngfst		
86								
85								
84							8	
83								
82		fst						
81					rng	fst		
80			4		sth			
79					fst		11	
78	rng		8, 11		ref, ord		4, 6	

continues

193

Table 13–5. continued

Overall % IT	16 Consonants Male				16 Consonants Female			
	6 chan	*n*-of-*m*	n chan	clin	6 chan	*n*-of-*m*	n chan	clin
77	fst, ord, sth							
76	slo		21		pol, slo			
75	ref	slo	6	SPEAK				
74								
73	els, pol	rngfst	6'				21	
72					els		6'	SPEAK

*All abbreviations are the same as those used in Table 13–1, except for the 6' abbreviation used in the "n chan" columns of the present figure. The 6' abbreviation is a further abbreviation of 6els.

Table 13–6. Protocol Processor Rankings, Subject NP4*

Overall % IT	16 Consonants Male				16 Consonants Female			
	6 chan	*n*-of-*m*	n chan	clin	6 chan	*n*-of-*m*	n chan	clin
89			8					
88	pol		11†					
87	fst, rng		21†			rngfst		
86	els, sth		4, 4†, 6'					
85	ref, ord		6, 6†, 8†			slo, rngslo		
84								
83		fst, rngfst		SPEAK				
82	slo	slo			rng			
81						fst		
80		rngslo						
79								

continues

Table 13-6. *continued*

Overall % IT	16 Consonants Male				16 Consonants Female			
	6 chan	*n*-of-*m*	n chan	clin	6 chan	*n*-of-*m*	n chan	clin
78								
77								
76								SPEAK
75					els		6'	
74								
73					fst			
72					ref, ord		6	
71							4, 6†, 21†	
70					pol, sth		4†, 8†	
69								
68					slo		8, 11†	
67								

*All abbreviations are the same as those used in Table 13–1, except for the 6' abbreviation used in the "n chan" columns of the present figure. The 6' abbreviation is a further abbreviation of 6els.

†Threshold amplitudes decreased by 3 dB.

Table 13–7. Protocol Processor Rankings, Subject NP5*

Overall % IT	16 Consonants Male				16 Consonants Female			
	6 chan	n-of-m	n chan	clin	6 chan	n-of-m	n chan	clin
96	pol							
95								
94								
93	ord							
92								
91								
90	sth, els		4, 6'					
89								
88	rng							
87	slo							
86								

continues

Table 13–7. continued

Overall % IT	16 Consonants Male				16 Consonants Female			
	6 chan	*n*-of-*m*	n chan	clin	6 chan	*n*-of-*m*	n chan	clin
85	ref	rngfst	6					
84		rngslo				rngslo		
83	fst							
82		fst						
81	els'	slo	6", 11			rngfst		
80								
79					rng			
78			8, 21					
77				SPEAK				
76								
75					pol			
74								

198

	16 Consonants Male				16 Consonants Female			
Overall % IT	6 chan	n-of-m	n chan	clin	6 chan	n-of-m	n chan	clin
73						fst		
72					sol			
71								
70					sth			
69					els		6'	
68					ref, ord, els'		6, 6"	
67					fst	slo	4	
66								SPEAK
65							8, 11	
64								
63							21	

*All abbreviations are the same as those used in Table 13–1, except for (1) the 6' and 6" abbreviations used in the "n chan" columns of the present figure and (2) the els' abbreviation used in the "6 chans" columns of the present figure. The 6' abbreviation is a further abbreviation of 6els, and the 6" and els' abbreviations both denote another separate set of selected electrodes.

Only the overall % IT scores are presented in Tables 13–3 through 13–7, because those scores are highly correlated with the percent-correct scores, although the relationship is a slightly nonlinear one (see Chapter 5 and also the scatter plots in Appendix 2 in QPR 5:3). In general, and over most of the range, a 1 to 2% difference in overall % IT scores corresponds to a significant difference in the percent-correct scores for the same tests. Thus, a 1% difference in the IT scores in Tables 13–3 through 13–7 sometimes corresponds to a significant difference in percent-correct scores for the compared processors for a given subject, whereas a 2% difference in the tables usually corresponds to a significant difference.

Specific evidence of test-retest reliability for the overall % IT scores is included for subject NP4 in Table 13–6. For that subject, apparent nonsimultaneous channel interactions forced us to reduce the minimum stimulation levels in order to fit 11- and 21-channel CIS processors without the perception of background noise. These arbitrary minimum levels were set 3 dB below the single channel thresholds normally used, and processors with these altered levels are labeled with the dagger symbols (†) in Table 13–6. Otherwise identical 4-, 6-, and 8-channel processors with both sets of minimum stimulation levels were compared to assess the magnitude of the interaction effects. Although a significant difference was noted between the two 8-channel processors for the male voice, evaluations of the two versions of the 4- and 6-channel processors — on different days — yielded overall information transmission scores that were identical for the male voice consonants and differed by only one percent for the female voice.

Although the protocol study is not yet complete, and important comparisons lack statistical significance in the absence of data from the final two subjects, some strong patterns have emerged already. Such findings need not await the additional year and a half required to complete the study.

All five subjects studied thus far enjoy good to excellent performance in terms of the cochlear implant population as a whole, as indicated by standard measures of open-set speech recognition. Nevertheless, Tables 13–3 through 13–7 reflect substantial variation among the subjects: in median level of performance with the protocol processors (from 77% overall IT for 16 consonants by subject NP3 to 86% overall IT for 24 consonants by subject NP2); in range of performance variation across the protocol processors (from a range of 13% in overall IT for subject NP1 to a range of 33% for subject NP5); in performance differences between male and female voices (e.g., little difference for subject NP1 to relatively large differences for subject NP5); and in the rankings of relative performance among the protocol processors. In the remainder of this report we shall discuss some patterns emerging from these various data, generally following the order of the four comparison groups represented by the columns in Tables 13–3 through 13–7.

SINGLE PARAMETER VARIATIONS WITH RESPECT TO A REFERENCE 6-CHANNEL CIS PROCESSOR

In Table 13–8 we have collected the changes in overall information transmission associated with changes in each of six CIS processor parameters. The reference processor for each subject is the **6ref** processor. Data for male and female voice medial consonant tokens are presented separately for each of the five subjects studied thus far. A positive change indicates that the parametric variation produced an improvement in performance with respect to the reference processor.

In terms of *average* change in overall % IT across these ten conditions (male and female speakers for each of the five subjects), the six parametric changes rank as follows: **rng** (+4.7), **ord** and **pol** (+0.9), **sth** (+0.6), **fst** (−0.4), and **slo** (−2.1), suggesting that the **rng** change is likely to produce a significant improvement in processor performance, whereas the **slo** option is likely to reduce performance.

If we assume that 2% approximates the minimum significant difference in overall information transmission for these comparisons, we obtain the results shown in Table 13–9 for the proportion of cases in which each parametric manipulation produced a significant change. As indicated in the table, extending the overall

Table 13–8. Changes in Overall % IT with Changes in Single CIS Parameters

	NP1		NP2		NP3		NP4		NP5	
	m	f	m	f	m	f	m	f	m	f
rng	+7	+9	+1	+1	+3	+3	+2	+9	+3	+9
sth	–3	–2	+2	–1	+2	+2	+1	–2	+5	+2
ord	+2	+3	–2	–3	+2	0	0	0	+7	0
fst	–1	–1	–3	–2	+2	+1	+2	+1	–2	–1
pol	+1	+2	–2	–6	–2	–2	+3	–2	+11	+6
slo	–6	–2	–6	–3	+1	–2	–3	–5	+2	+4

Table 13–9. *Prevalence of Changes in Performance Due to Parametric Manipulations*

	Improvement	Decrement
rng	80%	0
sth	50%	30%
ord	40%	20%
fst	20%	30%
pol	40%	50%
slo	20%	70%

frequency range analyzed by a 6-channel CIS processor (from 350 to 5500 Hz to 350 to 9500 Hz) produced an improvement in performance in 8 of the 10 cases. On the other hand, reducing the pulse rate (from 833 to 250 pulses/s on each channel) had a 70 % likelihood of reducing processor performance. (We note that even if the criterion for a significant difference were increased to 3% in overall IT, significant improvements would be found for **rng** in 70% of our cases and significant decrements in performance for **slo** in 60% of the cases.)

In terms of seeking an optimal fitting under the time constraints of a clinical setting, the extended overall frequency range clearly would be one parametric setting to try. After that, these results might suggest increasing the upper frequency cutoff point for the envelope smoothing filter from 200 to 400 Hz (**sth**), which produced an overall average change in IT of +0.6%, and an average change of 2.6% in the 50% of cases for which a significant improvement was obtained. Both changing from staggered to apex-to-base order of stimulation (**ord**) and reversing the polarity of the biphasic pulses (**pol**) produced +0.9% changes in IT overall and a 2% or greater improvement in 40% of the cases. For **ord** the average improvement when a significant improvement was obtained was 3.5%, and for **pol** the corresponding value (strongly influenced by the results for subject NP5) was 5.5%.

VARIATIONS AMONG *N*-OF-*M* PROCESSORS

Certain processors from this group have not yet been evaluated with subjects NP2 and NP3. One comparison for which the full 10 conditions are in hand is the effect of extended frequency range for the 833 pulses/s *n*-of-*m* processors (**nmrngfst** versus **nmfst**). For three of the subjects (NP2, NP4, and NP5) the extended frequency range version performed as well or significantly better for both male and female voices; the average improvement in those cases was 3.7%. For subject NP1 the extended range resulted in poorer performance for both male and female voices; the average decrement was 2.5%. For the remaining subject, NP3, extending the overall frequency range produced a marked (6%) improvement for the female voice, but an even larger (8%) decrement for the male voice.

Nine of the intended ten comparisons are available at present between the 833 pulses/s normal frequency range *n*-of-*m* processor (**nmfst**) and the corresponding 250 pulses/s version (**nmslo**). Use of the slower pulse rate produced a significant decrement in performance in six of the nine conditions tested, with an average decrement of 5.3% for those six conditions. The slower rate produced a significant improvement in performance (4%) in one case of the nine.

PROCESSOR PERFORMANCE VERSUS THE NUMBER OF CIS CHANNELS AND ELECTRODE SELECTION

The set of protocol processors designed to be as similar as possible except for number of CIS channels includes processors using 4, 6, 8, 11, and 21 channels. The data are complete for the first five subjects, except for the 21-channel processor condition for subject NP2. As the number of channels decreases, the number of options for assignment of channels to electrodes increases. For 4- and 6-channel processors there are many potential choices.

In selecting electrodes for 4-, 6-, and 8-channel processors, we were guided by data from formal electrode discrimination tests in which each subject was asked to rank sequential stimuli from various pairs of electrodes in terms of perceived pitch. We also consulted dynamic range data for each electrode at the appropriate pulse rate(s) and pulse duration. In order to obtain some indication of the sensitivity of processor performance to the exact choice of electrodes, we tested at least two different sets of 6 electrodes for each subject. (These are identified as **6** and **6'** in the "n chan" columns of Tables 13–3 through 13–7. They are the same processors identified as **ref** and **els** in the "6 chan" columns. A third case was tested for subject NP5, labeled **6"** and **els'**, respectively.) In selecting sets of 11 electrodes, the choice between all even and all odd-numbered electrodes was made on the basis of which involved fewer limitations in terms of available dynamic range and channel discrimination data. Selection of the single electrode to be omitted from the 21-channel CIS processors was based on similar criteria. With the exception of one alternative set of six electrodes for subject NP3, every processor's channels spanned at least 15 electrodes, with most spanning 19 or more. The choices we have made for each of the first five subjects in this study are tabulated in Appendix 3 in QPR 5:3. The electrode numbering system used in this study is apex-to-base, with electrode number one assigned to the apical-most electrode in the array.

Only for subject NP1 did we observe any performance advantage in using more than eight CIS channels.

Figures 13–1 through 13–5 show overall % IT scores for male and female voice medial consonant data as a function of the number of CIS channels. There is a separate plot for each of the five subjects. Notice that the differences in the IT scores associated with different choices of 6-electrode sets typically are comparable to the differences associated with varying the number of CIS channels between 4 and 21. Those processor pairs corresponding to statistically significant differences in performance are identified in Appendix 4 in QPR 5:3 (based on ANOVA analyses of the block percent-correct scores and post hoc comparisons among the means, as indicated by a significant ANOVA result for each of the five subjects).

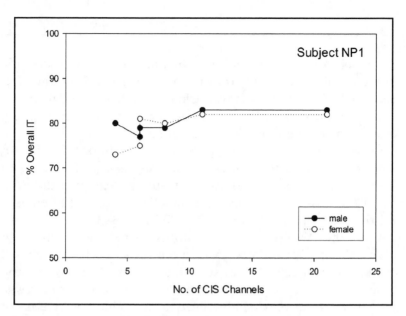

Figure 13–1. Overall information transmission (IT) scores for subject NP1 as a function of the number of CIS channels and for alternative choices of electrodes for the 6-channel processors.

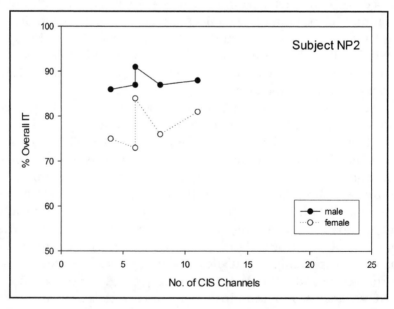

Figure 13–2. Overall information transmission (IT) scores for subject NP2 as a function of the number of CIS channels and for alternative choices of electrodes for the 6-channel processors.

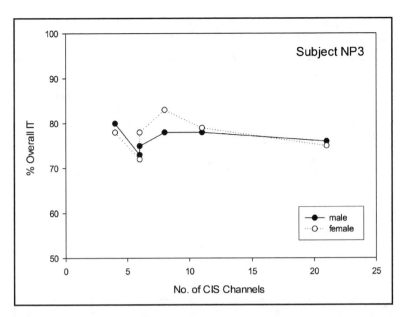

Figure 13-3. Overall information transmission (IT) scores for subject NP3 as a function of the number of CIS channels and for alternative choices of electrodes for the 6-channel processors.

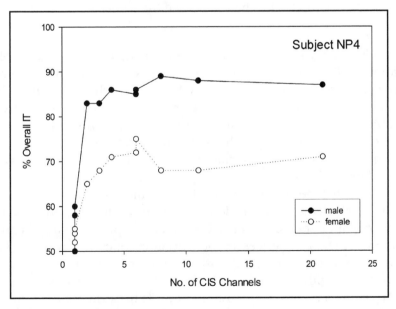

Figure 13-4. Overall information transmission (IT) scores for subject NP4 as a function of the number of CIS channels and for alternative choices of electrodes for the single- and 6-channel processors.

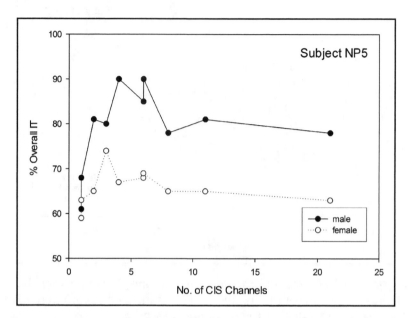

Figure 13–5. Overall information transmission (IT) scores for subject NP5 as a function of the number of CIS channels and for alternative choices of electrodes for the single- and 6-channel processors.

Based on the results of these comparisons, we evaluated some additional processors with subjects NP4 and NP5: otherwise similar CIS processors with 1, 2, and 3 channels. In each case the selected electrodes were subsets of those used in the subject's 4-channel processor. More than one of those electrodes was evaluated in single channel processors for both subjects, to gauge performance sensitivity to electrode choice vis-à-vis number of channels.

Taken together, these results (for monopolar stimulation via the Nucleus 22 electrode array) indicate that: (1) additional CIS channels become much less likely to produce significant improvements in processor performance once the number of channels exceeds four, (2) different choices of electrodes can produce significant differences in performance for CIS processors with as many as 6 channels, and (3) the principal potential benefit of additional implanted electrodes (beyond 4 to 6) may be the availability of alternative sites of stimulation rather than the availability of additional channels.

RELATIVE PERFORMANCE OF CIS, *N*-OF-*M*, AND MONOPOLAR SPEAK PROCESSORS

For two of these five subjects a 6-channel CIS processor performs significantly better than the best *n*-of-*m* processor tested (the **6rng** processor was better for the female voice for subject NP1 and better for the male voice for NP2). For subject NP3, *n*-of-*m* processors were at least as good as any of the protocol CIS processors. For each of the remaining two subjects, CIS processors tended to be better for the male voice, whereas an *n*-of-*m* processor was better for the female voice. Among current high-speed pulsatile processors, then, both CIS and *n*-of-*m* processors offer significant benefits to some patients.

As mentioned previously, the monopolar version of the clinical **SPEAK** processor had been used on an everyday basis for an extended period by each of the five subjects. Its performance was compared with the protocol CIS and *n*-of-*m* processors with which the subjects had had only limited experience in the laboratory. It is hoped that wearable hardware can be supplied to one or more of the subjects of this study to allow extended daily use of a CIS and/or an *n*-of-*m* processor.

Thus far in our study, one or more of the protocol CIS or *n*-of-*m* processors has performed significantly better than the chronic use monopolar **SPEAK** processor in nine of the ten conditions (NP2's SPEAK processor supported her best performance with the female voice, although the **nmrngfst** protocol processor produced equivalent or nearly equivalent results). A comparison of **6rng** and **nmrngfst** with **SPEAK,** for instance, yields the differences in percent overall information transmission shown in Table 13–10 (a positive difference corresponds to a higher score for **6rng** or **nmrngfst**). The average difference in overall IT is +6.4% for **6rng** and +5.7% for **nmrngfst**.

We conducted a one-way control ANOVA analysis comparing the relative overall IT performance of four processors: **6ref**, **6rng**, **nmrngfst**, and **SPEAK**. The analysis was based on differences in overall % IT among the processors for each of the five subjects. The ANOVA indicates significant differences ($p < 0.01$), and post hoc comparisons of the means indicates that performance is significantly better with **6rng** than with **SPEAK**, signifi-

Table 13–10. Differences in Overall % IT versus SPEAK

	NP1		NP2		NP3		NP4		NP5	
	m	f	m	f	m	f	m	f	m	f
6rng	+9	+11	+4	−2	+3	+8	+4	+4	+12	+11
nmrngfst	+5	+7	+1	−1	−2	+14	0	+10	+9	+14

cantly better with **nmrngfst** than with **SPEAK**, and significantly better with **6rng** than with **6ref**. These results are consistent with there being benefits to the faster pulse rates of **6rng** and **nmrngfst** compared to **SPEAK**, and to the extended frequency range of **6rng** compared to **6ref**.

Acknowledgments. We thank subjects NP1, NP2, NP3, NP4, and NP5 for their participation in the studies described in this report. We also gratefully acknowledge the support by Cochlear Corporation of the device, and surgical, audiological, and subject travel and per diem costs associated with the studies.

Part II

ELECTRICAL STIMULATION ON BOTH SIDES WITH COCHLEAR IMPLANTS

Our studies with recipients of bilateral cochlear implants (bilateral CIs) began in 1995 with a patient implanted at the Duke University Medical Center by Dr. John T. McElveen, Jr. In 1997 we initiated a long and productive collaboration with Dr. Joachim M. Müller of the Julius-Maximilians-Universität in Würzburg, Germany, and about a year later we began another long and productive collaboration with Dr. Bruce J. Gantz and his team at the University of Iowa in Iowa City, IA, USA. In later years the teams at the Manchester Royal Infirmary in the UK, the Medical University of Vienna in Austria, and the University of North Carolina at Chapel Hill in the USA each referred patients to the Research Triangle Institute (RTI).

In our studies, we asked, in very broad terms,

- Do recipients of bilateral implants have access to the principal binaural cues of interaural timing and amplitude differences?
- If so, can coordinated stimulation of the two sides restore binaural hearing and the signal-to noise advantages associated with binaural hearing?
- Can bilateral implants be exploited in other ways, for example, through use of additional distinct electrodes?
- Can independent processors confer any advantage, for example, through presentation of redundant information to the two sides or through a partial representation of interaural amplitude differences?

We found that: (1) subjects with bilateral CIs show a wide range of sensitivities to interaural timing differences, with some subjects having sensitivities as good as 25 μs or better, which approaches the sensitivities of subjects with normal hearing, but with other subjects having sensitivities of 300 μs or worse; (2) the sensitivity to interaural timing differences depends in many cases to matching sites of stimulation across the two sides, as determined by pitch matching, and the sensitivity is generally worse for unmatched than for matched pairs of electrodes; (3) sensitivities to interaural amplitude differences generally are excellent, with most tested subjects having a sensitivity that is at least as good as the smallest change in amplitude that can be produced by the implants; (4) independent processors, each stimulating one of the implants, confer significant advantages for many of the tested subjects for speech reception in quiet and in noise, particularly for different locations of the speech and the noise and particularly for highly adverse speech-to-noise ratios; (5) most subjects using independent processors benefit from head-shadow effects and some benefit as well from binaural squelch and/or summation effects; (6) for the strategies tested, no clear advantage is observed with coordinated stimulation across the two sides; and (7) bilateral CIs might be used in other ways to confer advantages, for example, by assigning a different bandpass range of sounds to each electrode within and between the two implants that can be discriminated on the basis of pitch, or by using a monaural sound processor that delivers the outputs from its odd-numbered channels to one of the implants and the outputs from the even-numbered channels to the other of the implants. Results from the studies at the RTI with recipients of bilateral CIs are reported in QPRs 5:5, 6:1, 6:4, 6:9, 6:12, 7:1, 7:2, 7:4, and 7:10, and in Lawson et al. (1998) and Wilson et al. (2003). The principal sections from QPRs 6:4, 7:4, and 7:10 are reproduced in this book, and the paper by Wilson et al. provides a summary of the studies up through 2002 and QPR 7:2.

In most cases, investigators from our collaborating institutions actively participated in the studies at the RTI. These investigators included Joseph Farmer, John McElveen, and Patricia Roush from Duke; Stefan Brill, Joachim Müller, and Franz Schön from Würzburg; Richard Tyler and Paul Abbas from Iowa; Martin O'Driscoll from Manchester; and Christoph Arnoldner, Wolf-Dieter Baumgartner, and Stefan (Marcel) Pok from Vienna. In addition, Peter Nopp and Raymond Mederake from the MED-EL companies in Innsbruck, Austria, and Starnberg, Germany, respectively, participated as co-investigators in some of the studies with recipients of MED-EL implants on both sides. We also received essential technical support from the Cochlear Pty. Ltd. in Sydney, Australia; the University of Innsbruck in Austria; and the MED-EL GmbH in Innsbruck. Most of this support was in the design and construction of interface systems for laboratory control of bilateral CIs.

One of the joys of our bilateral studies was the collaboration with Dr. Müller and his colleagues at the Julius-Maximilians-Universität. Our collaboration began in 1997 when Dr. Müller asked the RTI team to evaluate his first bilateral patient. The results from the initial studies at the RTI with this first patient (RTI subject ME2) confirmed and extended the findings from the prior studies with the same patient in Würzburg. The confirmation encouraged the Würzburg team to implant additional patients bilaterally. Results from the first nine patients implanted in Würzburg are reported in Müller et al. (2002). All of those patients were adults. Many more patients were implanted in Würzburg subsequently, including children. The results were positive and they helped to establish bilateral cochlear implantation as a standard procedure for the treatment of deafness or severe losses in hearing.

Chapter 14

SPEECH RECEPTION WITH BILATERAL COCHLEAR IMPLANTS[*]

Dewey T. Lawson, Blake S. Wilson,
Mariangeli Zerbi, and Charles C. Finley

Coordinated stimulation of bilateral cochlear implants might support a useful representation of the interaural timing and amplitude cues used by listeners with normal hearing to lateralize sounds in the horizontal plane. An ability to lateralize and separate sources of sound allows listeners to attend to a desired talker in environments with noise or competing talkers from other directions. The signal-to-noise advantages of binaural hearing can be quite large.

An alternative approach for coordinated stimulation of bilateral implants might be to utilize additional electrodes, compared with the unilateral case, to: (a) increase the number of effective channels, (b) increase rate of stimulation for a given number of channels, or (c) reduce electrode interactions for a given number of channels and rate of stimulation. In this alternative approach, no attempt would be made to represent or preserve interaural timing and amplitude cues.

Either approach might confer important advantages to recipients of bilateral implants. Some patients might enjoy the greatest advantage with one of the approaches, while others might benefit

*From QPR 6:4, July 1, 1999, through September 31, 1999.

more from the other approach. For example, a patient with poor sensitivities to the interaural cues might not receive much benefit from the first approach, aimed at representation of those cues, but might well benefit from one or more of the changes in processing supported through use of the second approach.

In addition, even uncoordinated stimulation of bilateral implants, using independent processors for the two implants, might be better than stimulation of either implant alone. Such independent processors would be expected to present redundant or strongly overlapping information across the two sides. Presentation of redundant information could be helpful for listening to speech in adverse situations. Independent processors also might preserve a representation of interaural amplitude differences, especially if the microphones for the two sides are at ear level, even while not preserving interaural timing differences.

In our view, the key questions in research on bilateral implants include the following:

■ Do recipients of bilateral implants have access to the principal binaural cues of interaural timing and amplitude differences?

■ If so, can coordinated stimulation of the two sides restore binaural hearing and the signal-to-noise advantages associated with binaural hearing?

■ Can bilateral implants be exploited in other ways, for example, through use of additional distinct electrodes?

■ Can independent processors confer any advantage, for example, through presentation of redundant information to the two sides or through a partial representation of interaural amplitude differences?

We have begun to address some of these questions in studies with three subjects having the same type of cochlear implant on both sides.

SENSITIVITIES TO INTERAURAL TIMING AND AMPLITUDE DIFFERENCES

Measures of sensitivities to interaural timing and amplitude differences were presented in QPR 6:1. Tables 14–1 and 14–2 pro-

Table 14–1. *Sensitivities to Interaural Time Delays (ITDs) Between Trains of Pulses Delivered to Pitch- and Loudness-Matched Pairs of Electrodes*

Laboratory	Subject	Minimum ITD
RTI	NU-4	150 μs
	ME-2	450 μs, 40 pulses/s >1 ms, other conditions
	NU-5	50 μs or less
MEEI*	1	150–200 μs
Melbourne†	P1	1 ms
	P2	500 μs, 200 pulses/s >1 ms, other conditions

*Massachusetts Eye and Ear Infirmary
†The University of Melbourne

Table 14–2. *Sensitivities to Interaural Amplitude Differences (IADs) Between Trains of Pulses Presented Simultaneously to Pitch-Matched Pairs of Electrodes*

Subject	Clinical Units	Fraction of DR
NU-4	1 (best) 4 (worst among 3 pairs)	1/75
ME-2	5	1/30
NU-5	1 3 (worst among 4 pairs)	1/75

vide summaries of the results. Table 14–1 shows the measured sensitivities to interaural timing differences (ITDs) for our three subjects and also for one subject studied at the Massachusetts Eye and Ear Infirmary (MEEI; Long et al., 1998, 1999) and for two subjects studied at the University of Melbourne (van Hoesel et al., 1993; van Hoesel & Clark, 1995, 1997). As described in detail in QPR 6:1, subject NU-4 has a full insertion of a Nucleus CI-22 implant on one side and a partial insertion of a CI-22 implant on the other side; subject ME-2 has full insertions of MED-EL COMBI 40 implants on both sides; and subject NU-5 has full insertions of Nucleus CI-24M implants on both sides. The subject in the MEEI study has an Ineraid implant on one side and a Clarion implant on the other side. The subjects in the University of Melbourne study both have Nucleus CI-22 implants on both sides.

Sensitivities to ITDs have been measured using bilateral pairs of electrodes that elicit the same pitch and loudness percepts. Three such pairs were included in our studies with NU-4, and four such pairs were included in our studies with NU-5. One pair was included in the studies with ME-2. Multiple pairs of pitch- and loudness-matched electrodes have been included in the studies of Long et al. (1998) and of van Hoesel and Clark (1997). In all studies trains of unmodulated pulses were delivered to the two implants (some of the studies also used additional stimuli, such as sinusoidally amplitude modulated trains of pulses). For measures of sensitivity to ITDs, one train was delayed with respect to the other.

As is evident from Table 14–1, a wide range of sensitivities is found for these subjects. Subject NU-5 was able to lateralize reliably a sound image toward the ear with the leading pulse train at a delay of 50 μs. We were unable to evaluate possible sensitivity to delays below 50 μs because that was the smallest delay our equipment and controlling software could support at the time of the studies.

In contrast, subject ME-2 in our studies, and both subjects in the Melbourne studies, had much poorer sensitivities. Under a particular condition, subject ME-2 had a sensitivity of 450 μs, but much worse sensitivities for other conditions. Similarly, subject P2 in the Melbourne studies had a sensitivity of approximately 500 μs at the pulse rate of 200/s, but much worse sensitivities for the other tested rates (50, 100, and 300 pulses/s). Subject P1 had quite poor sensitivities for all tested conditions (including two pitch- and loudness-matched pairs of electrodes and the rates of 50, 100, 200, and 300 pulses/s).

The maximum delay between ears for an adult human head in a sound field is about 680 μs. Thus one would expect that sensitivity to ITDs of 680 μs or less is necessary for utility of such cues in real acoustic environments (in the absence of some special processing to exaggerate ITD cues). A time difference of 50 μs, for instance, corresponds to an incidence from only about 5 degrees to one side of the midline. The intermediate sensitivities demonstrated by subject NU-4 in our studies and the subject in the MEEI studies correspond to an incidence from about 15 degrees to one side. Even a sensitivity as poor as 450 μs, which corresponds to an incidence angle of about 45 degrees, might be of some use in real acoustical environments.

A good sensitivity to interaural timing differences indicates that central auditory processing of binaural inputs is intact. Because differences in loudness between the two sides can be determined with monaural processing, sensitivities to interaural amplitude differences do not necessarily demonstrate integrity of the binaural system.

In our studies, subjects NU-5 and NU-4 had good sensitivities to ITDs. Subject ME-2 had only poor or quite poor sensitivities depending on the stimuli used. These and the other findings summarized in Table 14–1 suggest that at least some recipients of bilateral implants have functional binaural systems.

Sensitivities to interaural amplitude differences (IADs) have been measured in our studies by determining the point at which a reduction in the amplitude of pulses for one of the pulse trains shifts a sound image reliably toward the ear receiving the unaltered stimulus. (In this report, the term IAD is used rather than the more traditional term, interaural level difference or ILD; IAD is synonymous with ILD.) Table 14–2 shows generally good sensitivities to IADs for each of our three subjects. Subjects NU-4 and NU-5 could reliably lateralize a sound image with the smallest possible change in amplitude between the two sides (one clinical unit for the CI-22 or CI-24M devices, respectively), for at least one pair of pitch-matched electrodes. This change corresponded to about 1/75th of the dynamic range for each of these subjects. Subject ME-2 required a greater change for reliable judgments (five clinical units for the COMBI 40 device, which corresponded to about 1/30th of his dynamic range). In all cases, only relatively small changes in the amplitude were required for a reliable shift in the sound image toward the side with the greater amplitude compared to the loudness-balanced control condition.

As noted above, a good sensitivity to IADs might be achieved by purely monaural processing. Subjects with good sensitivities to IADs but poor sensitivities to ITDs may not enjoy great benefits from strategies designed to restore binaural hearing.

INTEGRATION OF INPUTS FROM THE TWO SIDES

We have conducted a variety of studies to evaluate potential benefits of various strategies for assigning channels across bilateral implants. The questions included: (a) whether bilateral stimulation might be distracting to a subject or otherwise reduce the performance of processors using bilateral stimulation compared with processors using unilateral stimulation; (b) whether an additional contralateral channel might be equivalent to an additional ipsilateral channel in terms of speech reception performance; and (c) whether the availability of bilateral electrodes under control of a single speech processor might support higher speech reception scores through changes such as an increase in the number of effective channels or a reduction in electrode interactions for a fixed number of channels. In these particular studies, no attempt was made to represent the lateralization cues of interaural timing and amplitude differences.

Results from studies with subject NU-4 are presented in Figures 14–1 and 14–2. Figure 14–1 shows consonant identification scores for various assignments of channels to electrodes between the two implants. Results for unilateral stimulation are presented in the first two bars, for stimulation of the left (processor 11) and right implant (processor 12), respectively. The electrodes selected for each side elicited similar ranges of pitch percepts and spanned the same cochlear distance.

The two right-most bars show results for assignments of channels across the implants. In one variation channels 1, 3, and 5 were directed to the left implant and channels 2, 4, and 6 were directed to the right implant. In the other variation the converse was done, with channels 1, 3, and 5 directed to the right implant and channels 2, 4, and 6 directed to the left implant.

The scores for either processor using bilateral stimulation are significantly higher than for either processor using unilateral stimulation. The left unilateral processor produced a higher score than the right unilateral processor.

The comparisons in Figure 14–1 indicate an advantage of "interlacing" channels across the two sides. For a fixed number of channels and for the same distance across the electrodes addressed in the electrode array(s), such interlacing increases the distance between stimulated electrodes on each side, and halves the aggregate stimulation rate to each ear. (The rate of stimulation on each active electrode, of course, remains constant.) The increases in distance may reduce electrode interactions.

Figure 14–2 shows results for additional assignments of channels within or across the implants. In the leftmost processor (processor 5) six channels are assigned to more widely spaced electrodes in the left implant. In the next processor (processor 6) those same channels are assigned across the implants, with channels 1 through 3 directed to the same electrodes in the left implant and channels 4 through 6 directed to similarly spaced electrodes in the right implant. In the third and fourth processors eight channels are assigned to widely spaced electrodes in the left implant (processor 10) or across the two implants (processor 13). As in the second processor (processor 6), the channel assignments in the fourth processor are equally divided between implants, with channels 1 through 4 directed to the left implant and with channels 5 through 8 directed to the right implant.

The scores for the two 6-channel processors are not statistically different; nor are the scores for the two 8-channel processors. This result shows that speech reception is not damaged even when the represented spectrum of speech sounds is split at the middle between the two implants.

Although the aggregate stimulation rate to each ear is again halved, the distance between stimulated electrodes within an implant is not changed with the unilateral versus bilateral manipulations in the processors of Figure 14–2. Thus, a reduction in the electrode interactions might not be expected for either the 6- or 8-channel comparisons.

Anecdotally, the subject was well aware of the bilateral nature of the processors stimulating both implants. However, she had no greater difficulty in recognizing speech compared with the control processors stimulating one implant only.

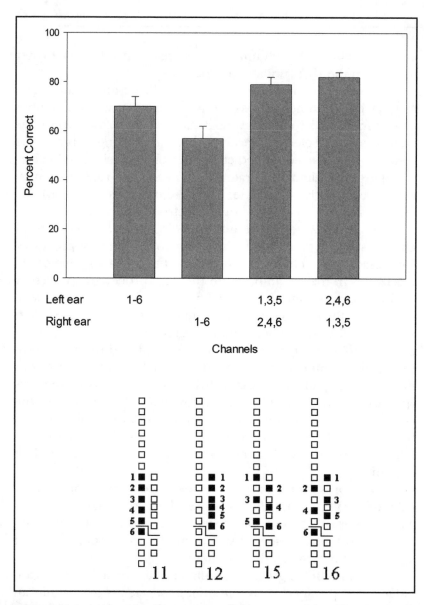

Figure 14–1. Results from tests of consonant identification with subject NU-4. The pulse rate was 480/s, the pulse duration was 80 μs/phase, and the frequency range was 350 to 5500 Hz. The squares in the bottom panels indicate, along the vertical direction, relative pitch ranking of "bipolar-plus-one" pairs of electrodes. Filled squares indicate activated pairs and are labeled by channel numbers ascending from the lowest to highest bandpass center frequency. Apical electrode positions are at the top of each array.

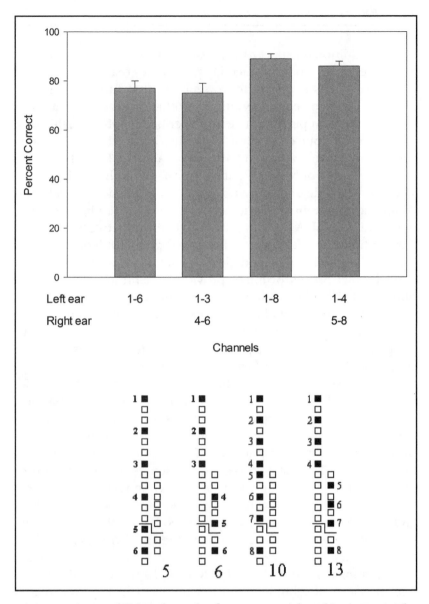

Figure 14–2. Additional results from tests with subject NU-4. The organization of the bottom panels is the same as that in Figure 14–1. The processors for both figures shared the same pulse rate, pulse duration, and frequency range.

An additional aspect of the results in Figure 14–2 is that the 8-channel processors produced higher scores than the 6-channel processors. This suggests the possibility that further increases in the number of channels might produce further increases in speech reception performance. As described in QPR 6:1, this subject can rank a total of 14 stimulation sites across the two implants according to pitch. This compares with a total of 13 such sites for the left implant only and 4 such sites for the right implant only. The additional distinct site of stimulation available with bilateral stimulation, as compared with stimulation of the left implant only, might be helpful. Also, a number of channels between 8 and 13 may optimize performance, through a good tradeoff between the number of channels and electrode interactions. For example, a 10-channel processor might provide a useful increment in the number of channels while still minimizing electrode interactions (with choices of channel-to-electrode assignments that maximize the distances between stimulating electrodes in each implant). We plan to evaluate these possibilities in future studies with this subject and in future studies with other subjects.

Similar studies also have been conducted with subject ME-2 to evaluate whether assignment of a fixed number of channels to electrodes across implants produces a decrement in performance compared with assignment of those channels to electrodes within one implant only. The results are presented in Figure 14–3. The first two bars show scores for stimulation of the right and left implants only, using 6-channel CIS processors. Channels 1 through 6 were assigned to electrodes 2, 3, 4, 6, 7, and 8, respectively, for both processors. Bars 3 through 6 show the scores for various assignments of the six channels across the two implants. The processors of bars 3 and 4 split the channels, with channels 1 through 3 directed to electrodes in the apical half of one of the implants and channels 4 through 6 directed to electrodes in the basal half of the other implant. Bars 5 and 6 show scores for alternating assignments of channels to electrodes across the implants. The processor of bar 5 directed the odd-numbered channels to electrodes 2, 4, and 7 in the left implant, and the even-numbered channels to electrodes 3, 6, and 8 in the right implant. The processor of bar 6 did the converse. The final condition involved two identical 6-channel processors, stimulating electrodes 2, 3, 4, 6, 7, and 8 in each implant.

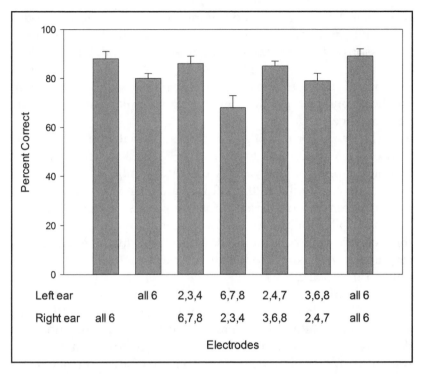

Figure 14-3. Results from tests of consonant identification with subject ME-2. The pulse rate was 1000/s, the pulse duration was 70 μs/phase, and the frequency range was 350 to 5500 Hz. Fullwave rectifiers and 200 Hz lowpass filters were used in the envelope detectors. Monopolar electrodes were used. The electrodes are numbered from apex to base (opposite to the numbering for the Nucleus implants). The identifying numbers for the processors are, from left to right, 13, 14, 5, 7, 9, 11, and 15.

Comparison of the scores for stimulation of either implant only indicates that stimulation of the right implant is better than stimulation of the left implant. In addition, comparisons among the scores for processors that present six channels across implants show a sensitivity to the way in which channels are assigned to electrodes. The processor that directs channels 1 through 3 to electrodes in the left implant (third bar in Figure 14–3) is better than the processor that directs those channels to electrodes in the right implant (fourth bar). However, the processor that directs the odd-numbered channels to electrodes in the left implant (fifth bar) is not statistically better than the processor that directs those channels to electrodes in the right implant (sixth bar). These findings suggest that inclusion of one or more of the electrodes in the right implant, or use of certain combinations of electrodes in the right implant, may degrade performance.

The score for the bilateral processor that directs channels 1 through 3 to the left implant (bar 3), and the score for the bilateral processor that directs the odd-numbered channels to electrodes 2, 4, and 7 in the left implant (bar 5), are not statistically different from the score for the processor that stimulates the left implant only (bar 1). This result shows that inputs from the two sides can be combined, without producing a decrement in performance compared with the performance of the better unilateral implant.

Unlike the results for subject NU-4, increasing the distance between stimulated electrodes within each implant (through assignment of alternating channels to each side) did not produce an improvement for ME-2. Possibly, electrode interactions were already low with the 2.7-mm spacing of adjacent electrodes in the MED-EL implants used by ME-2. A greater spacing may not have produced a significant reduction in interactions and therefore may not have enhanced the representation of channel-related cues. In contrast, the distance between adjacent bipolar electrode pairs in the Nucleus implants used by NU-4 is only 0.75 mm. Reductions in interactions would seem more likely with the tested increases in the distance between stimulating pairs in the Nucleus implants than with the tested increases in the distance between stimulating monopolar electrodes in the MED-EL implants.

In the final condition of Figure 14–3 both implants were stimulated with identical 6-channel processors. The score for this condition was not statistically higher than the score for stimulation of the left implant only (or for other conditions in Figure 14–3). The presentation of redundant information to the two sides did not improve speech reception scores, at least for conditions of these tests.

Like subject NU-4, ME-2 did not experience any difficulty in combining inputs from the two sides. He knew when both implants were activated, but also described unitary percepts of speech sounds. His scores in tests of consonant identification were not different among unilateral stimulation of his better (left) implant and two of the tested variations of bilateral stimulation that assigned either alternating channels to each implant or directed the outputs of channels 1 through 3 to one implant and the outputs of channels 4 through 6 to the other implant.

Results from the above studies with NU-4 and ME-2 demonstrate that inputs from the two sides can be integrated into single auditory percepts and also that presentation of channels across implants can be equivalent to or better than unilateral stimulation with the same number of channels, even when information is allocated between the two sides in arbitrary ways. In these studies the assignments of channels to electrodes for the bilateral processors did maintain a monotonic ordering of increasing pitch with increasing channel number.

A question not addressed by the results from the studies with NU-4 and ME-2 is whether a monotonic ordering must be maintained to support speech reception scores that are at least as good as unilateral stimulation with the same number of channels. Possibly, binaural processing might allow separation of channels on bases other than differences in pitch.

In studies with subject NU-5 we asked this question by comparing 8-channel processors that assigned channels across the two sides either to produce distinct pitches among all of the selected electrodes or to produce the same pitches for channels 1 and 2, the same pitches for channels 3 and 4, and so forth. This second variation of an 8-channel processor used pitch-matched pairs of electrodes between the two implants.

The results are presented in Figure 14–4. The first variation of 8-channel processors is labeled as "8 ch distinct" and the second variation is labeled as "8 ch matched pairs." As a control, 4-channel processors stimulating either the left or right implants also were tested. The tests included consonant identification in quiet and at the speech-to-noise ratios (S/Ns) of +10 and +5 dB.

As is evident from the figure, the first of these 8-channel processors produced significantly higher scores than the second processor for consonant identification in quiet and consonant

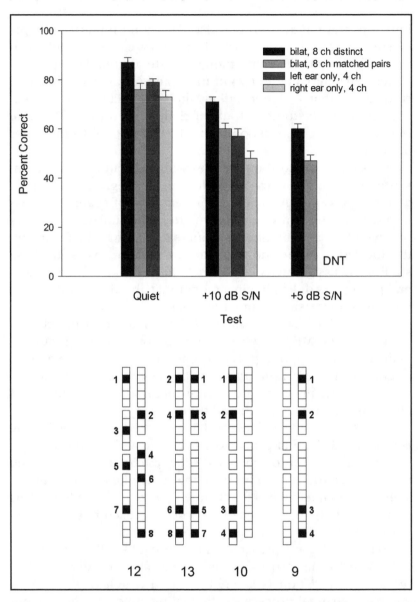

Figure 14-4. Results from tests of consonant identification with subject NU-5. The pulse rate was 750/s, the pulse duration was 25 µs/phase, and the frequency range was 350 to 5500 Hz. Fullwave rectifiers and 200 Hz lowpass filters were used in the envelope detectors. Monopolar electrodes were used. In the bottom panels, apical electrode positions are toward the top. The identifying numbers for the processors are, from left to right, 12, 13, 10, and 9.

identification at both S/Ns. This indicates that, for a given number of channels, speech reception scores may be maximized through channel-to-electrode assignments that produce distinct pitches among all of the electrodes, and that a lateral distinction without an associated pitch difference is not as effective as a pitch distinction.

The additional results in Figure 14–4 also indicate that a 4-channel processor stimulating one implant only can be equivalent to the 8-channel processor with channel-to-electrode assignments using matched pairs of electrodes between the implants on both sides. This finding suggests that the central auditory system integrates the information presented to the pitch-matched pairs of electrodes into a single percept. Thus, for example, the information in the bandpass of channel 1, presented to an electrode in one implant, may be combined with the information in the bandpass of channel 2, presented to an electrode in the other implant that elicits the same pitch percept. Such combinations would produce a total of only four information channels for the "8 channel, matched pairs" condition. Apparently, information is sorted according to pitch or pitch regions and not according to side of stimulation, at least for identification of consonants by this subject.

INDEPENDENT PROCESSORS

One of the key questions in research on bilateral implants is whether use of independent processors for the two sides is any better than use of a single processor, stimulating only one of the implants. This question was addressed in studies with subjects ME-2 and NU-5.

Results for ME-2 are presented in Figures 14–5 and 14–6. Figure 14–5 shows scores from tests of consonant identification for stimulation of the left implant only with one of the subject's clinical MED-EL (CIS) processors, stimulation of the right implant only with the second of the subject's MED-EL processors (programmed separately for that implant), and stimulation of both implants with both processors. In this last condition, the processors run independently of each other and may not preserve

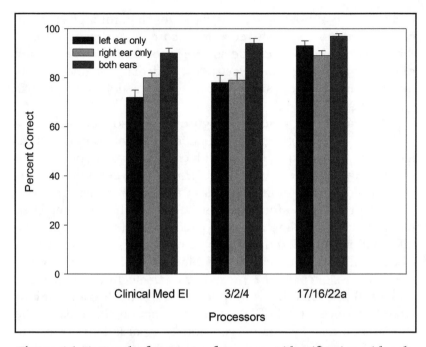

Figure 14–5. Results from tests of consonant identification with subject ME-2. The tests included 16 consonants presented from recordings in randomized orders and in an /a/-consonant-/a/ context. Multiple exemplars of the test tokens were produced by a male talker. CIS processors were used. The clinical MED-EL processors for the two implants each used seven channels and 40 µs/phase pulses. Laboratory ME-2 processors 3, 4, and 5 each used six channels and 70 µs/phase pulses, presented at the rate of 1000 pulses/s/electrode. Laboratory ME-2 processors 17, 16, and 22a each used six channels and 100 µs/phase pulses, presented at the rate of 823 pulses/s/electrode. Each of the laboratory processors assigned channels 1 through 6 to electrodes 2, 3, 4, 6, 7, and 8 in the one implant used for unilateral stimulation or in both implants for bilateral stimulation. A staggered order of electrode stimulation was used for each of the laboratory processors.

fine timing differences between the ears that would be present in normal hearing.

Figure 14–5 also shows scores for laboratory processors applied in these three ways: stimulation of the left implant only, stimulation of the right implant only, and stimulation of both

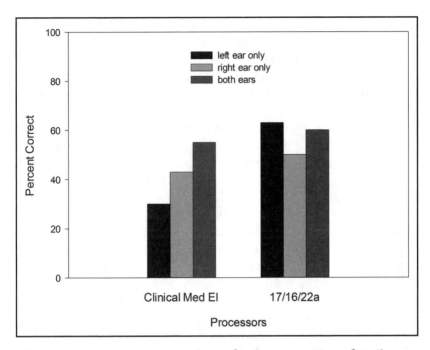

Figure 14-6. Percent correct scores for the recognition of Freiburger monosyllabic words by subject ME-2. The processors are the same as those described in the caption for Figure 14–5.

implants with two separate processors. Processors 3, 2, and 4 presented 70 μs/phase pulses at the rate of 1000 pulses/s/electrode, and processors 17, 16, and 22a presented 100 μs/phase pulses at the rate of 823 pulses/s/electrode. The clinical MED-EL processors used seven channels and electrode positions for each implant, whereas the laboratory processors used six channels and electrode positions for each implant.

The results show that bilateral stimulation with independent processors can be better than stimulation of either implant alone. That is true for the pair of MED-EL processors, where the score for bilateral stimulation is significantly higher than the scores for stimulation of either implant alone. Also, in the case of the MED-EL processors, the score for stimulation of the right ear alone is significantly higher than the score for stimulation of the left ear alone.

Similarly, the score for stimulation of both implants with laboratory processor 4 is significantly higher than the scores for stimulation of the left or right implants only, with processors 3 and 2, respectively. Among processors 17, 16, and 22a, the score for stimulation of both implants with 22a is significantly higher than the score for stimulation of the right implant only with processor 16. However, the score for bilateral stimulation with 22a is not significantly different from the score for stimulation of the left implant only with processor 17. Given the very high score for processor 22a, ceiling effects may have masked a possible difference between it and processor 17.

Scores from tests of monosyllabic word recognition for the clinical MED-EL processors and for laboratory processors 17, 16, and 22a are presented in Figure 14–6. The scores for these tests mirror the scores for consonant identification, presented in Figure 14–5. In both sets of data bilateral stimulation with the two MED-EL processors is better than stimulation of either implant alone, and unilateral stimulation of the right implant is better than unilateral stimulation of the left implant. Also, bilateral stimulation with laboratory processor 22a is better than unilateral stimulation of the right implant with processor 16, but not better than unilateral stimulation of the left implant with processor 17. The scores for monosyllabic words are in the sensitive range (i.e., well below the ceiling) for each of these processors, reducing the possibility that a difference between processors 22a and 17 was masked by a ceiling effect in the tests of Figure 14–5.

These findings for ME-2 do not indicate any destructive effect of bilateral stimulation that might be produced by the presentation of conflicting information between the two sides or an inability to integrate inputs from the two sides. In the comparisons involving the clinical MED-EL processors and those involving laboratory processors 3, 2, and 4, bilateral stimulation is clearly better than unilateral stimulation of either ear. In the comparison involving processors 17, 16, and 22a, bilateral stimulation is not worse than stimulation of the left implant only and is better than stimulation of the right implant only.

Results from tests with subject NU-5 are presented in Figures 14–7 and 14–8. Figure 14–7 shows scores from tests of consonant identification for stimulation of the left implant

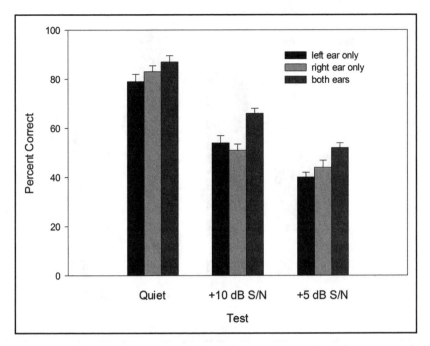

Figure 14–7. Results from tests of consonant identification with subject NU-5, using clinical SPEAK processors for either or both implants, as indicated in the legend. The tests included 24 consonants presented from recordings in randomized orders and in an /a/-consonant-/a/ context. Multiple exemplars of the test tokens were produced by a male talker. The consonants were presented in quiet or in conjunction with CCITT noise, which has a spectrum that matches the long-term spectrum of speech.

only with one of the subject's clinical SPEAK processors, stimulation of the right implant only with the second of the subject's SPEAK processors, and stimulation of both implants with both processors. Again the processors run independently of each other. Because of the nature of the SPEAK processing strategy, and the use of pulse burst length to convey information between the speech processor and implanted stimulator in the Nucleus devices, fine timing differences between the ears are not preserved. Figure 14–8 shows scores from additional tests for these same processor and implant conditions. The additional tests included recognition of consonant-nucleus-consonant (CNC)

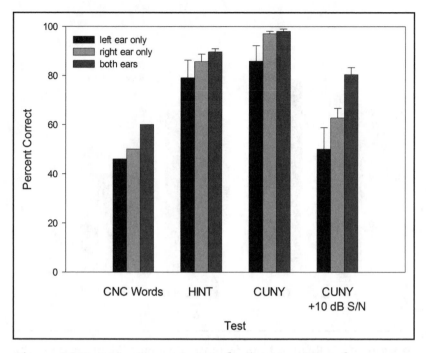

Figure 14-8. Percent correct scores for the recognition of consonant-nucleus-consonant (CNC) monosyllabic words and key words in the Hearing in Noise Test (HINT) and City University of New York (CUNY) sentences by subject NU-5. The HINT and CUNY sentences were presented in quiet. In addition, separate lists of the CUNY sentences were presented in conjunction with noise, at the speech-to-noise ratio of +10 dB. The subject's clinical SPEAK processors were used for either or both implants, as indicated in the legend. These tests were conducted at the University of Iowa. (Data kindly provided by Richard S. Tyler, University of Iowa.)

monosyllabic words, recognition of key words in the Hearing in Noise Test (HINT) sentences (presented here in quiet), recognition of key words in the City University of New York (CUNY) sentences, and recognition of key words in additional CUNY sentences presented in conjunction with noise at the S/N of +10 dB. These additional tests were conducted at the University of Iowa (data kindly provided by Richard S. Tyler, University of Iowa).

Scores from tests of consonant identification in quiet are not different among the three tested conditions: stimulation of the left implant only, the right implant only, or both implants. However, the scores from tests of consonant identification in noise show a large advantage of bilateral stimulation, at both S/Ns (+10 and +5 dB).

Scores from the remaining tests (Figure 14–8) also show an advantage of bilateral stimulation for speech reception in noise. In particular, recognition of CUNY sentences in competition with noise at the S/N of +10 dB is better with bilateral stimulation than with stimulation of either implant alone. Also, recognition of the monosyllabic CNC words appears to be better with bilateral stimulation than with stimulation of either implant alone. The scores for HINT sentences presented in quiet are not different among stimulation of either implant alone or bilateral stimulation. The scores for CUNY sentences presented in quiet are not different between bilateral stimulation or stimulation of the right implant only. However, possible differences among processor and implant conditions may have been masked by likely ceiling effects in these latter tests (the scores for two of the conditions are close to 100% correct).

The findings for NU-5 indicate an equivalence or superiority of bilateral stimulation compared with stimulation of either implant alone. Bilateral stimulation appears to be especially helpful to this subject for listening to speech presented in competition with noise.

SUMMARY

In response to the key questions listed at the beginning of this section, we now can say the following:

- Subjects with bilateral implants show a wide range of sensitivities to interaural timing differences, with some subjects having sensitivities that correspond to angles of sound incidence of 15 degrees or less from the midline.
- In general, sensitivities to IADs are good or even excellent.

- We do not yet know whether coordinated stimulation of the two sides can restore binaural abilities for patients with good sensitivities to ITD and IAD cues.
- Recipients of bilateral implants can integrate information from the two sides, even when that information is allocated between the two sides in arbitrary ways, for example, odd-numbered channels on one side and even-numbered channels on the other side, or the low-frequency half of channels on one side and the high-frequency half on the other side.
- Independent processors, each stimulating one of the implants, can confer an advantage for at least some patients, especially in the presence of competing noise.

FUTURE STUDIES

Our plans for the near future include further studies with subjects NU-4 and NU-5 and initiation of studies with additional subjects having CI-24M implants on both sides, referred to us from our colleagues at the University of Iowa, and with additional subjects having COMBI 40 or COMBI 40+ implants on both sides, referred to us from our colleagues at the Julius-Maximilians-Universität in Würzburg, Germany. The results collected to date are most encouraging. We now know that some patients have a good sensitivity to ITDs as well as a good sensitivity to IADs. Restoration of sound lateralization abilities, and the signal-to-noise advantages that accompany such abilities, is a realistic possibility for these patients. In future research we will evaluate that possibility. We also will collect results for additional subjects using the tests described in this report, including tests to evaluate various alternative representations of speech information with bilateral implants. Such alternative representations may be more effective for some patients than representations designed to preserve the interaural difference cues. Bilateral stimulation appears to offer important advantages for some patients even in the absence of any special processing. We expect that use of special processing, selected for the individual, may push scores higher.

Acknowledgments. We thank subjects NU-4, ME-2, and NU-5 for their participation in the studies described in this report. We also are grateful to Stefan Brill, Joachim Müller, Chris van den Honert, and Robert Wolford for their expert assistance in the studies, and to Richard Tyler for supplying the data presented in Figure 14–8.

Chapter 15

SENSITIVITIES TO INTERAURAL TIMING DIFFERENCES*

Robert D. Wolford, Dewey T. Lawson, Reinhold Schatzer, Xiaoan Sun, and Blake S. Wilson

BACKGROUND

In QPR 6:12 we summarized minimum interaural timing difference (ITD) values obtained for a variety of stimuli, including testing with unmodulated pulse trains, and with continuous pulse trains modulated by envelopes offset in time. In both cases the stimuli usually were delivered to pitch-matched, loudness-balanced pairs of electrodes, and occasionally to adjacent pitch-distinct, loudness-balanced electrode pairs. One electrode in each of the pairs was in one of the cochleas, and the other electrode in the pair was in the other cochlea. The minimum ITD is the lowest ITD that can produce a reliable shift in the perceived

---

*From QPR 7:4, January 1, 2003, through March 31, 2003. (The original title for this excerpted section from QPR 7:4 was "Measurements of Interaural Timing Difference.")

lateral location of the sound image from the midline for a given subject and test condition.

Also included in the summary of QPR 6:12 were the minimum ITDs obtained using trains of brief modulation envelopes, repeated at a rate of 50/s, produced by inputting pulses at that rate to CIS processors. These latter measurements, using independent non-synchronized CIS processors for the two ears, provided some of the shortest minimum ITDs measured in our laboratory, 25 μs for each of two tested subjects, which approaches the minimum ITDs for listeners with normal hearing (as low as about 10 μs for certain test conditions).

Further analysis of the data collected using unmodulated pulse train stimuli to selected pairs of electrodes showed that occasionally the minimum ITD was obtained for pitch-distinct electrode pairs rather than for pitch-matched electrodes in the same region of the cochlea. (A detailed description of our formal pitch ranking procedure is presented in QPR 6:12.) Also, ITD sensitivity seemed to be independent of the region within the cochlea that was chosen for stimulation. These observations differed from results obtained with normal hearing subjects for similar measures. In normal hearing, the minimum ITD for low- to mid-frequency signals shows sharp increases as the tones presented to each ear are separated in frequency. In addition, and consistent with the duplex theory of sound localization, the human auditory system is regarded as unable to utilize acoustic ITD information to localize high frequency tones (Nuetzel & Hafter, 1981; Tobias, 1972.) For listeners with normal hearing, the sites of cochlear excitation matter, and the "tuning" of minimum ITDs for apical and middle sites is sharp.

These apparent differences between normal and electrically elicited hearing prompted us to conduct additional experiments to confirm the differences and to elucidate further the factors that may affect minimum ITDs for users of bilateral cochlear implants. Trains of unmodulated pulses were used (as before), and the factors that were manipulated included: (1) the general region of the cochlea stimulated on each side (using electrodes in either the basal, middle, or apical parts of the electrode array on both sides); (2) the degree of pitch matching between single intracochlear electrodes on the two sides; and (3) the rate at which the pulses were presented within the unmodulated pulse trains. The purpose of this report is to present the results from these experiments with the seven subjects tested to date.

METHODS

Prior to any ITD measurements, each subject undergoes a multi-stage pitch ranking procedure. First, amplitudes corresponding to most comfortable loudness (MCL) are determined for each stimulating electrode at the selected pulse rate, and balanced for loudness. Next an informal pitch ranking is completed to identify a putative list for the order of the electrodes. Then the pitch ranking for each electrode is determined on the basis of electrode pair comparisons using an adaptive forced choice procedure (see, for instance, Bross, 1952.) A pitch ranking summary for the subjects participating in the studies described in this report is presented in Figure 15–1. Left ear electrodes are shown on the left side of each column, and right electrodes on the right. Vertical position differences denote differences in pitch, with higher pitches toward the top. Pairs that cannot be discriminated on the basis of pitch are highlighted, and electrodes that were intentionally omitted are indicated by an asterisk (*). The manufacturer of each subject's implanted electrode array is indicated by a code prefix: "NU" for Nucleus, and "ME" for MED-EL. Individual electrodes are numbered according to the conventions used by each manufacturer.

Based on these pitch ranking results, pairs of electrodes are selected for ITD evaluation. Prior to initiating the ITD trial, the two chosen electrodes are stimulated simultaneously at MCL (delta t = 0) and the subject is asked to report if the sound came more from the right or more from the left. The amplitude for one of the electrodes is then adjusted, if necessary, to provide a signal at the midline, that is, indiscriminable between right and left. The ITD trial is begun with an ITD offset of 2000 μs as the starting point. The signals used were unmodulated pulse trains consisting of three identical 300 ms pulse bursts with 500 ms gaps between them. The biphasic pulse width was 27 μs/phase,

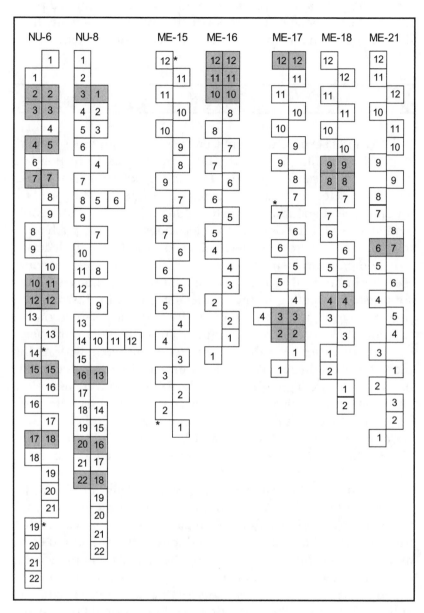

Figure 15–1. Formal pitch ranking results for each subject.

and the pulses were presented at the rate of 100 pulses/s for the first set of measures and at 100 or 1515 pulses/s for the second set of measures. The pulse trains were delivered in a random order. Subjects were instructed to select between two possibilities: more to the right or more to the left. A sufficient number of trials are completed at each ITD interval to obtain a statistically significant result, after which the ITD is progressively shortened until subject responses approach 50%. Occasionally, during this procedure, the subject will begin to lateralize to only one side. Such cases usually are due to a loudness imbalance that must be corrected. Accordingly, when such a pattern is encountered, the pulse amplitude on the side receiving the disproportionate number of responses is reduced until responses are equally divided between right and left. Once that is accomplished, the particular trial is aborted and started over with the new MCL values.

The offset of the pulse train is illustrated in Figure 15–2, with delta t representing the prescribed interaural delay.

Percent correct scores are recorded for each of the ITD intervals evaluated and fit to a weighted logistic function. The 75% crossing of the function is recorded as the minimum ITD for the selected electrode pair (for examples of logistic function fits and additional details, see QPR 6:12, p. 11).

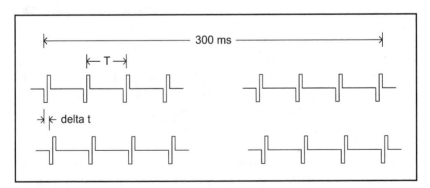

Figure 15–2. Interaural Timing Difference (ITD) stimuli using unmodulated pulse trains. The stimuli are shown as current versus time. The lower stimulus, to a chosen electrode in one ear, is delayed with respect to the upper stimulus to a chosen electrode in the other ear.

STUDIES OF ITD SENSITIVITY USING UNMODULATED PULSE TRAINS FOR DIFFERENT ELECTRODE PAIRS

Having occasionally obtained better ITD sensitivity for electrode pairs that were not pitch matched than for pitch-matched pairs differing by a single electrode location on one side, we designed a study with several subjects in which we recorded minimum ITDs while keeping the electrode on one side fixed and roving the electrode on the other side. In Figure 15–3, we show such results for two Nucleus subjects, with the left electrode 10 (pitch matched to right electrode 11) held constant for subject NU-6 and the right electrode 13 (pitch matched to left electrode 16) for subject NU-8 held constant while the test electrode in the opposite ear was moved either apically or basally for completion of ITD measures. As expected, deviation from the pitch-matched pairs is associated with decreases in sensitivities to ITDs. These differences are very gradual, however, and for subject NU-8 there is a broad region—from electrode 16 through electrode 10—where there is little change in ITD sensitivity. This span along the electrode array is approximately 4.5 mm in length (.75 mm between adjacent electrodes), corresponding to a range in characteristic frequency along the normally excited basilar membrane of about 1700 Hz (Greenwood, 1990), far from the sensitivity of 5 Hz expected for listeners with normal hearing (Tobias, 1972).

In Figure 15–4 are results from the same experiment conducted with two MED-EL subjects. For subject ME-15, the results of the pitch ranking procedure provided no matched pairs for the entire range of electrodes. For subject ME-21 the one pitch–matched pair is L7/R6. As was observed for subject NU-8, for both of these MED-EL subjects we see a broad range—from electrodes 5 through 7—over which the ITD sensitivity shows only a small variation. For the MED-EL device, this separation of electrodes corresponds to a longitudinal distance of approximately 4 to 5 mm (2.25 to 2.4 mm between electrodes).

Among the possible causes of essentially constant ITD sensitivity over such a long distance along the cochlea are: (1) the

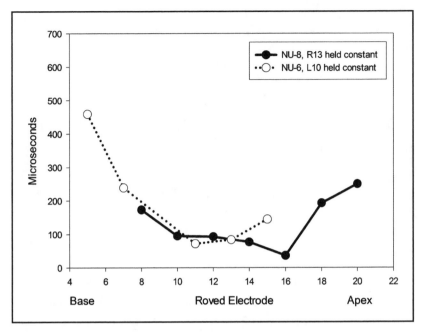

Figure 15–3. Minimum Interaural Timing Differences (ITDs) needed to produce a reliable shift in the perceived sound location from the midline for two Nucleus subjects. The stimulated electrode on one side is held constant and the one in the opposite ear is varied, including the pitch-matched electrodes as well as electrodes displaced various distances in both directions. Electrode 13 on the right side was held constant for subject NU-8, and electrode 10 on the left side was held constant for subject NU-6. Multiple ("roved") electrodes on the contra-lateral side were paired one at a time with the fixed electrode for each subject and the sensitivity to ITDs was measured for each pair. The numbers for the roved electrodes can be read from the horizontal scale.

fixed electrode's happening to be located in a region of the cochlea not associated with ITD sensitivity in normal hearing, and (2) neural elements over a large portion of the cochlea responding to stimuli from any of the involved electrodes.

We also looked for systematic variations in minimum ITDs as a function of location along the cochlea. For these studies, we selected electrode pairs from different regions of the electrode array, again based on a prior formal pitch ranking evaluation. As

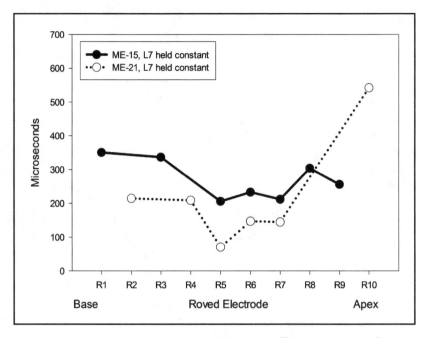

Figure 15–4. Minimum Interaural Timing Differences (ITDs) for two MED-EL subjects with the stimulated electrode on one side held constant and the electrode in the opposite ear varied. Subject ME-15 has no pitch-matched pairs, whereas for subject ME-21 electrodes L7/R6 form the only pitch-matched pair. The number of the roved right electrode is indicated on the horizontal axis. Electrode 7 on the left side formed the other member of the pair for both subjects.

can be seen in the pitch-ranking summary (see Figure 15–1), it was not possible to find pitch-matched pairs across the different regions of the cochlea for the majority of these subjects.

The minimum ITDs as a function of cochlear region for five subjects are shown in Figure 15–5. The electrodes on the right side for each subject that were pitch matched to electrodes on the left side are marked with asterisks.

The results in Figure 15–5 demonstrate that, as the selected pairs move from the apical region of the cochlea to the basal end, there is a gradual increase in the minimum ITD for these subjects. Such a pattern might be seen as consistent with the frequency-dependent utility of ITD information in normal acoustic hearing. A concern for this interpretation of these results is

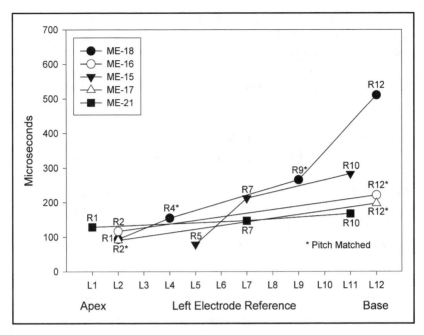

Figure 15-5. Minimum Interaural Timing Differences (ITDs) for electrode pairs in different regions of the cochlea. The horizontal axis identifies the electrodes on the left side that were paired with the electrodes on the right side, as indicated by labels adjacent to each data point. Pitch-matched pairs are indicated by an asterisk (*) where available for a given subject and region of the electrode array.

that there were an insufficient number of pitch-matched pairs in the different regions to address adequately the possibility that the minimum ITD was not obtained for certain pairs due to the mismatches in pitch. However, it is worth noting that: (1) for subjects ME-18 and ME-17, whose measures did include ITDs for pitch-matched pairs from two different regions, the more basal pairs showed larger minimum ITDs than those obtained from the more apical region, and (2) subject ME-16, whose pitch-matched pair was for the most basal electrodes, still showed a better ITD sensitivity for the apical region.

In order to understand better the importance of selecting only pitch-matched pairs for obtaining the optimum ITD sensitivity, we completed a comprehensive evaluation of roving ITDs across the electrode array for subject ME-16. For these studies, we held each of the six even-numbered left electrodes constant while roving the right electrodes in the same regions of the cochlea. For each condition the roved electrodes for the right ear spanned a region of three or four electrodes depending on the rate of change in ITD sensitivities. Figure 15–6 shows the results for this evaluation.

Comparisons of the roved ITD results for this subject indicate that for reference electrodes L2, L4, and L6 there is a broad region for which the minimum ITD shows no significant changes, with values approximating 100 µs. In contrast, the minimum ITD for reference electrodes L8, L10, and L12 is very sensitive to place of stimulation of the opposite ear. Comparison with the pitch ranking data for ME-16 in Figure 15–1 indicates that the minimum ITDs observed for L10 and L12 occurred when the paired

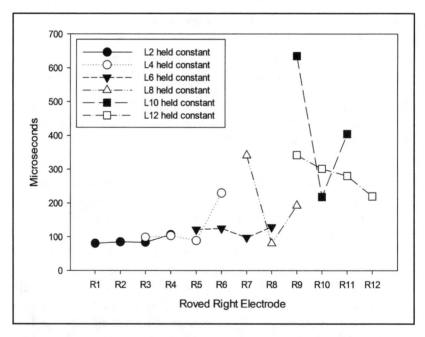

Figure 15–6. Minimum Interaural Timing Differences (ITDs) for roved electrodes in different regions of the cochlea. Results for subject ME-16 are shown. Each even-numbered electrode on the left side was paired with a range of contiguous electrodes on the right side in the same general region of the electrode arrays.

right side electrode was the pitch matched one. (Stimulation of R10 elicits the same pitch as stimulation of L10, and stimulation of R12 elicits the same pitch as stimulation of L12.)

The most sensitive ITDs, however, were obtained for the electrode pairs in the middle or at the apical end of the electrode array, despite the fact that the only pitch-matched pairs for this subject are found at the basal end of the cochlea (see Figure 15–1). This finding provides additional support to the indication from the data of Figure 15–5 that the apical to middle portions of the electrode array provide the best ITD sensitivities for unmodulated pulse bursts.

So, on the one hand, we observe sensitivity to smaller ITDs for stimulation from sites toward the apical end of the electrode array (approximately 1.5 turns into the cochlea), consistent with the greater reliance on ITD localization cues at lower frequencies in normal hearing. But on the other hand we find that ITDs are much more sensitive to pitch matching between contralateral sites of stimulation toward the basal end of the array (and of the cochlea), the region least associated with the use of ITD information in normal hearing.

Just as the response of neural elements over a wide range of the cochlea to stimuli from a given electrode is a possible cause of the effects seen in Figures 15–2 and 15–3 above, we note that asymmetry in current spread (apically versus basally) is a possible contributor to the trends seen in Figures 15–5 and 15–6.

STUDIES OF ITD SENSITIVITY USING UNMODULATED PULSE TRAINS: RATE EFFECTS

We also have completed a set of experiments in which the rate of pulses within the bursts was changed from either 50 or 100 pulses/s to 1515 pulses/s for specific electrode pairs. Minimum ITDs were obtained for electrode pairs L2/R2 and L12/R12 for both subjects ME-17 and ME-16 and for L2/R1 for subject ME-18. The minimum ITD increases strongly with increased pulse rate (Figure 15–7).

This finding is consistent with results obtained by van Hoesel and Tyler (2003). Those authors described lateralization of

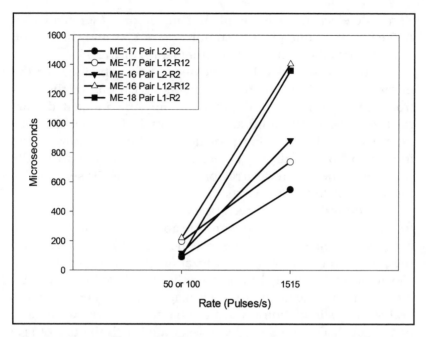

Figure 15–7. Effects of pulse rate on minimum Interaural Timing Differences (ITDs) for two subjects. The measurements included multiple pairings of electrodes for each of the subjects, as indicated in the legend. Unmodulated pulse trains were used.

unmodulated pulse trains only when using a low pulse rate and reported that when the rate exceeded 800 pulses/s, none of their subjects was successful at lateralizing for ITDs of up to the tested limit of 400 μs. Only one of our subjects, subject ME-16, showed an ITD sensitivity better than 400 μs at the rate of 1515 pulses/s, and that best sensitivity happened to be for the apical, pitch-distinct electrodes L2/R2.

SUMMARY

- Stimulation in the apical and middle portions of the implant array provides the greatest sensitivities to ITDs for unmodulated pulse trains.

- The minimum ITD is not sensitive to pitch matching of electrode pairs for those portions of the electrode array. In particular, there seems to be a broad range of stimulation sites, 4 to 5 mm along the electrode array that can support similar sensitivities to ITDs. This finding suggests the possibility that pitch matching is not important for the lateralization of low frequency sound—typically attributed to ITD sensitivity in normal hearing listeners—by users of cochlear implants.

- Stimulation from sites near the basal end of the electrode array is more sensitive to departures from the pitch-matched location for minimum ITDs, and typically provides less sensitive ITDs than the areas stimulated by the other two-thirds of the electrode array.

- The minimum ITDs for unmodulated pulse trains are sensitive to the rate at which the pulses are presented, with ITD sensitivity decreasing as the rate is increased.

Acknowledgments. We thank volunteer research subjects NU-6, NU-8, ME-15, ME-16, ME-17, ME-18, and ME-21 for their participation in the studies described in this report.

Chapter 16

PITCH RANKING OF ELECTRODES FOR 22 SUBJECTS WITH BILATERAL COCHLEAR IMPLANTS*

Dewey T. Lawson, Blake S. Wilson, Robert D. Wolford, Xiaoan Sun, and Reinhold Schatzer

Our group now has studied a total of 22 subjects with bilateral cochlear implants. The studies have included investigations of sensitivity to interaural time and amplitude differences, and of reception of speech in competition with noise from various directions, using a wide variety of candidate stereophonic speech processing strategies. Other studies have assessed potential benefits of additional contralateral stimulation sites to the performance of monophonic processors.

*From QPR 7:10, July 1, 2004, through September 30, 2004. (The original title for this excerpted section from QPR 7:10 was "Pitch Ranking of Electrodes for 22 Subjects with Bilateral Implants.")

Tables 16–1 and 16–2 summarize some attributes of our 22 subjects. Table 16–1 identifies each subject's bilateral cochlear implant devices, the number of electrodes available for stimulation on each side, the approximate number of years each subject went without bilateral stimulation, the number of years each went without any significant auditory stimulation, the month and year of each subject's most recent visit to the Research Triangle Institute (RTI), and the total number of days each has served as a research subject at the RTI. Table 16–2 lists what is known about the etiology of each subject's deafness or severe loss in hearing.

Central to all our studies with this group of subjects has been a knowledge of differences in perceived pitch across all available stimulating electrodes. After initial determination of threshold and most comfortable loudness (MCL) stimulation levels for a pulse rate and duration to be used in psychophysical studies and with speech processors, the MCL levels across both sides are carefully loudness balanced in preparation for pitch ranking.

Three different techniques have been employed in obtaining pitch ranking data: (1) an initial informal ranking to obtain a putative list of electrodes in pitch order, (2) a formal matrix survey comparing randomized pairs of electrodes in a specified range within such a putative list, and (3) a sequential analysis of selected pairs, guided by a chart that embodies a statistical standard and terminated as soon as that standard is met.

INFORMAL RANKING

Pulse bursts were played sequentially to pairs of electrodes at the loudness balanced MCL levels to obtain an indication of pitch ranking of the percepts within and across the two arrays and to identify potential contralateral pitch-matched pairs for studies of other variables. The number of trials with each pair varied. The result was a list of both sides' electrodes in a putative pitch order and a list of potential pitch-matched pairs.

Table 16–1. Subjects. The data include the devices used by each subject (Devices); the numbers of available electrodes (Avail. Els) on the left (L) and right (R) sides for each subject; the duration in years that each subject went without bilateral electrical stimulation (no bilat.) or no stimulation in either ear (no stim.); and the participation by each subject in studies at the RTI including the starting date of the most recent visit (Last Visit) and the total number of accumulated days (Tot. days).

Subject	Devices	Avail. Els		Duration (yrs)		Studies at RTI	
		L	R	no bilat.	no stim.	Last Visit	Tot. Days
NU4	N22	16	8	1	0	12/01	37
NU5	CI24M	20	20	0	0	3/99	9
NU6	CI24M	22	20	2	1	6/02	19
NU7	CI24M	22	22	20	6	3/02	20
NU8	CI24M	20	19	0	0	11/00	10
ME2	C40C	8	8	3	2	10/97	15
ME3	C40P	12	12	5	2	8/03	20
ME4	C40P	12	12	2	2	7/00	13
ME5	C40P	12	12	3	2	8/00	15

continues

Table 16–1. continued

Subject	Devices	Avail. Els		Duration (yrs)		Studies at RTI	
		L	R	no bilat.	no stim.	Last Visit	Tot. Days
ME7	C40P	9	12	0	0	9/01	14
ME8	C40CS, C40P	8	11	9	3	1/01	14
ME9	C40C	7	8	32	0	3/01	10
ME10	C40P, C40C	12	8	31	11	9/03	30
ME12	C40P	12	12	2	1	6/03	17
ME14	C40P	12	12	6	0	10/03	11
ME15	C40P	11	11	13	0	7/03	25
ME16	C40P	12	12	10	0	12/03	23
ME17	C40P	12	12	12	0	9/02	5
ME18	C40P	12	12	20	0	5/03	18
ME21	C40P	12	12	0	0	2/03	7
ME22	C40P	12	11	0	0	6/03	4
ME24	C40P	11	12	0	0	1/04	2

Table 16-2. *Etiology of Deafness or Severe Loss in Hearing for Each of the Subjects*

Subject	Etiology of deafness
NU4	Listeria rhomboencephalitis
NU5	acute noise exposure, further loss during subsequent pregnancy
NU6	onset coincident with poliomyel(oencephal)itis, familial history
NU7	Ménière's disease
NU8	Ménière's disease
ME2	gradual progressive
ME3	sudden loss of unknown cause
ME4	bilateral basal skull fractures
ME5	otosclerosis
ME7	bilateral temporal bone fractures
ME8	Ménière's disease
ME9	measles, familial history
ME10	right skull fracture, later sudden and progressive losses
ME12	20 years noise exposure as military pilot, familial history
ME14	genetic
ME15	sudden onset, each side separately
ME16	unknown, sudden, familial history
ME17	Ménière's disease
ME18	noise exposure, familial history
ME21	meningitis
ME22	early, likely genetic
ME24	left head trauma, progressive, familial history

MATRIX METHOD

A pair of loudness-balanced MCL pulse bursts separated by 0.5 s was delivered sequentially to two different electrode sites. The subject was asked to indicate whether the second sound was higher or lower in pitch (two alternative forced choices). Initially, each comparison was for electrodes separated by a fixed, relatively large distance, specified by an initial offset in position along the putative list. After a specified number of randomized comparisons of each pair of electrodes sharing that separation (equal number of presentations of each pair in each order) the separation within the putative list was reduced by one and the process repeated. Thus a subject typically would experience clear pitch contrasts early in the test, gradually becoming more subtle. The percentage of responses consistent with putative list order could then be displayed in a matrix of absolute electrode position versus offset within the list. Based on early comparisons, rearrangement of the list could be followed by additional comparisons, eventually resulting in a map of pitch discrimination across the electrode array against which various proposed subsets of electrodes could be considered for assignment to processor channels, or for use in psychophysical studies. Further details about the matrix method have been presented in QPR 6:1.

SEQUENTIAL ANALYSIS

Based on earlier work on sequential analysis (Wald, 1947), model procedures were developed for determining whether two conditions are discriminable or indiscriminable under selected statistical criteria (Bross, 1952). The procedures, embodied in graphic charts for recording the results of successive trials with randomized presentation order, were designed to be terminated as soon as the statistical criteria are met, rather than requiring a fixed number of trials in each case. Plan A as presented in Bross's paper—designed to ensure a correct determination of discriminability 90% of the time—was selected for use in formal pitch ranking determinations in our laboratory. The associated chart and a discussion of its use have been presented in QPR 6:12.

The statistical criteria contained within this sequential analysis procedure require a minimum of seven trials with each stimulus pair. Seven trials are sufficient only if the subject identifies the same stimulus as being higher in pitch in every case. Similarly, agreement in 9 out of 10 trials (90%) meets the statistical criterion for discrimination, and the minimum required percentage drops slowly as the number of trials increases (72% is sufficient after 25 trials, 66% after 35 trials, and 60.4% after 48 trials). On the other hand, a minimum of 22 trials (divided at 50% with 11 instances of each response) is required to establish that two stimuli are statistically indistinguishable, and the maximum percentage consistent with that verdict increases slowly after more trials, for example, 58.3% after 48 trials. In our practice, several different electrode pairs are evaluated as a group, with separate charts for each pair and with the order of successive trials randomized among the pairs. These statistical criteria are summarized in Figure 16–1.

Sequential analysis has particular advantages when the task is to identify pairs that are indistinguishable on the basis of pitch. Some candidate pairs can be eliminated after only 7 to 10 trials, for instance. And the more thorough exploration required to reach the conclusion that a pair of electrodes are truly pitch matched is built into the procedure. Once a limited number of such pairs has been identified in a subject using sequential analysis, relatively little further effort is required to extend the number of trials and to reduce the roughly 10% chance of error remaining inherent in Bross's Plan A chart.

An extended matrix procedure may be superior to sequential analysis, however, for identifying electrodes to support independent channels of stimulation for speech processors. While a contralateral pair of electrodes determined to be rankable on the basis of pitch with a 61% score after 48 trials has passed the same statistical test as a pair ranked the same way on all of an initial 7 trials or 9 of an initial 10, such a pair would not necessarily support independent channels as well as a pair that,

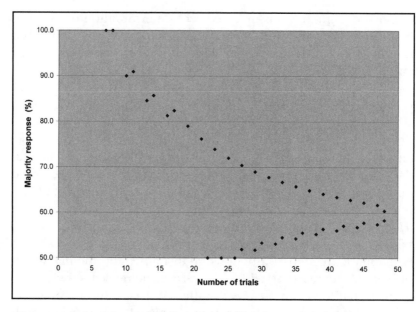

Figure 16-1. Criteria for discriminability between two alternatives, expressed as the percentage of the majority response as a function of the number of trials. The upper group of points indicates the minimum percentage to determine discriminability after a given number of trials (a minimum of 7 trials are required for such a determination). The lower group of points indicates the maximum percentage of responses for one alternative consistent with a determination of indiscriminability after a given number of trials (a minimum of 22 trials are required for such a determination). Values derived from the Plan A chart (Bross, 1952).

say, maintained a 90% ranking score consistently through many more trials.

Alternative sequential analysis designs (e.g., Armitage, 1957) may offer some advantages for future use.

In all three pitch ranking procedures, 300 ms bursts of pulses were presented, with pulse rates and phase durations appropriate to the speech processing strategies used by each subject. The interval between bursts in a paired comparison was set at 500 ms in the automated matrix procedure and was approximately the same under manual control in the other two procedures.

RESULTS

Our pitch ranking data for all 22 bilaterally implanted subjects are summarized in Figures 16–2 and 16–3.

The rankings shown in Figure 16–2 are based on sequential analysis. Eleven of the 22 subjects were studied using this approach. In the case of some subjects, matrix studies preceded the sequential ones and data from the matrix studies have been used where available to improve our judgments as to the ability of electrode pairs to support independent channels.

The rankings shown in Figure 16–3 are based on matrix comparisons for subjects NU4, NU5, NU8, ME2, ME3, ME4, ME5, and ME8, and on initial, informal comparisons or relatively few comparisons within a matrix algorithm for the remaining three subjects. The full matrix comparisons typically included 10 to 20 comparisons of each regional pair. Further testing with sequential analysis might well have indicated significant pitch distinctions between additional pairs but, as discussed above, might not have represented the availability of additional independent channels of stimulation. The matched pairs indicated in these matrix rankings may not be as well established as those using the sequential technique. In addition, results from the informal or relatively crude comparisons for subjects ME14, ME22, and ME24 (shown in the final three columns of Figure 16–3) should be regarded as preliminary indications only.

Side-by-side pitch-matched pairs as determined with the sequential analysis or the full matrix method are indicated in Figures 16–2 and 16–3 by the gray shadings in the aligned boxes. These pairs were used subsequently by us in formal studies such as interaural time delay and interaural amplitude difference detection.

A number of patterns that emerge in Figures 16–2 and 16–3 have implications for research possibilities and clinical expectations.

Pitch ranking patterns and apparent relative insertion depths are generally quite similar across sides in the same subject, even for ME8 where a shorter, higher-density array was implanted on one side (see Figure 16–3). A possible exception is the case of ME10,

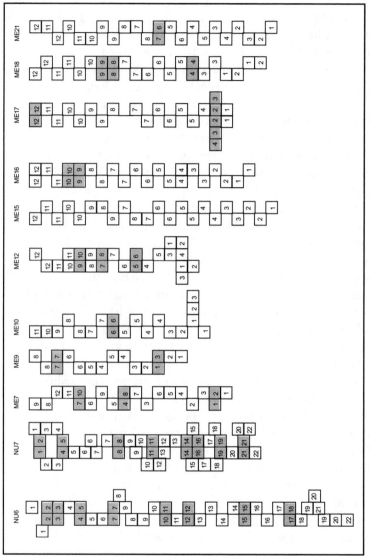

Figure 16–2. Pitch ranking data using the sequential analysis approach. Each cell corresponds to a ranked electrode, with numbering from the basal end of the array for the Nucleus devices and from the apical end for the MED-EL devices; in each case, electrodes associated with the highest pitch percepts are shown at the top of the figure. Only relative pitch ranking is conveyed. No significance should be attached to the degree of vertical displacement or extent. Cells shown side by side for the same subject could not be discriminated on the basis of pitch.

264

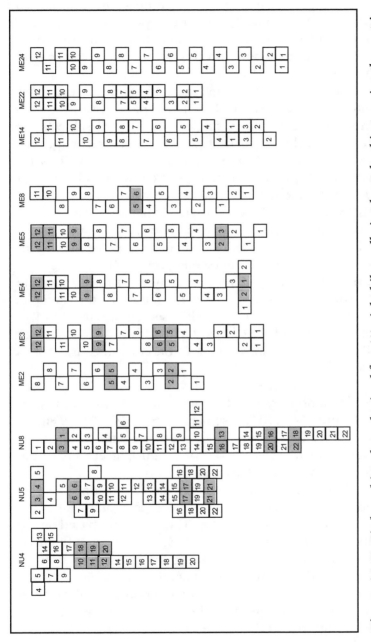

Figure 16–3. Pitch ranking data obtained for: (1) eight bilaterally implanted subjects using the matrix comparison approach (subjects NU4, NU5, NU8, ME2, ME3, ME4, ME5, and ME8) and (2) three additional bilaterally implanted subjects from preliminary informal assessments (subjects ME14, ME22, and ME24). The organization of this figure is the same as that for Figure 16–2.

also involving different implanted electrode arrays on the two sides (see Figure 16–2). Finally, a clear exception is seen for NU4, for whom the electrode array on one side was inserted only about halfway due to a bony obstruction in the scala tympani (see Figure 16–3).

The data for NU6 and NU7 in Figure 16–2 provide examples of a wealth of contralateral pitch-matched pairs at various locations across the cochleas of a single subject. Such subjects are particularly valuable for such studies as interaural amplitude difference and interaural time delay detection, as well as for studying binaural speech processing strategies with channels of stimulation that are pitch identical on the two sides.

In ME15 we have a subject for whom all of the electrodes on both sides are pitch discriminable; potentially supporting twice as many independent channels of stimulation as the number of electrodes on either side alone (see Figure 16–2).

The pitch ranking results for many of our subjects indicate tonotopic consistency along each electrode array, for example, subjects ME2 (see Figure 16–3), ME5 (see Figure 16–3), ME15 (see Figure 16–2), and ME16 (see Figure 16–2). In other cases (e.g., ME3, ME14) occasional marked tonotopic inconsistencies were observed (see Figure 16–3).

The results for some subjects show regions of relatively poor pitch discrimination across electrodes, such as the results for NU4 (see Figure 16–3), NU5 (see Figure 16–3), ME17 (see Figure 16–2), and ME12 (see Figure 16–2), perhaps reflecting regions of relatively poor neural survival, or distant placements of the electrodes with respect to excitable tissue.

Table 16–3 indicates the number of pitch-distinct sites of stimulation available for each subject, on each side alone and with both sides considered together. These data are based on the pitch rankings of Figures 16–2 and 16–3, and may be influenced to some extent by differences among the techniques used to obtain those rankings. Rankings obtained with sequential analysis, for instance, may tend to indicate additional significant distinctions beyond those based on the matrix comparisons.

The average bilateral channel advantage—defined as the number of pitch discriminable sites available across both sides divided by the maximum number of pitch discriminable sites available on one side in the same subject—has average and

Table 16-3. Subjects and Pitch-Discriminable Sites of Stimulation

		Pitch-Discriminable Sites			
Subject	Devices	Left	Right	Both	Advantage
NU4	N22	13	6	13	1.00
NU5	CI24M	13	14	15	1.15
NU6	CI24M	20	18	28	1.40
NU7	CI24M	15	17	20	1.18
NU8	CI24M	22	19	26	1.18
ME2	C40C	8	7	13	1.63
ME3	C40P	12	12	19	1.58
ME4	C40P	11	11	18	1.63
ME5	C40P	12	12	19	1.58
ME7	C40P	9	10	16	1.60
ME8	C40CS, C40P	8	11	18	1.64
ME9	C40C	7	8	12	1.50
ME10	C40P, C40C	11	6	16	1.45
ME12	C40P	11	10	15	1.36
ME14	C40P	12	11	20	1.60
ME15	C40P	11	11	22	2.0
ME16	C40P	12	12	21	1.75
ME17	C40P	9	11	17	1.55
ME18	C40P	12	12	21	1.75
ME21	C40P	11	12	22	1.83
ME22	C40P	11	11	14	1.27
ME24	C40P	11	12	21	1.75

267

median values of about 1.6 across the 17 MED-EL subjects. This result provides some indication of the potential clinical benefits of additional independent stimulation channels for monophonic speech processor use.

Among the 11 cases investigated with sequential analysis, the ratio of the number of contralateral pitch-matched electrode pairs at distinct pitches to the lesser of the numbers of electrodes available on each side provides some indication of the incidence of such opportunities for psychophysical comparisons controlled for pitch. The average of that ratio for these 11 subjects is 0.24. It is 0.38 for the two Nucleus subjects and 0.18 for the nine MED-EL subjects.

DISCUSSION

Searches for pitch-matched pairs of electrodes can be made more efficient through the use of sequential analysis procedures, allowing the elimination of some candidates after only 7 to 10 trials. Additional testing of those pairs identified as pitch indiscriminable by sequential analysis on the basis of relatively few trials (e.g., 22) can further improve the 90% accuracy of the technique's determinations.

Those pairs of electrodes determined by sequential analysis to be pitch discriminable only after many trials (e.g., 45) are not likely to be good choices to support independent channels in a speech processor. Among the pairs determined to be discriminable on the basis of 90% or better scores after only 7 to 10 trials, there may be some that would continue to yield such high scores through more extensive testing. Such pairs would be good choices to support possibly highly independent channels in a processor, or in a pair of processors (with one processor for each side), and the further testing required to identify them should be considered.

In some circumstances, such as a simultaneous need to identify both pitch-matched pairs for research and sets of pitch-distinct electrodes for independent processor channels, the additional testing described in the previous two paragraphs may effectively cancel any efficiency gained through the use of a sequential technique rather than an extended matrix survey.

Acknowledgments. We thank subjects NU4, NU5, NU6, NU7, NU8, ME2, ME3, ME4, ME5, ME7, ME8, ME9, ME10, ME12, ME14, ME15, ME16, ME17, ME18, ME21, ME22, and ME24 for their participation in the studies described in this report.

Part III

COMBINED ELECTRIC AND ACOUSTIC STIMULATION (EAS) OF THE AUDITORY SYSTEM

Our studies of combined electric and acoustic stimulation (EAS) of the auditory system began with a meeting among Christoph von Ilberg, Ingeborg Hochmair, and Blake Wilson at the J. W. Goethe Universität in Frankfurt, Germany. This meeting took place in early December 1999 and was very kindly arranged by Dr. Hochmair.

In the meeting, Prof. von Ilberg described his experience with the first patient who was implanted in Frankfurt—and worldwide—with the intention to preserve residual hearing at low frequencies in the implanted cochlea and to use that residual hearing in conjunction with the electrical stimuli provided by the implant. The initial experience was encouraging and is described in von Ilberg et al. (1999). (Combined EAS of same cochlea also was described by Gantz and Turner in 2003 [Gantz & Turner, 2003].)

The findings prompted Prof. von Ilberg to ask whether the team at the Research Triangle Institute (RTI) might be willing to conduct studies with this same patient, to learn whether the same or similar results would be obtained in other hands and to extend the scope of the prior studies in Frankfurt. This request led to a series of studies at the RTI with that first patient from Frankfurt (subject ME6 in the RTI studies) plus six others as referred to us by groups at the International Center of Hearing and Speech in Poland; the Medical University of Vienna in Austria; and the University of North Carolina at Chapel Hill in the USA. The studies were joint studies among these various institutions, and the participating investigators included Blake Wilson, Robert Wolford, Dewey Lawson, Reinhold Schatzer, and Stefan Brill from the RTI; Wolfgang Gstöttner, Jan Kiefer, Thomas Pfennigdorff, Stefan (Marcel) Pok, and Christoph von Ilberg from Frankfurt; Wolf-Dieter Baumgartner from Vienna; Oliver Adunka, Carol Higgins, and Harold Pillsbury from Chapel Hill; and Artur Lorens from Warsaw. The first visit by the first patient to the RTI was in August 2000.

Results from these collaborative studies at the RTI are reported in QPRs 6:8, 6:11, 6:13, and 7:3, and in Wilson et al. (2003) and Wilson (2010). In addition, these and other results from studies of combined EAS are summarized in recent reviews by Dorman et al. (2007); Dorman and Gifford (2010); and Wilson and Dorman (2008a, 2008b, 2009, 2011).

In broad terms, the results from the RTI studies affirmed the initial findings from Frankfurt. In addition, the studies included a wide range of new psychophysical and speech reception measures and a higher number of subjects.

The principal sections from two of the QPRs are included in this book: the section in QPR 6:11 on "Further Studies to Evaluate Combined Electric and Acoustic Stimulation," and the section in QPR 7:3 on "Additional Perspectives on Speech Reception with Combined Electric and Acoustic Stimulation." The first of these sections describes detailed psychophysical studies with subject ME6, including: (1) measures of masking by one mode of stimulation on the other and vice versa, and (2) pitch ranking of electric and acoustic stimuli presented to the same cochlea for the different implanted electrodes and for different frequencies of acoustic tones, respectively. To our knowledge, these were the first studies on these topics. The second of the sections describes speech reception studies with the first five subjects, including: (1) comparisons among scores for acoustic stimulation only, electric stimulation only, and combined EAS, and (2) comparisons of the efficacy of combined EAS for some of the subjects between ipsilateral versus contralateral delivery of the acoustic stimulus.

Results from our studies have recently been summarized in Wilson (2010), on behalf of the investigator team. The results show, among other things: (1) large benefits of combined EAS across most of the subjects and across a broad range of residual hearing; (2) a "synergistic" effect for many of the subjects, in which the speech reception score for combined EAS is greater than the sum of the scores for electric stimulation only and acoustic stimulation only; (3) relative immunity from noise interference for sentence understanding with combined EAS, which is in sharp contrast to the extreme sensitivity to noise interference typically observed with electric stimulation only; and (4) an equivalence in benefits of ipsilateral versus contralateral acoustic stimulation for subjects with comparable levels of residual hearing on the two sides.

Chapter 17

PSYCHOPHYSICAL STUDIES RELATING TO COMBINED EAS*

Stefan Brill, Dewey T. Lawson, Robert D. Wolford, Blake S. Wilson, and Reinhold Schatzer

Until recently, people with any significant amount of residual hearing were not considered candidates for cochlear implantation. Recently, cochlear implant (CI) candidates with a significant degree of residual hearing in one ear either would be implanted in the other ear or—if specifically electing to implant the "better ear"—expect to sacrifice the residual acoustic hearing in hope of greater potential for CI performance. Published reports have indicated the destruction of usable residual hearing capacity in a majority of such intracochlear implantations, at least over the range of frequencies corresponding to the length of the inserted electrode array (Bogess, Baker, & Balkany, 1989; Brimacombe, Arndt, Staller, & Beiter, 1994; Hodges, Schloffman, & Balkany, 1997; Rizer, 1988; Shin, Deguine, Laborde, & Fraysse, 1997).

---

*From QPR 6:11, April 1, 2001, through June 30, 2001. (The original title for this excerpted section from QPR 6:11 was "Further Studies to Evaluate Combined Electric and Acoustic Stimulation.")

In studies presently under way at the Johann Wolfgang Goethe University in Frankfurt (von Ilberg et al., 1999) and at the University of Iowa, electrode arrays are being inserted a relatively short distance into the scala tympani in an effort to preserve residual low frequency acoustic hearing (apical to the apical-most position of the arrays) while allowing high frequency speech information to be conveyed to the basal end of the cochlea by electrical stimulation. A traditional hearing aid and a CI speech processor then are employed simultaneously and cooperatively to convey speech to the same ear.

As detailed previously in QPR 6:8, we began studies with Frankfurt subject ME6 during a 2-week visit to our laboratory beginning late in August 2000. In a recent second visit by ME6 (June 4–15, 2001), we conducted a series of psychophysical studies focused on the possible interaction of acoustical and electrical stimulation of the same ear. Additional studies of speech reception in noise also were carried out during that second visit.

In daily life, ME6 wears both a Resound hearing aid and a Tempo+ BTE external speech processor, the latter for her CI. The stimulation strategy employed in the CI is CIS at a high stimulation rate (2273 pulses/s/channel), using envelope extractors based on the Hilbert transform. One of the key questions in the psychophysics of combined electric and acoustic stimulation is whether the presence of ongoing electrical stimulation affects acoustical hearing.

The recent psychophysical studies consisted of:

■ Acoustic pure-tone up-down-tracking audiogram in the presence of a steady state electrical masker
■ Mixed electric and acoustic pitch ranking and scaling
■ Threshold of an acoustic probe in the presence of an electric masker at varying masker levels
■ Effects of phase relationship between electric and acoustic stimulation
■ Threshold of an electric probe in the presence of an acoustic masker at varying masker levels
■ Speech reception for combined electric and acoustic stimulation.

1. ACOUSTIC PURE-TONE UP-DOWN TRACKING AUDIOGRAM WITH ELECTRICAL MASKER

Acoustic pure-tone thresholds were measured with an up-down tracking algorithm. Using a 0.1 dB step size, the pure-tone level was increased until audible. Then the direction was reversed and the level decreased until inaudible, whereupon the direction was reversed again and increased. For each condition, we collected 16 reversals and assumed the mean value of the last 10 reversals as the resulting threshold value. With this procedure we were able to achieve a repetition accuracy of 1.1 dB in the range of good residual hearing below 500 Hz.

An electric masker stimulus, consisting of an ongoing non-modulated pulse train of 1515 pulses/s on electrode 1 was used, at the three following stimulus levels:

1. Not activated
2. Set to threshold level, equaling 0 on a 0 to 50 subjective loudness scale
3. Set to subjective loudness level 10 on a 0 to 50 subjective loudness scale.

The first condition is the control condition without the electrical masker, corresponding to the everyday situation with the CI not activated. The second condition corresponds to the CI activated at threshold levels, mimicking an external CI processor without an incoming signal from the microphone. In this configuration the CI is activated, but inaudible. The third condition corresponds to an everyday situation where the CI is activated and audible at a low level, for example, as with a steady state input signal like a low-level background noise. It should be noted though, that in an everyday situation, we would expect any incoming signal from the external processor to exhibit some temporal structure, which is different from the setup used here.

Figure 17–1 shows the pure tone audiogram of ME6 under the three different electrical masker conditions. Thresholds were measured for all three masker conditions from 250 Hz up to

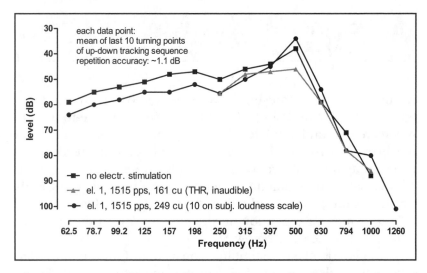

Figure 17–1. Up-down tracking audiograms for different values of electrical masker loudness. Abbreviations include electr. for electrical, el. for electrode, pps for pulses/s, cu for clinical unit, THR for threshold, and subj. for subjective.

1260 Hz in steps of musical thirds. At 1260 Hz under conditions 1 and 2, an acoustic sensation could not be reached before the subject reported tactile sensation. For conditions 1 and 3, the covered frequency range was extended down to 62.5 Hz.

In Figure 17–2, the differences between threshold levels under conditions 1 and 3 are highlighted for the lower frequencies. The biggest threshold shift of 5.9 dB was observed at 157 Hz, and the reversal of threshold shift at 500 Hz was due to a "nondisappearing" acoustic sensation when lowering the level in the up-down-tracking procedure. That effect remains unexplained, but one might speculate that in the region of best residual hearing around 500 Hz, the presence of the electrical stimulus caused a minor short-lived "tinnitus-like" ringing.

For the higher frequency range above 500 Hz, additional reversals can be seen and we assume the thresholds to be unreliable, on one hand because of the precipitous drop toward high frequencies, and on the other hand because of the possibility of an effect similar to that observed at 500 Hz.

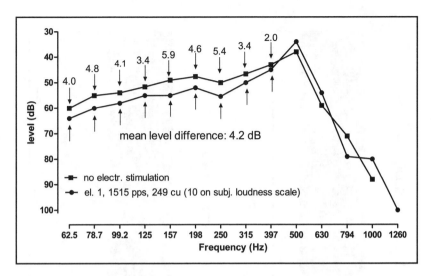

Figure 17–2. Difference between up-down tracking audiograms: no masker present versus masker loudness 10. Abbreviations are the same as in Figure 17–1.

2. MIXED ELECTRIC AND ACOUSTIC PITCH RANKING AND SCALING

During the subject's previous visit (see QPR 6:8), we conducted a pitch comparison study across ears, using the frequency range of residual hearing common to both ears. With the second visit by this subject, we extended our studies of pitch perception in the implanted ear, within both electric and acoustic domains, employing pitch ranking and pitch scaling procedures.

To exclude possible influences from different loudness levels, a 300 ms stimulation burst at 1515 pulses/s was adjusted to most comfortable loudness (MCL), and then used as a reference to adjust sound pressure levels (SPLs) of 300 ms acoustic pure tone bursts to the same perceived loudness. The resulting equal-loudness levels for frequencies 100 Hz through 600 Hz are listed in Table 17–1.

For all loudness judgments, a scale ranging from 0 to 50 was used, where 0 corresponded to the threshold level, 25 to the MCL, and 50 to intolerably loud.

Table 17–1. *Equal–Loudness Levels (at MCL) for Acoustical Pure–Tone Stimulation, Lower Frequency Range*

	Pure–Tone Frequency [Hz]						Electrical Reference Stimulus	
	100	200	300	400	500	600	Perceived Loudness	Stimulus Amplitude [cu]
level [dB]	–15	–15	–15	–10	–5	0	25 (= MCL)	633

Table 17–2. *Equal-Loudness Levels (at MCL) for Acoustical Pure-Tone Stimulation, Higher Frequency Range*

	Pure–Tone Frequency [Hz]					Electrical Reference Stimulus	
	500	630	794	1000	1260	Perceived Loudness	Stimulus Amplitude [cu]
level [dB]	—	—	> 0	—	—	25 (= MCL)	633
level [dB]	–15	–5	–4	0	> 0	20	555
level [dB]	—	–18	–12	–10	0	12	428

For higher frequencies ranging from 500 Hz through 1260 Hz, we tried to adjust the sound pressure level to match the loudness of the electrical reference stimulus, but did not succeed due to limited residual hearing at higher frequencies. As can be seen in line 1 of Table 17–2, this was already the case at 794 Hz, where MCL could not be reached. Readjusting the reference stimulus to a loudness of 20 and eventually 12 (lines 2 and 3 of Table 17–2), allowed us to find a set of equal-loudness SPLs for frequencies from 630 Hz through 1260 Hz, providing loudness matches to the softer reference stimulus.

Using the thus found stimulation levels, acoustic pure-tone bursts were pitch ranked to the electric reference stimulus on electrode 1, the most apical electrode of the array. Stimuli were randomized across frequencies and stimulation order. Individual judgments are listed in Tables 17–3 and 17–4, where each entry displays the order of stimulation and whether the electric (e) or acoustic (a) stimulus was perceived higher in pitch. The last line of each table lists the number of judgments in which the electric stimulus was ranked higher. This was the case for each single judgment and for all frequencies, suggesting that the apical-most electrode, which we would expect to exhibit the lowest pitch perception among the set of usable electrodes, is judged to be higher in pitch than the pitches elicited with the whole available frequency range of the residual hearing.

Table 17–3. Pitch Ranking: Acoustical Pure Tones Versus Electrical Stimulation on Electrode 1—Frequencies of 100 to 600 Hz at Perceived Loudness Level 25 (MCL)

Pure-Tone Frequency [Hz]					
100	200	300	400	500	600
e > a	e > a	a < e	e > a	a < e	a < e
a < e	a < e	e > a	a < e	e > a	e > a
e > a	a < e	a < e	a < e	e > a	a < e
a < e	e > a	e > a	e > a	a < e	e > a
4 / 4	4 / 4	4 / 4	4 / 4	4 / 4	4 / 4

Table 17–4. Pitch Ranking: Acoustical Pure Tones Versus Electrical Stimulation on Electrode 1—Frequencies of 630 to 1260 Hz at Perceived Loudness Level 12

Pure-Tone Frequency [Hz]			
630	794	1000	1260
e > a	a < e	a < e	a < e
a < e	a < e	e > a	a < e
e > a	e > a	e > a	e > a
a < e	e > a	a < e	e > a
4 / 4	4 / 4	4 / 4	4 / 4

In a second pitch judgment study, we asked the subject to scale the perceived pitch of each stimulus on a range of 0 to 100. The combined set of acoustic pure-tone burst stimuli at frequencies 100 Hz through 600 Hz and electric stimuli on all usable electrodes 1 through 8 was offered at equal-loudness levels and in randomized order. Ten judgments were collected for each stimulus condition. Individual single judgments and mean values are displayed in Figure 17–3.

Surprisingly, a wide range of conditions, namely frequencies 300 Hz through 600 Hz and electrodes 1 through 3, seem to elicit indistinguishable pitch percepts. This seems to contradict the findings from the ranking study. After completion of both the pitch ranking and the pitch scaling studies, we carefully interviewed the subject about differences in perception under the two study paradigms. She described the perception of the electrical stimulus as a tone that was accompanied by an additional "electric" component, and which conveyed a high pitch sensation. Under the ranking paradigm, one of the two stimuli to be compared always was an electric stimulus, while the other was acoustic. This pairing of stimulus types made it easy for her to always identify the electric stimulus of the two and rank it higher due to the said "electric" perception component. Under the scal-

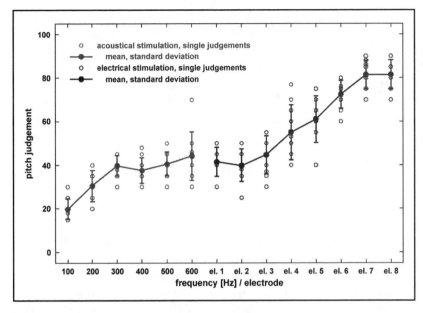

Figure 17-3. Acoustic and electric pitch scaling, subject ME6. Abbreviations include el. for electrode.

ing paradigm, though, the order of stimuli was randomized, so that after a short while she "lost track" of whether a stimulus was accompanied by the "electric" component, and eventually ended up ignoring it.

Whether this description can be accepted as offering sufficient explanation for the observed differences between the ranking and the scaling studies is questionable. An additional factor may have been the number of judgments per condition (10), which is relatively small for a scaling study.

3. THRESHOLD OF AN ACOUSTIC PROBE IN THE PRESENCE OF AN ELECTRIC MASKER

In a three dimensional simultaneous masking study, we assessed interaction between electric and acoustic domains for short stimuli. Under all conditions within the study, the electrical stimulus served as the masker and was presented on electrode 1. This electrode was used because, being the most apical one, it is located most closely to the region of residual hearing in the cochlea. Until recently, interactions between electric and acoustic stimulation had not been demonstrated in human subjects (von Ilberg et al., 1999), and we therefore sought to increase the likelihood of detecting such interactions if they are present, by using electrode 1 and including a greater number of stimulation parameters.

To maximize the precision with which we could measure sensation thresholds and thus observe masking effects, a four alternative forced choice (4AFC) test was used in an up-down tracking procedure. The stimulus pattern we used is depicted in Figures 17–4 and 17–5. A sequence of six electrical masker stimuli (marked "M") 300 ms each in duration and 400 ms apart was presented. Simultaneous with any one of the embedded 4 (i.e., 2, 3, 4, or 5) masker stimuli, the acoustic probe tone (marked "P") was presented. The duration of the probe was 20 ms, plus a linear ramp of 11 ms duration at the beginning and end, summing to a total length of 42 ms for the stimulus. The probe was placed in the middle of the masker, beginning at 129 ms and ending at 171 ms after the onset of the masker burst.

ME6 was instructed that the probe could occur only in one of the middle 4 masker tones. The task was to detect which of these sounded different from the others. In the up-down tracking procedure, the probe level was decreased upon correct recognition of the masker that was accompanied by the probe, and was increased upon incorrect selection. Initially using modification steps of 6 dB, then 3 dB, and finally 1 dB, we collected 16 reversals and assumed the mean value of the last 10 reversals as the resulting perception threshold. The repetition accuracy we achieved with this procedure was about 1 dB; 4 repeated measurements of the perception threshold yielded a maximum difference of 0.9 dB.

The parameters varied in the three-dimensional study were:

1. Stimulation rate of the electric masker stimulus: 200, 500, or 1515 pulses/s
2. Pure-tone frequency of the acoustic probe: 157, 500, or 630 Hz

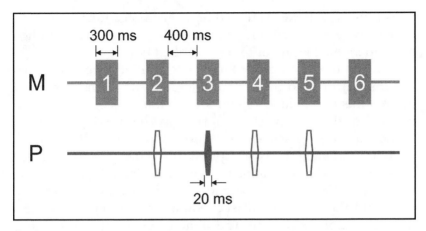

Figure 17–4. Stimuli for psychophysical procedure: 4AFC (out of 6) test, simultaneous.

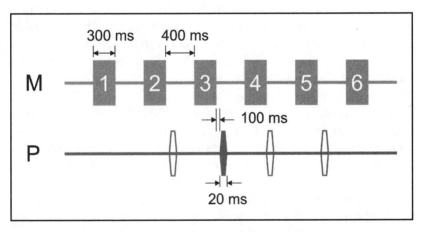

Figure 17–5. Stimuli for psychophysical procedure: 4AFC (out of 6) test, nonsimultaneous.

3. Subjective loudness level of the electric masker: 0 (i.e., not present), 10, 20, or 30 on a loudness scale of 0 to 50.

This resulted in a 3 × 3 matrix of stimulation rate versus frequency conditions. However, the 500 pulses/s, 500 Hz condition was not tested because we suspected that varying phase relations between electric and acoustic stimulation might affect perception thresholds. Thus, 8 different combinations of rate and frequency were tested. Phase relationship effects were studied in a separate experiment to be described below.

One of the four masker loudness conditions presents a special case and has to be treated differently. If the masker is not present it is not audible, of course, and the subject cannot identify one of the four masker intervals as the one including the probe. In order to assess the threshold of the probe in quiet, while reproducing the psychophysical task as it was performed in the three other conditions as closely as possible, the probe was placed 100 ms *after* the end of the respective masker tone burst and thus in quiet. Masker loudness was set to a subjective perception level of 10. The stimulus pattern for this case is shown in Figure 17–5. The large offset of 100 ms is sufficient to avoid forward or backward masking effects, yet the subject is asked to perform basically the same task.

Results for the 8 combinations of masker stimulation rate and probe frequency conditions are displayed in the 8 plots of Figure 17–6. Each plot shows perception threshold levels versus the subjective loudness of the masker. Each point is the mean value of the last 10 reversals in the up-down tracking procedure and the error bars indicate the standard errors of the means. A one way analysis of the variance (ANOVA), which was performed with each of the eight data sets, indicated significant ($p < 0.05$) differences for all sets but the 630 Hz, 1515 pulses/s condition. For the other seven rate versus frequency conditions, post-hoc comparisons of all pairs within the set were performed, employing both the Fisher least significant difference (LSD) method and the more conservative Tukey test. Statistically significant differences between adjacent conditions are indicated by the filled triangles at the top of the graph. Significant differences are indicated by an upright triangle for the Tukey test, and by a downward pointing triangle for the Fisher LSD test.

A condensed overview of the results from the simultaneous masking study is given in Figures 17–7, 17–8, and 17–9. In each figure, a matrix of the 8 tested rate and frequency combinations is displayed. Each of the matrices shows the change of the perception thresholds when going from one to the next of two adjacent masker loudness conditions: Figure 17–7 for 0 to 10, Figure 17–8 for 10 to 20, and Figure 17–9 for 20 to 30.

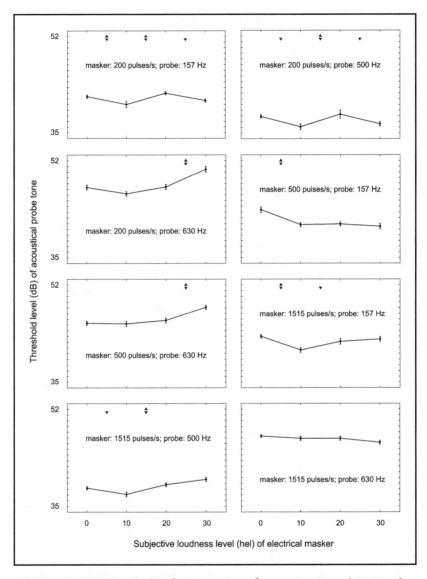

Figure 17-6. Thresholds for detection of an acoustic probe stimulus presented in conjunction with an electric masker. The probe was a tone burst and the masker was a train of electric pulses directed to the most apical electrode in the implant. The frequency of the tone was varied, as were the levels and pulse rates of the masker. The probe and masker were presented to the same ear. Means and standard errors of the means are shown.

287

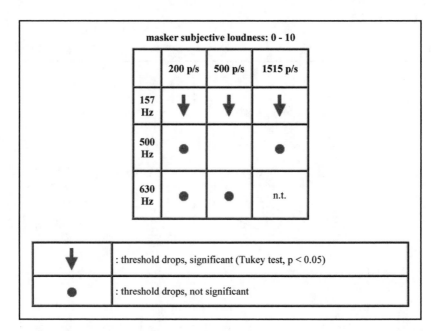

Figure 17–7. Overview: acoustical threshold changes for an increase in the loudness of the electrical masker from 0 to 10. Abbreviations include p/s for pulses/s and n.t. for not tested.

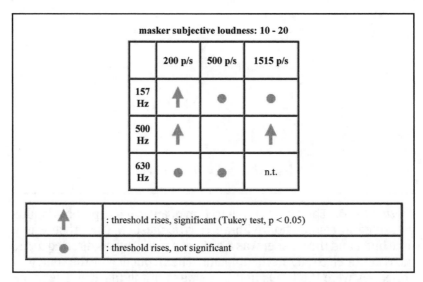

Figure 17–8. Overview: acoustical threshold changes for an increase in the loudness of the electrical masker from 10 to 20. Abbreviations include p/s for pulses/s and n.t. for not tested.

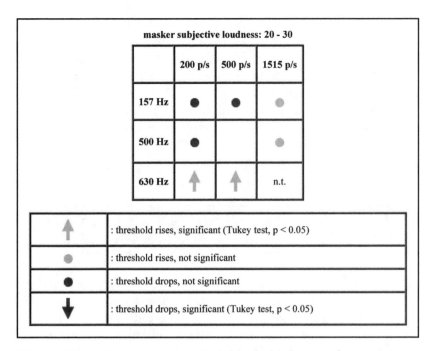

Figure 17-9. Overview: acoustical threshold changes for an increase in the loudness of the electrical masker from 20 to 30. Abbreviations include p/s for pulses/s and n.t. for not tested.

The matrix elements symbolize the respective changes. Arrows indicate significant differences, with a light gray upward arrow standing for an increased threshold and a dark gray downward arrow indicating a threshold drop. The circles indicate nonsignificant differences: light gray for increased, and dark gray for decreased, thresholds. Post hoc analysis was not performed for the 630 Hz, 1515 pulses/s condition (n.t.: not tested).

Comparing perception thresholds when no electrical stimulus is present versus a masker present at a loudness of 10, we found a decrease for all conditions (see Figure 17-7), although it is significant only for a probe frequency of 157 Hz. We consider this to be an "enhancement" effect, where the acoustic probe becomes more audible due to the presence of the (low level) electric stimulation.

We observed the opposite effect when we increased the masker level from loudness 10 to 20 (see Figure 17-8). For all conditions, the threshold rises, although the increase is significant for only a subset of the conditions, for the probe frequencies of 157 Hz and 500 Hz. We consider this to be a masking effect, where the acoustic probe becomes less audible with an increasing level of electric stimulation.

When further increasing the level of the masker, the pattern becomes erratic. Both enhancement and masking effects occur in particular conditions (see Figure 17–9), with no clear pattern of occurrence.

4. EFFECTS OF PHASE RELATIONSHIP BETWEEN ELECTRIC AND ACOUSTIC STIMULATION

When the stimulation rate of the electrical stimulus and the frequency of the acoustic pure-tone probe are set to the same value, one might expect the phase relation between the two stimuli to have an influence on the perception threshold. The acoustic pure-tone stimulation elicits a peak amplitude at some specific location along the basilar membrane, and we would expect the psychophysical perception threshold of the stimulus to be predominantly defined by the sensitivity of the nerve population around this location. Assuming that some kind of interaction between electric and acoustic stimulation exists, we would further expect to observe a difference in the perception threshold depending on the exact time at which an electric biphasic stimulus pulse occurred in relation to the acoustic sine wave signal. For instance, a pulse coincident with the peak of the sine wave period should have a different probability either to mask or enhance nerve activity than a pulse that occurs at the valley of the sine wave period.

The phase relationship of interest is subject to a number of parameters that lie beyond our control and whose values are essentially unknown. (There are phase delays, for instance, between the electric signal to the headphones and the vibration of the tympanic membrane, and between that oscillation and the location of peak amplitude along the basilar membrane.) Therefore, instead of being able to concentrate on a (hypothetical) phase region where we would expect the largest interaction effects, we must measure the perception threshold for several phases over the complete range, that is, sample the threshold perception function.

Figure 17–10 shows two periods of a combined electric-acoustic stimulus of the same frequency. In the top row, two biphasic stimulus pulses of the electric stimulus are plotted as a solid line. Again, as in the study described in section 3 above, the electric stimulus is the masker (marked "M"), whereas the acoustic pure tone is the probe stimulus (marked "P"). The basic timing parameters, such as stimulus and ramp durations, are also identical to those of the setup as described in section 3. The phase relationship is shown here as the distance between the positive zero-crossing of the pure tone signal and the onset of the negative phase of the biphasic electric stimulation pulse, however the absolute position is in fact unknown (as described above, only the relative timing is known). Altogether, 8 different phase conditions have been tested, at 8 uniformly distributed phase positions within one period. Each of the dotted lines in the top row of Figure 17–10 shows the position of a biphasic pulse for one of those phase conditions.

A frequency of 500 Hz would have been the natural extension of the previous study (center in the 3 × 3 matrix of rate/

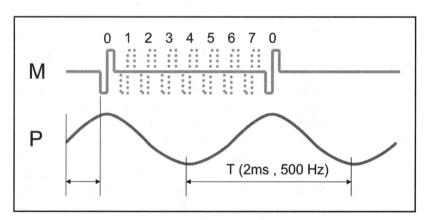

Figure 17-10. Stimuli for the assessment of phase relation effects. The frequency and stimulation rate are depicted here are 500 Hz and 500 pulses/s, for the acoustic and electric stimuli, respectively, whereas in the study a much lower frequency and rate was used.

frequency conditions), but in the phase study, we chose a stimulation frequency near 157.5 Hz on the basis of two considerations: (1) that frequency exhibited the largest electric-acoustic interaction in the up-down tracking audiogram (see Figure 17–2), and (2) that frequency's period of over 6.3 ms would be expected to lie largely outside the refractory period of the nerve cells, a condition not achieved for a 500 Hz stimulus with its period of 2 ms.

The electric stimulus was generated by the implant manufacturer's clinical fitting device (i.e., MED-EL's diagnostic interface box, the "DIB"), which was set up as if being used for EABR stimulation with a clinical ABR recording machine. In this configuration, using special host PC software which also was provided by the manufacturer, the DIB was set up to send out a stimulus, for example, a train of biphasic stimulation pulses on a particular electrode. Then the predefined stimulus could be delivered by the implant in response to each external trigger signal input to the DIB.

As the DIB and the PC audio output do not share a common system clock, we couldn't assume that a nominally identical pure-tone frequency and stimulation rate were actually precisely matching and were not de-synchronizing toward the end of a longer stimulus. By carefully fine-tuning the pure tone frequency, we achieved reliable synchrony and controlled phase differences with a frequency of 158.1 Hz, very close to our 157.5 Hz target.

Both the trigger signal to the DIB and the acoustic signal that is played through headphones are generated at the standard stereo audio outputs of a PC. Precise relative timing between acoustic and electric stimulus is assured by using one stereo channel for the trigger signal and the other for the acoustic stimulus. Stimulation sound data files are generated offline in preparation for the psychophysical test runs. Amplitude modification of the acoustic signal, for example, for threshold detection, is done with an external precision attenuator later in the signal path, whereas the amplitude generated by the PC audio subsystem is never modified.

The perception thresholds were measured under the various phase conditions and masker levels. Embedded within the set of conditions, we also performed four repeated reference measurements of the pure-tone threshold in quiet, that is, without the electrical masker present. A one-way ANOVA of the four reference measurements exhibited no difference among them, and we therefore could pool these data to obtain a single reference value. The fact that the references did not exhibit any differences also confirmed repeatability of the measurements.

A further ANOVA was performed on the thresholds under phase conditions 0 to 7, together with the pooled reference set. Statistical significance ($p < 0.001$) was found for both masker level conditions 10 and 20. Post hoc comparisons of all pairs were performed with both the Fisher LSD method and the more conservative Tukey test. An overview over the results of all pairwise comparisons using the Tukey test is given in Table 17–5.

Perception thresholds under the various phase conditions are displayed in Figures 17–11 and 17–12, for masker loudness values of 10 and 20, respectively. Marked 0 through 7 on the abscissae, the two figures show perception thresholds (mean values of the last 10 reversals in the up-down procedure). For a better overview, the data are displayed twice, so that a full period is available without discontinuity for every starting phase.

Table 17-5. *Pair-Wise Post Hoc Comparisons of Phase Conditions 0 to 7 and Pooled Reference Set A for Subjective Masker Loudness Conditions 10 (above the diagonal) and 20 (below the diagonal)**

	A	0	1	2	3	4	5	6	7
A	—	X		X	X			X	X
0	X	—	X			X	X		X
1	X		—						
2				—			X		
3	X				—		X		X
4	X			X		—			
5	X						—	X	
6		X	X		X	X	X	—	
7		X	X			X	X		—

*Each cell in the table contains an "X" if the respective pair of results was significantly different (Tukey test, $p < 0.05$).

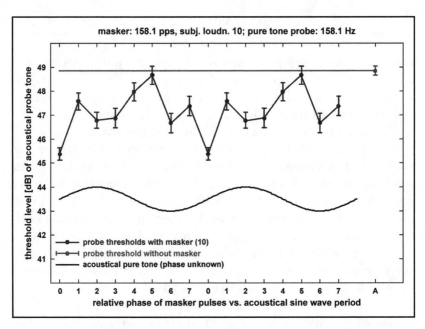

Figure 17–11. Phase relationship effects, electrical masker at loudness 10. Abbreviations include pps for pulses/s, subj. for subjective, and loudn. for loudness.

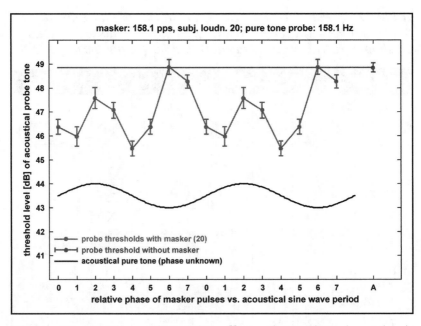

Figure 17–12. Phase relationship effects, electrical masker at loudness 20. Abbreviations are the same as those in Figure 17–11.

The sine waves below each data plot symbolically indicate two cycles of the acoustic pure tone (the absolute phase is unknown, of course). The horizontal rule on top indicates the pure-tone threshold in quiet, that is, the mean of the pooled set of the 4 repeated measurements. Error bars indicate standard errors of the means.

The statistical analysis indicates that the phase relation of the acoustic and the electric stimulus indeed does affect the perception threshold, yet the effect is not very big. Every threshold shift observed in this study was an "enhancement" effect, that is, the threshold was reduced with respect to the threshold in quiet.

For masker loudness 20, conditions 2 and 6 represent local maxima, whereas conditions 1 and 4 present local minima. According to the Tukey test, each maximum is significantly different from each minimum, with the exception of conditions 1 and 2, which are different only according to the Fisher LSD test. In comparison to the pure-tone sine wave, this pattern of results represents an effective doubling of the frequency, and the perception threshold as a function of the phase roughly resembles full-wave rectification of a sine wave.

For both masker loudness conditions, at least one phase condition is indistinguishable from that in quiet (clearly condition 5 for masker loudness 10 and condition 6 for masker loudness 20). It seems as if this point of non-interaction shifts to a later point on the time axis (i.e., from phase condition 5 to condition 6) with increasing masker loudness.

5. THRESHOLD OF AN ELECTRIC PROBE IN THE PRESENCE OF AN ACOUSTIC MASKER

In an additional study of electric-acoustic interactions, we reversed the roles of the electric and acoustic domains. In all the studies described thus far we had used the electric stimulation as the masker and the acoustic stimulation as the probe. One reason for this was the better control we have over the acoustic stimulation regarding the basic parameters of frequency and amplitude. It is much easier to control these in the acoustic domain than for the electric stimulation, which is always limited by the capabilities of the implant system. Here we used an acoustic broadband speech spectrum noise as the masker and an electric pulse train of 300 ms duration as the probe. The psychophysical procedures employed were the same as described in section 3 above: a 4AFC test in an up-down tracking procedure, where 16 reversals in stimulus amplitude were collected and the mean value of the last 10 reversals was assumed to be the perception threshold. In the amplitude modification, we were restricted to the minimum step size—a "current unit" (cu)—supported by the implanted electronics.

Again, this was a three-dimensional study, and the parameters under variation were:

1. Stimulation rate of the electric probe stimulus: 200 or 1515 pulses/s
2. Implant electrode used: electrode 1 or 2
3. Subjective loudness level of the acoustic noise masker: 0 (i.e., not present), 10, or 20 on a loudness scale of 0 to 50.

This resulted in a 2 × 2 matrix of electrode and stimulation rate conditions. Figure 17–13 displays the results for the 4 conditions. The plots show perception threshold current amplitudes versus the subjective loudness of the masker. Error bars indicate the standard error of the means. A one way ANOVA was performed on the 3 data sets of each of the 4 conditions. Neither of the 200 pulses/s conditions exhibited any significant differences, whereas both the 1515 pulses/s conditions did ($p < 0.001$ for both electrode 1 and electrode 2). Post hoc comparisons of all pairs within these two conditions were performed with both the Fisher LSD method and the Tukey test. Statistically significant differences between adjacent conditions are indicated by filled triangles at the top of the graph. Significant differences at a level of $p < 0.05$ are indicated by an upright triangle for the Tukey test, and by a downward-pointing triangle for the Fisher LSD test. The paired comparison for the loudnesses of 0 versus 20 exhibited no difference for electrode 1, whereas for electrode 2 it did.

The most conspicuous aspect of the data is that the perception threshold is affected only very little under the 200 pulses/s stimulation rate condition (i.e., no significant differences between any of the masker loudness conditions), whereas for the 1515

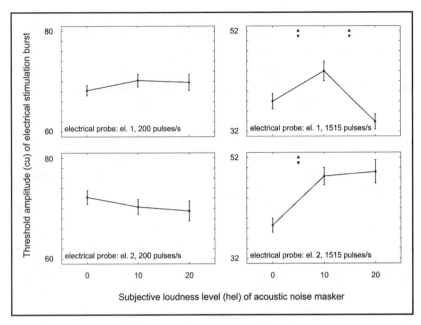

Figure 17–13. Thresholds for detection of an electric probe stimulus presented in conjunction with an acoustic broadband masker. The probe was a train of electric pulses delivered either to electrode 1 or electrode 2 in the implant. (Electrode 1 was the most apical electrode in the implant.) The rate of the pulses within the train was either 200 or 1515 pulse/s. The level of the masker was varied. The probe and the masker were presented to the same ear. Means and standard errors of the means are shown. Abbreviations include el. for electrode and cu for clinical unit.

pulses/s stimulation rate condition, we observed large effects. The amplitude differences between the two most extreme conditions were 10.1 cu (loudness 10 versus loudness 20) on electrode 1, and 10.6 cu (loudness 0 versus loudness 20) on electrode 2, for the 1515 pulses/s conditions. In contrast, the maximum threshold amplitude difference was only 2.0 cu (loudness 0 versus loudness 10) on electrode 1, and 2.7 cu (loudness 0 versus loudness 20) on electrode 2, for the 200 pulses/s conditions.

The obvious difference in behavior of the electric threshold between the 200 pulses/s and 1515 pulses/s conditions suggests a fundamental difference in the nerve behavior between the two situations. A possible explanation may involve how strongly neural activity is synchronized with the electrical stimulation pulses. At 200 pulses/s we would expect the majority of the nerve cells of the concerned population to be out of their refractory periods for each successive pulse, so that the cells would be available to respond to every pulse. At 1515 pulses/s we would expect many of the nerves to be still within a refractory period following a previous stimulation pulse, and thus unavailable to respond to a given later pulse. Due to individual variations among the nerves, we therefore would expect the involved nerve populations to desynchronize over time (see also Chapters 19 and 21).

An important factor in this model is the absolute amplitude of the electrical stimulus, which can be directly compared when looking at average perception threshold in quiet for the different stimulation rates. For electrode 1 it is 68.2 cu for 200 pulses/s compared to only 38.0 cu for 1515 pulses/s, and for electrode 2 it is 72.2 cu for 200 pulses/s compared to only 38.6 cu for 1515 pulses/s. The absolute amplitude level for the 1515 pulses/s condition is substantially lower than the level for the 200 pulses/s condition. This difference in levels again makes it more likely that the nerves will synchronize to the individual pulses at the lower rate. Comparing the two different "modes of operation" of the nerve, we might imagine the 200 pulses/s condition as being a mode were the majority of nerves closely synchronize to high amplitude stimulation pulses, and the 1515 pulses/s condition as being a mode were the nerve population as a whole is relatively desynchronized with respect to the electrical stimulation pulses. It seems reasonable to suppose that in the 1515 pulses/s condition the nerve population might be more sensitive to additional stimulation sources, such as the acoustical masker.

6. DISCUSSION OF ELECTRIC-ACOUSTIC PSYCHOPHYSICAL STUDIES

Looking back at the study described in section 3 (and also the pure tone audiogram study of section 1 and the phase relation study of section 4), where the electric stimulus served as the masker, we did *not* observe any significant differences in threshold behavior when comparing stimulation rate conditions of 200 pulses/s and 1515 pulses/s, in contrast to the observations just discussed in section 5. This may seem contradictory at first sight, but it actually represents a different case. In the study of section 3, the acoustic stimulus was a pure-tone probe, and therefore any effects we observed in that study concerned the region of residual hearing. Masking or enhancement interactions between electric and acoustic stimulation were predominantly effects of the electric stimulation reaching into and influencing the neural region involved in residual acoustic hearing.

However, in the study described in section 5, the situation was reversed, with a broadband acoustical masker and electrical stimulation as the probe. Generally, we have to assume the neural region of the cochlea affected by electric stimulation from a specific electrode to be much broader than that affected by a pure tone in the range of residual hearing. For electrical stimulation amplitudes at threshold level, however, we may think of the excited region as being more localized in the vicinity of the site of stimulation. In that case, the situation of section 5 might be analogous to that of section 3, but with interaction effects predominantly occurring near the site of electrical stimulation, to the extent that residual acoustical hearing mechanisms influence that neural region of the cochlea.

One of the main findings of our various interaction studies is that when looking at the size of both masking and enhancement effects, we find only small threshold shifts. The largest single shift we observed was the 5.9 dB masking at 157.5 Hz in the up-down-tracking audiogram (see Figure 17–2). Considering the fact that all other observed effects were even smaller, it is not surprising that no interactions had been observed previously. On the other hand, the surprisingly large influence of an acoustic broadband noise masker on the threshold of an electric probe stimulus, as described in section 5 (see Figure 17–13) may indicate a substantial effect. An amplitude difference of 10 current units is typically associated with a large difference in perceived loudness, if the electric stimuli are presented and compared in quiet. The dynamic range of electrical stimulation observed for CI subjects is typically only 15 to 20 dB. Given the different scales, of course, the size of this effect cannot be compared directly with the size of effects in the other studies.

7. SPEECH RECEPTION FOR COMBINED ELECTRIC AND ACOUSTIC STIMULATION

In an extension of the speech reception studies conducted during the subject's previous visit (see QPR 6:8), we were able to close many gaps in a systematic set of parametric combinations. A summary of the speech reception performance under various conditions is given in Figure 17–14. As one indicator, we used identification of 16 medial consonants, presented with both male and female talkers, in quiet and in competing speech spectrum CCITT noise at the speech-to-noise ratio (S/N) of +5 dB. As described in QPR 6:8, ME6 is a native German speaker, so our standard English set of consonants was modified and relabeled, with the English "y" sound substituted to correspond to the German pronunciation of the consonant "j," a new consonant "h" substituted for the English voiced "th," and the unchanged English consonants "f, v, s, z, and sh" relabeled as "v, w, ss, s, and sch," respectively.

ME6's considerable English skills made it possible to employ the English CUNY sentence lists, which were presented in competing CCITT noise at the S/Ns of +5 dB, +10 dB and in quiet. The three main rows in Figure 17–14 correspond to three different ranges of input frequencies represented by electric stimulation, that is, via the CI system. The frequency band conveyed acoustically was the same in every case: the upper cutoff frequency of the lowpass filter in the path of the acoustic signal was held constant at 1 kHz. (Comparisons during ME6's first visit had shown that speech reception was not improved by acoustic presentation of signals above 500 Hz.)

Each configuration was tested in three different conditions: CI alone (left-most of each set of three bars), amplified acoustic stimulation (hearing aid) alone (right-most bars), and the CI and the hearing aid together (middle bars). Use of the CUNY sentences in quiet resulted in scores limited by ceiling effects for this subject, so testing under that condition was suspended after obtaining those initial results.

Several strong patterns emerge immediately from these data. In quiet (see the first two columns of Figure 17–14), electric stimulation alone supports much better speech reception than aided acoustic stimulation alone.

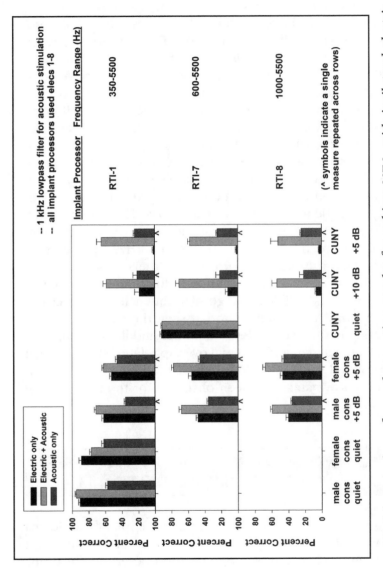

Figure 17-14. Overview of speech reception results for subject ME6, with ipsilateral electric and acoustic stimulation provided separately and in combination. Error bars indicate standard errors of the means. The tests included identification of consonants (cons) and recognition of the City University of New York (CUNY) sentences at the indicated S/Ns. Additional abbreviations include elecs for electrodes.

301

But the addition of speech spectrum noise has a much more severe impact on the electric-alone performance than on the acoustic-alone performance (columns 3, 4, 6, and 7).

Although there is no evidence from these data that combined electric and acoustic stimulation (EAS) improves speech reception in quiet, the combination is far superior to electric-alone stimulation in the presence of noise. The benefit of combined EAS is particularly striking in the CUNY sentence data.

The three rows in Figure 17–14 represent three different relationships between the frequency spectrum conveyed by the aided acoustic signal and the frequency spectrum on which the electrical stimulation is based. In all three cases the acoustic signal is limited by a 1 kHz lowpass filter; speech reception comparisons reported in QPR 6:8 found that ME6 gains no benefit from any acoustic information above 500 Hz. Thus, the top row of Figure 17–14, with electrical stimulation conveying information for the frequency range of 300 Hz to 5 kHz, represents an overlap in the representations provided by the acoustic and electric stimuli. Similarly, the bottom row in the figure corresponds to conveying a 1- to 5-kHz range of frequencies via electrical stimulation and represents a gap between the spectral regions represented by the two modes. It is in the middle row, approximating a minimal gap and minimal overlap relationship between the represented spectral regions, where the best overall speech reception performance has been observed for the tests to date with ME6.

8. POTENTIAL BENEFITS OF APPLYING THE SAME APPROACH CONTRALATERALLY

Evolving CI criteria have led to there being implant candidates with more residual hearing than was the case in the past. In a parallel trend, whereas not long ago the poorer ear (in terms of residual hearing, duration of deafness, or both) tended to be chosen for cochlear implantation, it is more common today to implant the better ear.

There is great interest currently in combined EAS as a therapy for hearing loss in patients who have some residual hearing but suffer from poor speech reception using available acoustic hearing aids alone. Such patients' residual acoustic sensitivity typically is at low frequencies. If it is possible to limit any trauma associated with careful cochlear implantation to the immediate vicinity of the implanted electrode array, then residual hearing may be preserved and simultaneous electrical and acoustic stimulation may be achieved in the same ear. The assumption is that a relatively shallow insertion of the electrode array from the basal end of the cochlea avoids damage to the more apical regions on which the low-pitch residual hearing depends.

Groups of patients in Iowa City, Iowa, and Frankfurt, Germany, currently are being treated in this way using, respectively, Nucleus and MED-EL CIs. ME6 is a member of the Frankfurt group.

There is concern among otologic surgeons about the most appropriate depth of electrode array insertion when combined EAS of the same ear is contemplated. Shallower insertions, although less likely to damage residual hearing, are also less likely to achieve the best possible performance with electrical stimulation alone. In the event that residual hearing eventually is lost, a second surgery might be required to fully insert the original electrode array—or even to substitute a longer one—in order to realize the full potential of electrical stimulation alone.

Insertions have been limited to 6 or 10 mm beyond the basal end of the cochlea for the Iowa City group, and have typically been 20 mm for the Frankfurt group. Although the numbers of patients remain too small to allow statistical conclusions, there has been some incidence of immediate loss of residual hearing among members of the Frankfurt group.

There also is concern among otologic surgeons about the possibility of long-term gradual loss of residual hearing as a result of an ipsilateral implant. Evaluating such a possibility may prove difficult, since progressive loss would be expected to occur in some ears even without surgical intervention.

Noting the generally high levels of performance of combined electrical-acoustic patients with electrical stimulation alone—despite relatively shallow electrode insertions—some observers suspect that the advantages of full insertion might outweigh any (perhaps temporary) benefit of preserving the possibility of some acoustic stimulation.

As described in detail previously, our studies with ME6 have indicated substantial improvements of speech reception in noise with the simultaneous use of both modes. Performance with electrical stimulation alone is far superior to that with acoustic amplification alone for that subject. Although she prefers the use of both modes in all circumstances, we observed no significant performance difference between electric stimulation only and both modes for speech reception in quiet. Performance in noise seems to be best when there is minimum overlap and a minimum gap between the input sound spectra assigned to the two modes.

Meanwhile, studies of subjects with bilateral CIs in our laboratory have shown that signals from monophonic speech processor channels can be redirected to contralateral cochlear electrodes without damage to speech reception performance. Improvements in speech reception in the presence of directionally distinct speech spectrum noise with stereophonic binaural stimulation have been a major focus of studies with those subjects, some of whom received bilateral MED-EL devices at Würzburg, Germany, and others Nucleus devices at Iowa City.

Given this combination of observations and circumstances, and access to a well-developed set of tools and techniques for assessing speech reception in noise, our laboratory is interested in exploring possible benefits of an alternative therapeutic approach: simultaneous electrical and acoustic stimulation combined contralaterally.

Such an approach would avoid all decisions about precise depth of insertion, and eliminate concerns about immediate and eventual surgical damage to residual hearing. In the event that residual hearing eventually was lost, a full-insertion CI would already be in place for stimulation in an electric-only mode. Initially, some of the apical-most electrodes might not be stimulated, depending on the nature and extent of the contralateral residual hearing. The hardware involved in simultaneous use of an acoustic aid and a CI would not have to compete for space at the same ear. Some degree of sound lateralization might even be obtained in some cases.

A potential problem with this approach might be the possibility of poorer CI performance in the ear with less or no residual hearing, perhaps correlated with differences in the durations of deafness and/or other differences in the hearing history of the two ears. Our studies demonstrating great freedom to assign electrodes to contralateral as well as ipsilateral electrodes happen to have involved early subjects from our bilaterally implanted group, each of whom had a relatively small difference in duration of deafness between ears; more recent bilaterally implanted subjects, with quite different histories and durations of deafness between ears, will be scheduled for similar electrode assignment studies. The series of patients implanted bilaterally at Iowa City were selected in part on the basis of large differences in history between ears, including both etiology and duration of deafness. The primary original goal of the studies there was to obtain information that might better guide selection of which ear to implant for purely electrical stimulation; the same information could be very useful in assessing the prospects for simultaneous contralateral electrical and acoustic stimulation involving implantation of only one ear.

Acknowledgments. We thank subject ME6 for her participation in the studies described in this report. We also are grateful to Jochen Tillein for his participation as a co-investigator in the studies.

Chapter 18

SPEECH RECEPTION
WITH COMBINED EAS*

*Blake S. Wilson, Robert D. Wolford,
Dewey T. Lawson, and Reinhold Schatzer*

BACKGROUND

Our investigation of combined electric and acoustic stimulation
of the auditory system (combined EAS) began in August 2000,
with initial studies with subject ME6, for whom an intentionally
shallow electrode insertion had preserved significant residual
hearing at low frequencies in her implanted ear. In the presence
of speech-spectrum noise, her speech reception scores were
significantly higher when ipsilateral acoustic stimulation was
added to electrical stimulation from her cochlear implant. The
combined mode also was associated with better performance
whenever any significant difference between combined and electric-only conditions was noted in quiet. Data in quiet and at the
speech-to-noise ratios (S/Ns) of +10 and +5 dB were consistent
with the combined mode being less sensitive than electric stimulation alone to the negative impact of increasing levels of noise

---

*From QPR 7:3, October 1, 2002, through December 31, 2002. (The original
title for this excerpted section from QPR 7:3 was "Additional Perspectives on
Speech Reception with Combined Electric and Acoustic Stimulation.")

on speech reception. Detailed descriptions of the studies to date with ME6 are presented in QPR 6:8 and Chapter 17.

In December 2001 we were able to study a second subject (ME14) with a similar pattern of residual acoustic hearing, but in this case contralateral to her cochlear implant. That subject showed even greater speech reception benefits from combined electric and contralateral acoustic stimulation in the presence of competing speech-spectrum noise than had been seen with ME6. The pattern of the combined mode being less sensitive than electric stimulation alone to the negative impact of increasing levels of noise on performance was affirmed. (For more detail, see QPR 6:13.)

SUBJECTS

Recently, we have conducted studies with three additional subjects, each of whom has significantly extended our perspective on combined EAS. Two of the new subjects were referred to us as having residual acoustic hearing both ipsilaterally and contralaterally with respect to their shallow-insertion cochlear implants (subjects ME19 and ME20). These subjects provided us with an opportunity to conduct within-subject comparisons of ipsilateral versus contralateral acoustic stimulation, in combination with the electric stimuli provided by the implant. Data for one of those subjects generally confirmed but also significantly refined the pattern seen in our previous studies, whereas results with the other subject presented a clear exception to that pattern. The third additional subject (SR3) had substantially less residual hearing than our other EAS subjects, but enough to prompt inclusion in these studies in the hope of obtaining similar performance improvements for her in the presence of noise. Unlike the other subjects in this group, SR3 had no chronic experience with combined EAS.

Subject ME19 was born in 1942 and experienced a sudden hearing loss during her first pregnancy in 1966. Progressive loss eventually forced her to retire from teaching in 1993 and continued until she became a candidate for a cochlear implant. She reports no family history of hearing loss. Her right ear was implanted in July 2001 by Dr. Wolf-Dieter Baumgartner of the Medical University of Vienna, Austria. In order to maximize the number of useable electrodes while limiting the depth of insertion to preserve residual hearing, a "short" MED-EL array was used—one designed to substitute for a standard length array when obstruction of scala tympani would prevent full insertion. ME19's clinical cochlear implant fitting utilizes nine of the twelve electrodes in the array. She also routinely uses bilateral hearing aids—Siemens Signia CT devices. She experienced an onset of both tinnitus and vertigo along with her hearing loss in 1966. Although the tinnitus remains unchanged, she has not experienced vertigo since her cochlear implant surgery. She reports that she routinely uses both hearing aids together with the cochlear implant. She also reports that she can make some use of the telephone, and that her residual hearing is better in the left ear than the right. Her speech reception performance was minimal immediately after surgery and has improved gradually over the period since implantation, but remains less than has been seen in the other EAS subjects we have studied. She still finds lipreading helpful in most circumstances.

There is neither a family history nor any other indication of a cause for the hearing loss that led to subject ME20's receiving a cochlear implant. Born in 1953, she first noticed a change in her hearing during high school. At age 26 she was fitted with a hearing aid on the right side, and added a second aid on the left at age 30. She was implanted on the right side in September 2001 by Dr. Jan Kiefer of the University of Frankfurt, Germany. A standard MED-EL electrode array was inserted 22 mm into scala tympani. SR20 experienced tinnitus bilaterally before cochlear implantation but only on the left side since then, and to a degree that she does not find bothersome. She denies any history of vertigo before or after implantation. She experienced good speech reception immediately upon first fitting of her clinical processor, and her overall performance is now excellent. She does report difficulty, however, using a telephone with either the left ear (residual hearing alone) or the right (residual hearing and implant), and switches to a different program whenever using her processor to carry on a telephone conversation.

Subject SR3 was born in 1937. She first noticed and documented a hearing loss in 1957, while training to become a nurse.

Over the next 15 years, fluctuations in her hearing—rapid drops followed by spontaneous recovery after one to two weeks—were superimposed on a slow deterioration. Attempts to correlate such episodes with a variety of things (diet changes, exposure to allergens, tension, barometric pressure, etc.) were unsuccessful. An extensive series of diagnostic procedures in 1973 failed to reveal any abnormality, after which vasodilation therapy seemed to slow the progressive loss until 1983 when it began to increase rapidly. Another extensive series of tests revealed only an abnormality in thyroid function that was quickly corrected by a change in chronic medications. The hearing lost during that period was never recovered. A left ear shunt was performed in 1984 for Mondini syndrome. Dr. Bruce Gantz of the University of Iowa implanted an Ineraid percutaneous electrode array on SR3's left side late in 1987. She was first seen in our laboratories in March 1990, when she volunteered to be a research subject in our first comparisons of CIS processors to the compressed analog strategy of the clinical Ineraid devices. Her performance was substantially improved with the use of a CIS strategy, and she subsequently used the MED-EL CIS-Link device as her clinical processor. She has returned to our laboratories on numerous occasions to take part in an exceptionally wide variety of studies. She is among our top several subjects in terms of the time she has contributed to participate in our research. We knew that some residual hearing in her right ear had led one physician to discourage her from having cochlear implant surgery in 1987, but in our laboratory studies we found that she didn't even notice normal conversation taking place in the testing room when her cochlear implant was turned off or was receiving signals via direct connection to a prerecorded source. In the light of the striking benefits seen recently for combined EAS in the presence of speech spectrum noise, we decided to assess SR3's contralateral residual hearing and its potential as an adjunct to her cochlear implant system. She has not used a hearing aid since receiving her cochlear implant.

We note that the previously studied subject ME6 also had and has some residual hearing in the ear contralateral to the implant. As indicated in Figures 18–1 and 18–2, that hearing was not as good as the hearing on the ipsilateral side. Our work to date with this subject has been limited to tests involving the implanted ear only.

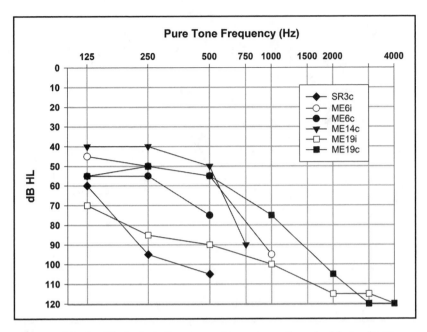

Figure 18–1. Clinical audiograms. Pure-tone thresholds in dB Hearing Level (db HL) versus frequency at standard audiometric frequencies for each ear with measurable residual hearing are shown. Symbol shapes are associated with individual subjects. Open and filled symbols indicate residual hearing that is ipsilateral and contralateral, respectively, to the cochlear implant. Six ears are represented, across four of the five subjects. Thresholds could not be measured at 750 Hz for the ears contralateral to the implant for subjects ME6 and SR3; at 1000 Hz for the ear contralateral to the implant for subject ME14; or at 1500 Hz for the ear ipsilateral to the implant for subject ME6.

STUDIES

Most of our subjects were able to provide us with copies of clinical audiograms obtained postimplantation, typically at the time of first fitting of a cochlear implant speech processor. The clinical audiograms we have available are summarized in Figure 18–1, where each subject has been assigned a unique symbol shape, and symbols corresponding to ears that are ipsilateral and contralateral to the side of electric stimulation are shown as open and filled, respectively. Included are a total of six

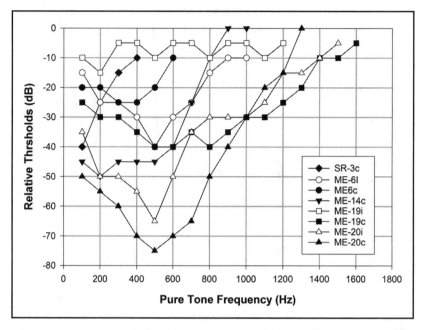

Figure 18–2. Detailed audiograms. Relative pure-tone thresholds versus frequency at 100 Hz intervals for each ear with measurable residual hearing are shown. Thresholds were obtained under earphones. Symbol shapes are associated with individual subjects, and are consistent with the symbols used in Figure 18–1. Open and filled symbols indicate residual hearing that is ipsilateral and contralateral, respectively, to the cochlear implant. Eight ears are represented, across the five subjects. Note that better hearing corresponds to points nearer the bottom in Figure 18–2, but nearer the top in Figure 18–1.

ears, across four of our five subjects. (Audiograms for each of the fifth subject's ears have been requested from the referring clinic.)

The overall pattern was one of various degrees of residual hearing for pure tone frequencies below about 1 kHz. An audiogram, of course, provides only a partial indication of the nature of any residual hearing. Also important are the degree of frequency discrimination across the residual spectrum, and the nature of loudness growth and recruitment.

To better characterize and compare the individual degrees and patterns of residual hearing, we obtained our own high-resolution audiograms for each of the subjects at the outset of the EAS studies with him or her. These audiograms document relative thresholds for pure tones at 100 Hz intervals from 100 Hz to the upper limit of each subject's residual hearing. The data are displayed in Figure 18–2, for all eight ears with significant residual hearing across our five subjects. The symbols are consistent between Figures 18–1 and 18–2.

As shown in Figure 18–2, a wide range of degrees and spectral extents of residual hearing are represented among these eight ears. The thresholds span a 40 dB range at 100 Hz, and approach a 70 dB range at 500 Hz. The upper frequency limit of residual hearing varies from 1300 Hz to less than 250 Hz for a −20 dB threshold criterion for each subject's better ear, and from 1100 Hz to less than 200 Hz for a −30 dB criterion. Comparisons between the two figures indicate that a relative threshold of −20 dB in Figure 18–2 corresponds roughly to a hearing loss of 80 dB in Figure 18–1, and a −30 dB relative threshold to about 70 dB HL. Our initial two EAS subjects, ME6 and ME14, have very similar audiograms at and above 500 Hz, while below that frequency ME14 has substantially better hearing than ME6's better-hearing ear (ipsilateral to the implant). Between our two most recent subjects, one (ME19) has much more residual hearing contralaterally than ipsilaterally, whereas the other (ME20) has quite similar patterns of residual hearing on the two sides. The residual hearing of our long-term subject SR3 is limited to a narrower frequency range than any of the chronic EAS users. In some of the figures to follow, labeling will be used to distinguish between generally "good" and "poor" levels of residual hearing. In such cases, only the (contralateral) residual hearing of SR3 and the ipsilateral residual hearing of ME19 will be characterized as relatively poor.

Both consonant and sentence materials were used to compare speech reception with various combinations of electric and acoustic stimulation in these five subjects. Identification of medial consonants in an /a/-C-/a/ context was one measure used with all five subjects. The consonant tests used multiple exemplars and provided no feedback as to correct or incorrect responses, with the tokens randomized in sets to allow statistical analysis of uncertainty. Two of the subjects (ME14 and SR3) were tested with the corpus of 24 English consonants routinely used in our laboratories when overall performance levels are high. The other three subjects (ME6, ME19, and ME20), whose native language is German, were tested with a subset of 16 of the same consonants, selected and relabeled as appropriate to that language. ME6's command of English was good enough to allow use of the City University of New York (CUNY) sentence materials with her as well as with native English speakers ME14 and SR3. For Austrian and German subjects ME19 and ME20, the sentence test materials chosen were from the Oldenburger Satztest (Wagener et al., 1999a, 1999b, 1999c). Each of those sentences is composed of one word from each of five closed sets, in the order: name, verb, number, adjective, and noun. Each of the five closed sets contains ten words. Although not an open-set test as in the CUNY corpus, these materials are not contaminated by even extensive previous use, and do constitute natural connected speech. A minimum of four lists of the CUNY sentences (approximately 408 words) and a minimum of four lists of the Oldenburger sentences (200 words) were used for each condition. For both tests, the scores recorded were the percentages of correctly identified words in the sentences.

In all cases involving competing noise, CCITT noise (which approximates the long-term spectrum of speech) was added to the speech signals to produce a specified S/N. In these studies, all noise and speech signals were preprocessed using head-related transfer functions (HRTFs) to include cues that would be present for a sound source in front of the subject. These preprocessed signals were used as inputs for subsequent processing to produce the electric and/or acoustic stimuli presented to the subject, via a circumaural earphone or earphones for acoustic stimulation and via the transcutaneous or percutaneous link of the implant device for electric stimulation. The HRTFs did not include a simulation of frequency filtering imposed by the ear canal.

RESULTS

We begin with a comparison of results among the three subjects using residual hearing in only one ear. This comparison includes original subjects ME6 and ME14 and our long-term subject with relatively poor residual hearing contralateral to her cochlear implant (SR3). Figure 18–3 summarizes speech reception results for identification of consonants and recognition of key words in the CUNY sentences as a function of the S/N, and does so for electric stimulation only, for combined EAS, and for acoustic stimulation only. For the conditions involving electric stimulation, the frequency range represented by the implant processor was 350 to 5500 Hz in every case.

Among the scores shown in Figure 18–3, four of the scores for combined EAS are high enough to raise the possibility of differences being distorted because of ceiling effects. These four include the scores for consonant identification in quiet by subjects ME6 and SR3, and recognition of the key words in the CUNY sentences at the S/N of +10 dB by subjects ME14 and SR3. The corresponding electric only results for consonants in quiet are subject to the same possibility.

The data for ME14 and ME6 shown in Figure 18–3 have been discussed previously and were summarized in the background section of this report. Of particular interest, then, is whether subject SR3, our long-term cochlear implant subject with substantially less residual hearing than either ME6 or ME14 and no chronic experience with EAS, can achieve significantly better speech reception in noise with combined stimulation. Although her acoustic-only scores are, as expected, much lower for all combinations of test and S/N shown, the combined EAS mode does support significantly better scores than electric-only for consonants at the S/N of +5 dB. For CUNY sentences at the S/N of +10 dB, whereas the corresponding scores differ from each other by more than a standard deviation of the mean, the significance of the difference is not clear ($p = .054$). Electric-only and combined EAS results for the CUNY sentences clearly are not significantly different at the S/N of +5 dB, and combined EAS performance for SR3 does not seem to be any less sensitive to the impact of increased noise than her performance with the cochlear implant alone.

A similar summary is presented in Figure 18–4 for our two new subjects, each of whom has residual hearing both ipsilaterally and contralaterally with respect to her cochlear implant. Shown in the figure are speech reception results for identification of consonants and identification of words in the Oldenburger sentences as a function of S/N, again comparing scores for electric stimulation only, combined EAS, and acoustic stimulation only.

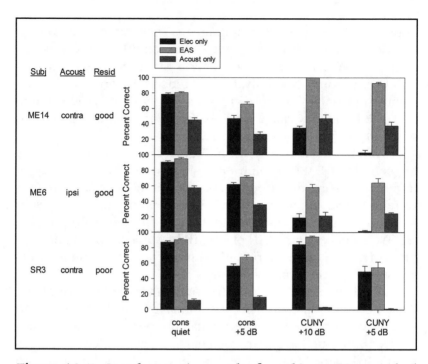

Figure 18–3. Speech reception results for subjects using residual hearing in one ear only. Percent-correct scores are shown for electric stimulation only (Elec only; *black bars*), combined electric and acoustic stimulation (EAS; *light gray bars*), and acoustic stimulation only (Acoust only; *darker gray bars*). The tests included: (1) identification of medial consonants (cons), with the consonant tokens presented in quiet and in conjunction with CCITT speech spectrum noise at the speech-to-noise ratio (S/N) of +5 dB, and (2) recognition of key words in the City University of New York (CUNY) sentences, presented in conjunction with the noise at the S/Ns of +10 and +5 dB. For the consonant tests, 24 medial English consonants were used in the measures with subjects ME14 and SR3, and 16 medial German consonants were used in the measures with subject ME6. Labels to the left indicate whether the residual acoustic hearing is ipsilateral (ipsi) or contralateral (contra) to the electrically stimulated ear, and the degree of that residual hearing for each of the three subjects. Error bars indicate standard deviations of the means. The frequency range analyzed and represented by the implant processor was 350 to 5500 Hz in every case. Additional abbreviations include: Subj for Subject, Acoust for Acoustic, and Resid for Residual Hearing.

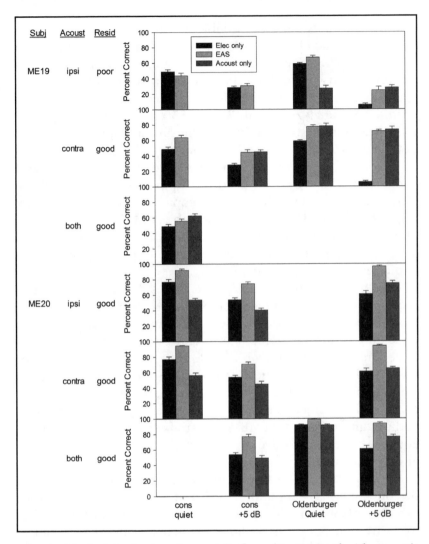

Figure 18–4. Speech reception results for subjects tested with acoustic stimulation of either ear or both ears. The organization and stimulus conditions for this figure are the same as those for Figure 18–3, except that German language materials were used throughout for the speech tests, including 16 medial German consonants and the Oldenburger formulaic sentences. Conditions shown in the present figure without bars were not tested.

Results are shown for each subject with acoustic stimulation ipsilateral to the electrical stimulation, contralateral to it, and to both ears. (The same electric-only data are reproduced across all three acoustic condition panels for each subject). As in the previous figure, the cochlear implant speech processors represented here analyzed a full 350 to 5500 Hz overall frequency range. Conditions without bars in the present Figure 18–4 were not tested because of time limitations.

As was the case in Figure 18–3, Figure 18–4 includes several comparisons that may be distorted by possible ceiling effects. This possibility seems likely for comparisons involving the six highest combined EAS scores for subject ME20. It also seems likely for comparisons involving either the electric-only or the acoustic-only scores for ME20's identification of words in Oldenburger sentences in quiet.

With her relatively poor ipsilateral residual hearing, ME19's scores show no advantage for combined EAS except for the single case of Oldenburger sentences in quiet. In noise, her residual hearing—whether ipsilateral or contralateral—seems in general to account fully for her EAS scores (i.e., the scores for combined EAS are statistically the same as the scores for acoustic stimulation only). This pattern is strikingly different from that of our other subjects, especially considering that our detailed audiograms indicate that ME19's contralateral residual hearing is equal to or more sensitive than ME6's ipsilateral residual hearing at all frequencies.

ME20's results—both with ipsilateral and contralateral acoustic contributions—are more consistent with those of our earlier subjects. Also, as might be expected on the basis of the similarity of her left and right audiograms, her ipsilateral and contralateral results are quite similar to each other. These results are consistent with earlier patterns in the superiority of electric-only over acoustic-only performance for consonants in quiet, and the superiority of combined EAS over either mode alone, especially for consonants or sentences in noise. Apparently inconsistent with patterns based on the earlier studies is performance with EAS not being markedly less sensitive than electric stimulation alone to the negative impact of noise, at least for consonants. (Results for the Oldenburger sentences are difficult to interpret due to possible ceiling effects.)

To facilitate comparisons of any advantage offered by combined EAS, in Figure 18–5 we have replotted the data of Figures 18–3 and 18–4 as differences between percent correct scores with combined EAS and the higher of the electric-only and acoustic-only scores under the same test conditions. These differences provide measures of EAS benefit with respect to the next best alternative.

The most obvious trend in these difference data is the general increase in EAS benefit with increasing noise (consonants in quiet at the top of the figure versus consonants at the S/N of +5 dB in the middle) and, in noise, the greater EAS benefit for recognition of words in sentences than for identification of isolated consonants (consonants at +5 dB S/N in the middle of the figure versus sentences at +5 dB S/N at the bottom). In the cases of the sentence data for subjects ME6 and ME14, the EAS benefit reflects scores for combined EAS that are greater than the sum of the scores for the electric-only and acoustic-only conditions (see Figure 18–3).

An additional pattern is the absence of any obvious advantage to either ipsilateral or contralateral acoustic stimulation. This lack of an effect can be seen by comparing the ipsilateral versus contralateral results for subjects ME19 and ME20 in each of the three parts (A, B, and C) of Figure 18–5.

Finally, no negative difference in Figure 18–5 is statistically significant, so we have found no evidence of any destructive interaction between the two modes of stimulation.

All of the data shown thus far have been for cochlear implant processors that analyzed and represented an overall frequency range of 350 to 5500 Hz, a range shared by many processors studied in our laboratories. Our previous EAS studies also included comparisons with processors restricted to ranges of 600 to 5500 Hz and of 1000 to 5500 Hz, which were designed to explore possible effects of overlap between the spectral ranges represented electrically and acoustically, or of a gap between those spectral ranges. Figure 18–6 compares speech reception data for electric stimulation only, using each of those electrical analysis ranges, for each of our five subjects.

As would be expected for electric stimulation alone, a performance advantage for the widest frequency range (350 to 5500 Hz) was seen for every subject.

Figure 18–7 shows similar comparisons for combined EAS.

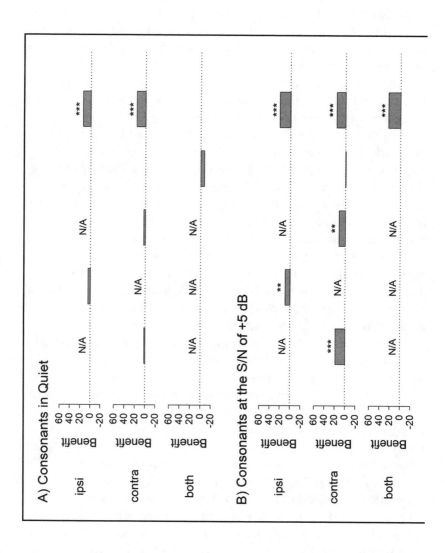

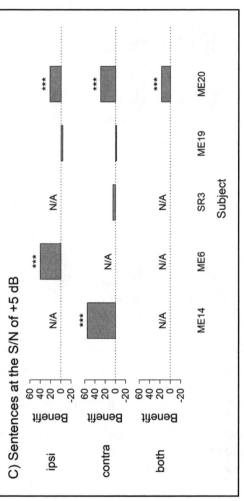

Figure 18–5. EAS benefit with respect to the next best alternative. The difference between the speech reception score obtained with combined EAS and that obtained with the better of the electric-only and acoustic-only scores is shown for each of the indicated conditions and subjects. Labels to the left indicate the ear(s) to which the acoustic stimuli were presented. Conditions marked "N/A" are those for which residual hearing was not available on the appropriate side. Double and triple asterisks mark differences that are significant at $p < 0.01$ and $p < 0.001$, respectively; all other differences are not significant. The data presented in this figure were derived from the data presented in Figures 18–3 and 18–4. Additional abbreviations in the present figure include: Benefit for % EAS benefit, and S/N for speech-to-noise ratio.

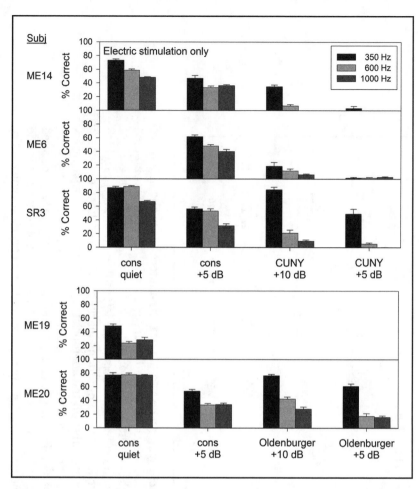

Figure 18-6. Effects of changes in the lower end of the frequency range analyzed and represented by the implant processor, for electric stimulation only. Percent-correct scores are shown by the black, light gray, and darker gray bars for the frequency ranges of 350 to 5500 Hz, 600 to 5500 Hz, and 1000 to 5500 Hz, respectively. Results for English-speaking subjects are presented in the top part of the figure, and results for German-speaking subjects in the bottom part. The tests are the same as those in Figures 18–3 and 18–4, except that the Oldenburger sentences were presented in noise at the speech-to-noise ratio of +10 dB rather than in quiet. Data were collected for all tests and frequency ranges for subject ME14, and included zero scores for the combinations for which no bar is visible. Consonant tests in quiet were not conducted with subject ME6 for the frequency ranges of 600 to 5500 Hz and 1000 to 5500 Hz. Similarly, those ranges were not included for any but the consonant tests in quiet for subject ME19. Error bars and abbreviations are the same as those in Figure 18–3.

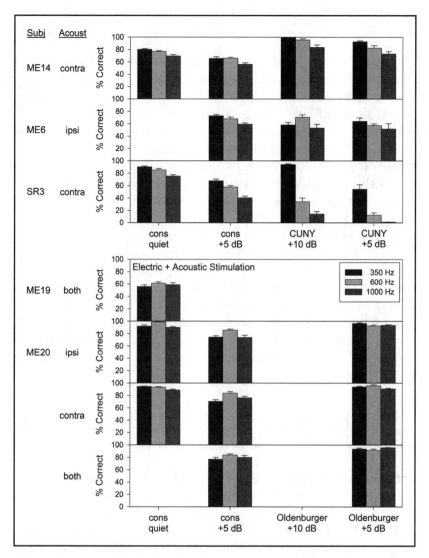

Figure 18–7. Effects of changes in the lower end of the frequency range analyzed and represented by the implant processor, for combined electric and acoustic stimulation. The organization of this figure is the same as that in Figure 18–6, except for the labels on the left in the present figure that indicate to which ear(s) the acoustic stimuli were presented. Bars are shown only for those combinations of tests, subjects, and acoustically stimulated ears for which all three frequency ranges were included. Error bars and abbreviations are the same as those in Figures 18–3 and 18–4.

There are several instances in which the percent-correct scores in Figure 18–7 are high enough that ceiling effects may distort differences among them. This is the case, for example, for ME14's sentence data at the S/N of +10 dB, and for ME20's consonant data in quiet and sentence data at the S/N of +5 dB.

For ME14 and SR3 there are clear advantages to the use of the widest frequency range, 350 to 5500 Hz.

Although there are significant performance differences among the three ranges for ME6's consonant data at the S/N of +5 dB, and for her CUNY sentence data at the S/N of +10 dB, there is no overall pattern of advantage across those conditions.

The limited data for ME19 show no significant differences.

For ME20, there are significant advantages for the 600 to 5500 Hz range wherever the scores are not clearly subject to ceiling effects (the data for consonants at the S/N of +5 dB are free of possible ceiling effects). Similar advantages are observed for both ipsilateral and contralateral acoustic stimulation for this subject, who has nearly equivalent patterns of residual hearing on the two sides.

SUMMARY

- For some subjects, speech reception scores in noise for combined EAS exceed the sum of their scores with electric stimulation alone and acoustic stimulation alone.
- Even an extremely limited range of residual hearing can support some improvement in speech reception in the presence of speech spectrum noise. SR3's residual pure tone threshold rises by 30 dB between 100 Hz and 400 Hz (see Figure 18–2). Yet, the addition of acoustic stimulation to the use of her contralateral cochlear implant produces significant improvements in her scores for identification of consonants at the S/N of +5 dB. Although her improvement with EAS is not significant for sentences at +10 and +5 dB, her results indicate potential for meaningful improvements in performance in the face of competing noise for cochlear implant users with relatively small amounts of residual hearing.

- Comparable ranges and degrees of residual hearing between subjects, however, do not ensure comparable benefits from combined EAS. Subject ME19's detailed audiogram indicates levels of residual hearing superior to those of subject ME6 at all frequencies; yet her scores in tests of consonant and word identification in speech spectrum noise show no EAS benefit.
- There is no indication of any difference in the EAS benefits to speech reception in noise depending on whether ipsilateral or contralateral residual hearing is used in conjunction with the electric stimulation. This lack of dependence now has been shown in within-subject comparisons as well as in comparisons across subjects.
- Our subjects typically show a decreased sensitivity to the negative effects of additional noise with combined EAS as compared to electric stimulation alone. Some subjects require higher levels of noise than others to demonstrate such an effect (e.g., subject ME20, in comparison with subjects ME6 and ME14).
- In some cases, speech reception performance is improved by raising the low-frequency boundary of the overall band analyzed by the cochlear implant speech processor, reducing the overlap with the range of frequencies conveyed via acoustic stimulation.

Acknowledgments. We thank subjects SR3, ME6, ME14, ME19, and ME20 for their participation in the studies described in this report. We also are grateful to Stefan (Marcel) Pok for his participation as a co-investigator in the studies with ME20.

Part IV

REPRESENTATIONS OF TEMPORAL INFORMATION WITH COCHLEAR IMPLANTS

Our work up until early 1994 had been largely directed at improving spatial representations with cochlear implants (CIs), for example, through elimination of simultaneous channel (or electrode) interactions with CIS processors (Wilson et al., 1991a) and through controlled shifts in sites of neural excitation with "virtual channel" interleaved sampling (VCIS) processors (Wilson et al., 1994). With the work reported in QPR 4:7 we turned our attention to representations of temporal information with CIs and how those representations might be improved. By temporal representations we mean the temporal patterns of responses evoked in the auditory nerve by electrical stimuli and the fidelity with which those patterns represent the time waveforms of the stimuli.

The work relating to temporal representations included:

■ The further development of a mathematical model to predict the population response of the auditory nerve to electrical stimulation, as described in QPR 4:7
■ Recordings of intracochlear evoked potentials (EPs) for a wide range of stimuli, as described in QPRs 4:7, 4:11, 5:6, 5:7, 5:8, and 7:9

■ Measurement of psychophysical responses to some of the same or similar stimuli, in tests with the same subjects, as described in QPRs 5:7 and 5:8

■ Comparisons of model predictions and the recorded intracochlear EPs, as described in QPR 4:7

■ Refinement of the model based on observed differences between the predictions and the data, as also described in QPR 4:7

■ Development of strategies for the repair of demonstrated deficits in temporal representations, as described in QPR 4:9.

We note that the initial development of the model is described in QPR 1:8, and the refined model was used as a tool to help develop the strategies just mentioned in the final point above.

The results from the work on temporal representations also are reported in Rubinstein et al. (1999), Wilson et al. (1997, 2003), and Wilson (1997, 2000). The papers by Rubinstein et al., Wilson (2000), and Wilson et al. (2003) describe the design and possible application of high-rate "conditioner pulses" that can improve the temporal representations of other stimuli presented in conjunction with the conditioner pulses. All of the papers by Wilson and Wilson et al. together describe recordings of intracochlear EPs for many different types of electrical stimuli, and the paper by Wilson (1997) describes relationships between temporal patterns of neural activity, as demonstrated in recordings of intracochlear EPs, and psychophysical scaling of pitches for the same stimuli and by the same subject.

We were assisted in these studies by Drs. Paul J. Abbas and Carolyn J. Brown from the University of Iowa in Iowa City, IA, USA. They served as consultants for our projects, and they were the first to record intracochlear EPs in CI subjects (e.g., Brown et al., 1990), using a masking and subtraction technique that allowed the recording of the EP in response to a second pulse of high amplitude following a masking pulse of the same amplitude.

We were able, with the help of Drs. Abbas and Brown and with the further substantial development of recording and analysis procedures, to extend greatly the repertoire of recordings. With the new procedures, we could and did record responses to: (1) pulses of much lower amplitudes than were required previously;

(2) trains of identical pulses with various pulse rates, pulse amplitudes, and burst durations; (3) pairs of pulses, including responses to both pulses, and with wide ranges of interpulse intervals and either identical or different amplitudes for the two pulses; (4) sinusoidally amplitude modulated (SAM) pulse trains with various carrier rates, modulation frequencies, modulation depths, and burst durations; (5) a single-pulse probe following pulse train or SAM pulse train maskers, with wide ranges of parameters for the maskers and with various delays between the offset of the masker and the onset of the probe; (6) pulse trains with either linear or exponential onset ramps of pulse amplitudes; (7) pulse trains with other manipulations in pulse amplitudes to evaluate some of the developed strategies for repairs in temporal representations with CIs; (8) the pulsatile outputs of a single-channel *continuous sampling* (CS) speech processor; and (9) "split phase" pulses in which the inter-phase gap was long enough to record a response to the first phase, approximating the presentation of a monophasic pulse, but also short enough to ensure full charge recovery and therefore safe stimulation for the subjects. Aspects of the further development of recording and analysis procedures are described in Wilson (1997), in Wilson et al. (1997), and in QPRs 4:7, 4:11, 5:6, 5:7, 5:9, and 7:9. The laboratory system for the EP studies is described in detail in QPR 5:9, as are various procedures for the recording, analysis, and interpretation of intracochlear EPs.

This part of the book includes a summary of major sections in QPRs 4:7 and 4:11, on recordings of intracochlear EPs to unmodulated and SAM pulse trains and to the outputs of the CS processor, which was originally presented in FR 4. In addition, this part includes the principal sections from QPRs 4:9 and 5:7, on strategies for the repair of deficits in temporal representations with implants and on recordings of responses to trains of modulated or unmodulated pulses with pulse rates exceeding 1000/s, respectively. The section from QPR 5:7 also describes: (1) a special deconvolution technique that was developed and used to separate EPs across rapidly presented pulses, and (2) the first of the psychophysical studies to relate perception to the recorded temporal patterns of nerve activity for the same stimuli and in tests with the same subject. Further psychophysical and electrophysiological studies are reported in QPR 5:8 for a much wider range of stimuli and for many more subjects.

Chapter 19

TEMPORAL REPRESENTATIONS WITH COCHLEAR IMPLANTS*

Blake S. Wilson, Dewey T. Lawson, Mariangeli Zerbi, and Charles C. Finley

A focus of recent work in our laboratory is the measurement and improvement, if possible, of temporal representations with cochlear implants. By temporal representations we mean the temporal patterns of responses evoked in the auditory nerve by electrical stimuli and the fidelity with which those patterns represent the time waveforms of the stimuli.

Studies of temporal representations have included: (a) development of a model to predict the population response of the auditory nerve to electrical stimulation, as described in QPR 4:7; (b) recordings of intracochlear evoked potentials for a wide range

---

*From a summary in FR 4 of sections in QPRs 4:7 and 4:11. The dates for these three reports are August 1, 1992, through July 31, 1995, for FR 4; February 1, 1994, through April 30, 1994, for QPR 4:7; and February 1, 1995, through April 30, 1995, for QPR 4:11. The authors for QPR 4:7 are Blake S. Wilson, Charles C. Finley, Mariangeli Zerbi, and Dewey T. Lawson, and the authors for QPR 4:11 are Blake S. Wilson, Charles C. Finley, Dewey T. Lawson, and Mariangeli Zerbi.

of stimuli, as described in QPRs 4:7 and 4:11; (c) measurement of psychophysical responses to some of the same or similar stimuli, as mentioned in QPR 4:7; and (d) development of strategies for the repair of demonstrated deficits in temporal representations, as described in Chapter 20. Work to develop the population model was supported under a separate NIH project, Project IV of NIH P01 DC00036. The remaining activities were supported by the present project.

Recordings of intracochlear evoked potentials (EPs) have been made with implant patients having percutaneous connectors, that is, patients with either the Ineraid device or an experimental version of the Nucleus device that includes a percutaneous connector. Potentials are measured at unstimulated electrodes in the implant array. An example is presented in Figure 19–1 for trains of identical pulses presented to electrode 3 in the implant array of Ineraid subject SR2. Potentials following the pulses were recorded differentially between intracochlear electrode 4 and a surface electrode secured with electrode paste at the ipsilateral mastoid. Body potential was measured with a reference electrode at the wrist. Additional details on the recording technique are presented in QPR 4:7.

Stimuli used for EP studies have included:

- Trains of identical pulses, with various pulse rates, pulse amplitudes, and burst durations.
- Pairs of pulses, including identical pulses with a wide range of interpulse intervals and pulses with fixed interpulse intervals and a wide range of amplitudes for the first pulse.
- Sinusoidally amplitude modulated (SAM) pulse trains, with various carrier rates, modulation frequencies, modulation depths, and burst durations.
- A single-pulse probe following pulse train and SAM pulse train maskers, with wide ranges of parameters for the maskers. The interval between the offset of the maskers and the onset of the probe pulse was varied over six logarithmic steps from 2.5 to 80 ms.
- Pulse trains with either linear or exponential onset ramps of pulse amplitudes.

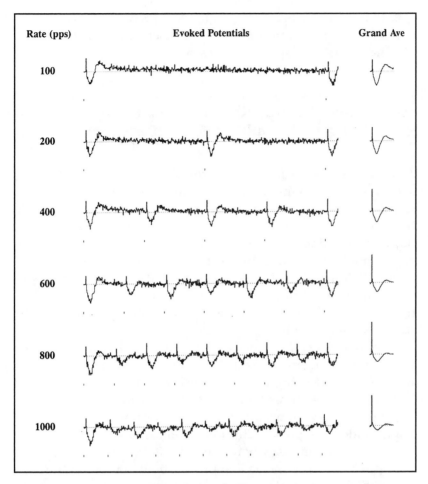

Rate (pps)	Evoked Potentials	Grand Ave

Figure 19-1. Recordings of intracochlear evoked potentials (EPs) for Ineraid subject SR2. Stimuli included 16.4 μs/phase pulses presented at the indicated rates to electrode 3 in the Ineraid array. The pulse amplitude was 750 μA. The times of pulse presentations are indicated with the short vertical lines beneath each EP trace. Potentials were recorded differentially between intracochlear electrode 4 and an external electrode at the ipsilateral mastoid. The average of EPs following each pulse for a given condition is shown in the right column, under the heading "Grand Ave." The horizontal dotted lines in the EP columns indicate zero potential. Note that EPs fail to follow pulses with equal EP magnitudes for rates of stimulation above 200 pulses/s (pps).

- Pulse trains with other manipulations in pulse amplitudes.
- The pulsatile outputs of a single-channel *continuous sampling* (CS) speech processor.

RESPONSES TO PULSE TRAINS AND SAM PULSE TRAINS

An example of one subject's patterns of responses to pulse trains and SAM pulse trains is presented in Figure 19–2. This figure shows the normalized magnitudes of the evoked potentials (measured as the difference in amplitudes of the first negative peak and the first positive peak in the EP waveforms, see QPR 4:7 for additional details) following each stimulus pulse for the entire 1000 ms of each record. The initial and final 100 ms of the records are shown in Figures 19–3 and 19–4, respectively. In addition to the EP magnitudes, normalized amplitudes of the stimulus pulses are indicated in Figures 19–3 and 19–4.

For reference, this subject (SR2) enjoys high levels of speech recognition with his implant. He obtains percent correct NU-6 word scores in the high 90s for a variety of CIS processors used in conjunction with his Ineraid electrode array.

Figure 19–2 shows a decrement in response over time for trains of identical pulses. This decrement is most evident for the 401 pulses/s stimulus, where the magnitudes of EPs following each pulse continue to decline out to about 300 or 400 ms.

Although small, decrements in response over time also can be observed for the 100 pulses/s stimulus. This is most easily seen by comparing the upper panels of Figures 19–3 and 19–4.

In contrast to the slow decrement in response observed for the 401 and 100 pulses/s stimuli, an alternating pattern of response is observed for the 1016 pulses/s stimulus. The difference between the relatively large EP magnitudes for odd-numbered pulses and the relatively small EP magnitudes for even-numbered pulses declines over time. Ultimately, the EP magnitudes for odd- and even-numbered pulses become indistinguishable, as may be seen in the middle panel of Figure 19–4. The average of EP magnitudes for sequential 1016 pulses/s pulses also declines over time. Most or all of the decrements

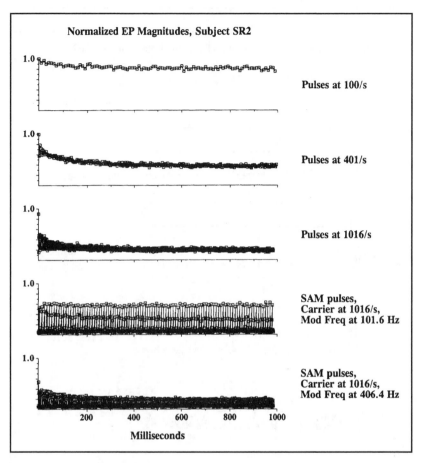

Figure 19–2. Normalized magnitudes of evoked potentials for Ineraid subject SR2. Stimuli were delivered to electrode 3 of the implant with reference to a remote electrode in the temporalis muscle. Potentials were recorded differentially between electrode 4 and an external electrode at the ipsilateral mastoid. The top three panels show EP magnitudes for trains of identical pulses with the indicated rates of pulse presentations within the trains. The bottom two panels show EP magnitudes for sinusoidally amplitude modulated (SAM) pulse trains with the indicated carrier rate and modulation frequencies. The level of the carrier, and the amplitude of the pulses in the trains of identical pulses, was 290 µA. The duration of all pulses was 32.8 µs/ phase. The condition involving the presentation of identical pulses at 1016/s produced a most comfortable loudness (MCL) percept for this subject. Lower loudnesses were produced for all other conditions. The maximum EP magnitude across these five conditions for this subject was 90.2 µV.

335

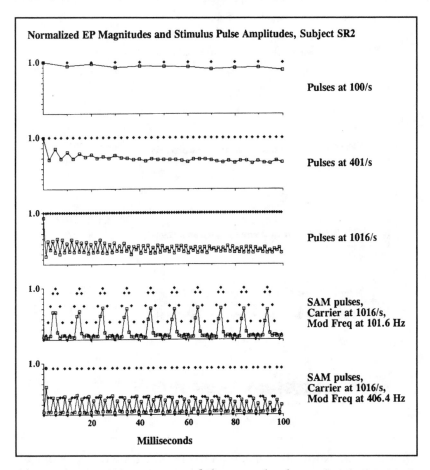

Figure 19–3. First 100 ms of the records shown in Figure 19–2. Open squares show normalized EP magnitudes and filled diamonds show normalized pulse amplitudes.

appear to occur within the first 300 to 400 ms, as with the 100 and 401 pulses/s stimuli.

Patterns of responses to SAM pulse trains reflect to some extent the modulation of pulse amplitudes. For the 101.6 Hz modulation, responses are in synchrony with the periodicity of the modulation waveform. A detectable response is observed for the fifth stimulus pulse in each cycle of 10 pulses. The normalized amplitude of this pulse is 0.905. A similar or larger response

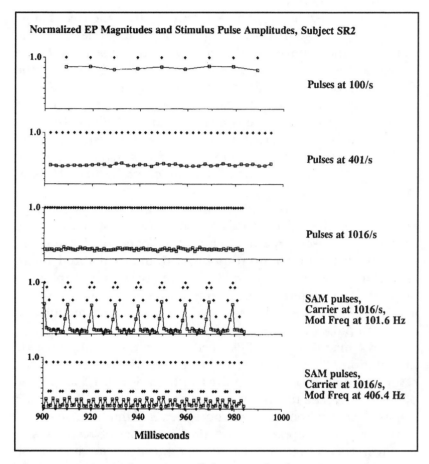

Figure 19–4. Final 100 ms of the records shown in Figure 19–2. Open squares show normalized EP magnitudes and filled diamonds show normalized pulse amplitudes.

is observed for the sixth pulse in each cycle. The normalized amplitude of this pulse is 1.0. A diminished or no detectable response is observed for the subsequent, lower amplitude pulses in each cycle.

Details in the patterns of response change over the first several cycles. A just detectable response is elicited by the fourth pulse (normalized amplitude of 0.655) in the first cycle (see Figure 19–3).

In addition, the responses to pulses five and six change somewhat over the first several cycles. EP magnitudes are quite similar for those pulses in the first cycle. In subsequent cycles the response to pulse five is progressively diminished over the first 200 ms of the stimulus, whereas the response to pulse six is slightly augmented for cycles two and three and then maintained for the remainder of the record (see Figures 19–3 and 19–4).

Although minor variations are observed in responses from cycle to cycle, the peak magnitudes of EPs across cycles are approximately uniform for the full duration of the 101.6 Hz SAM stimulus.

For the 406.4 Hz modulation condition, a relatively large response is elicited by stimulus pulse two, and little or no response by pulses three and four (bottom panel of Figure 19–3). Pulse two is the first nonzero pulse, with the normalized amplitude of 0.905. Pulses three and four have normalized amplitudes of 0.345. This pattern of pulse amplitudes—zero, 0.905, 0.345, and 0.345—is repeated across cycles for 406.4 Hz modulation of a 1016 pulses/s carrier.

Peak magnitudes of EPs decline over time with 406.4 Hz modulation. The response to pulse two is greater than the response to all subsequent pulses with a normalized amplitude of 0.905. Also, the responses to those subsequent pulses exhibit a slow decrease in magnitude thereafter. The time course of this slow component appears to be similar to that of responses to identical pulses presented at 401/s, quite near the modulation frequency of the present condition. However, the magnitude of the decrement appears to be somewhat less with SAM pulse trains than with identical pulses presented at the modulation frequency (compare second and fifth panels in Figure 19–2).

The overall response with 406.4 Hz modulation is somewhat lower than the overall response with 101.6 Hz modulation. This may reflect the difference in the peak amplitude of stimulus pulses for the two conditions. For the 406.4 Hz condition that amplitude was 0.905, whereas for the 101.6 Hz condition it was 1.0.

In general, these responses to SAM pulse trains reflect features of the modulation waveform. Unlike responses to identical pulses at the carrier rate, the responses to SAM pulse trains are sustained at a relatively constant level over one second of stimulation with the 101.6 Hz modulation frequency. At the higher modulation frequency a slow decrement is observed in the response over time, similar to but not quite as great as the decrement observed for identical pulses presented at the modulation frequency.

RESULTS ACROSS SUBJECTS

Results for SR3, using 1000-ms pulse trains and SAM pulse trains as above, were quite similar to those just described for SR2 (see QPR 4:11 for details). Recordings of responses to pulse trains have been obtained in studies with five additional subjects (SR10, SR14, NP1, NP2, and NP4). Burst durations always included 200 ms and, for some of the subjects, shorter durations. Pulse rates typically have included 100 to 1000 pulses/s, in steps of 100 pulses/s. The stimuli have been presented at levels corresponding to a "most comfortable loudness" judgment for each subject and electrode. Recordings of responses to SAM pulse trains have been obtained in studies with one additional subject (SR10). The burst duration for these latter studies was 200 ms. Carrier rates for the SAM pulse trains have included 1000, 500, and 250 pulses/s. Modulation frequencies have included 50, 100, 150, and 200 Hz for the two lower carrier rates and those frequencies along with 300 and 400 Hz for the 1000 pulses/s carrier rate.

In general and as described above for subject SR2, responses to trains of pulses show approximately equal magnitudes of EPs across pulses for low rates (e.g., 100 pulses/s). At higher rates an alternating pattern of response is observed, with a large EP in response to the first pulse, a diminished EP to the second pulse, a partially recovered response to the third pulse, and so on. Also, a gradual reduction in the average response across sequential pulses is observed over the duration of 200-ms bursts for rates at and above 200 pulses/s. The alternating response first appears at different rates for different subjects and for different electrodes within a subject. The rates were between 200 and 600 pulses/s, for the tested subjects and electrodes. It may be, as suggested in QPR 4:7, that the "pitch saturation limit" observed with implant patients is related to the inability of the auditory nerve to reflect fully the stimulus waveform for rates above 200 to 600 pulses/s.

In addition, differences among subjects and electrodes in the rate at which the alternating response first appears may reflect differences in the functional status of the population of auditory neurons excited by each electrode.

RESPONSES TO THE PULSATILE OUTPUTS OF A SINGLE-CHANNEL SPEECH PROCESSOR

To examine the neural representation of more complex stimuli with implants, we also have recorded EPs in response to the pulsatile outputs of a single-channel speech processor. The processor was a single-channel variation of CIS processors, which we call a *continuous sampling* processor, as interleaving is not relevant when there is only one channel. The CS processor uses the same front end as CIS processors, with a pre-emphasis filter (attenuation of 6 dB/octave below 1.2 kHz) and the same envelope detector and mapping function as in each CIS channel. The bank of bandpass filters is omitted in the CS processor, so the input to the envelope detector is the broadband speech signal, as modified somewhat by the pre-emphasis filter.

An example of the presented stimuli and recorded responses for one of the tokens in our consonant test, /asa/, is presented in Figure 19–5. The stimuli were delivered to electrode 3 in the Ineraid implant of subject SR2, with reference to a remote electrode in the temporalis muscle. Recordings were made differentially between the adjacent electrode 4 and an external electrode at the ipsilateral mastoid. Stimulus pulses were 32.8 μs/phase in duration, and were presented at the rate of 824/s. Normalized amplitudes of the pulses are shown in the top panel of Figure 19–5 and normalized magnitudes of the EPs following each pulse are shown in the bottom panel. The initial /a/ occurs during the first 140 ms of the records, the /s/ in the interval from about 190 to 330 ms, and the final /a/ in the interval from about 350 to 640 ms.

In broad terms, the neural response reflects the relatively deep modulations of pulse amplitudes during the /a/ segments and the relatively small differences among pulse amplitudes dur-

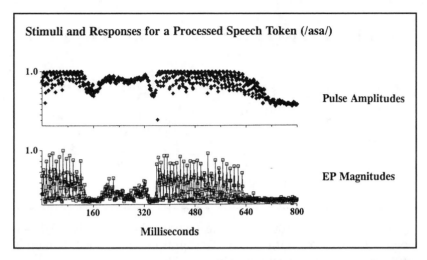

Figure 19-5. Normalized pulse amplitudes (*top panel*) and normalized EP magnitudes (*bottom panel*) for a processed speech token. A continuous sampling (CS) processor was used to process the speech token /asa/. Neural responses to the output of the processor were recorded for Ineraid subject SR2, as described in the text.

ing the /s/ segment. Peak magnitudes of the response are greatest during the /a/ segments, where the pulse amplitudes reach peak levels.

The pattern of response to the temporal fine structure of stimulus pulses during the initial 100 ms of the records is shown in Figure 19–6. Here, normalized pulse amplitudes and normalized EP magnitudes are plotted in the same panel to facilitate comparisons.

Although the pattern of responses reflect the fundamental frequency of the vowel, with peaks in the response at the first intense stimulus pulse in each (approximately 10 ms) period, other features in the stimulus are not represented. In periods two through eight, for instance, a series of three or more pulses with identical or nearly identical amplitudes is presented at the beginnings of the periods. The neural response to the first pulse in each of these periods is large, as noted before. However, the response to the second pulse is much smaller in all cases. Responses to subsequent pulses show an alternating pattern,

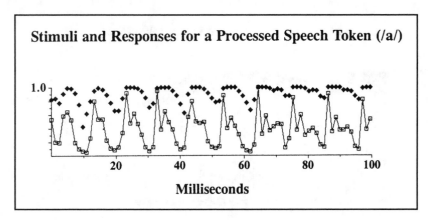

Figure 19–6. First 100 ms of the records shown in Figure 19–5. Open squares show normalized EP magnitudes and filled diamonds show normalized pulse amplitudes.

much like the one observed before for identical pulses presented at the rate of 1016/s for this subject (middle panel of Figure 19–3). Thus, the pattern of response to these subsequent pulses in each period appear to reflect primarily properties of the auditory nerve, as opposed to the pattern of stimulation (and intended pattern of response).

The overall level of response during the /s/ segment appears to be depressed in relation to the pulse amplitudes (see Figure 19–5). Figure 19–7 shows, however, that EP magnitudes for pulses of the same amplitudes are quite similar for the /a/ and /s/ segments. If any fatigue or accommodation occurs over the course of the /s/, it must be quite small.

Responses to SAM pulse trains demonstrate various distortions and ambiguities in the neural representation of the modulation waveform, depending on the carrier rate and modulation frequency. At low carrier rates, the patterns and magnitudes of EPs reflect features of both the modulation and carrier waveforms. At high carrier rates, EPs reflect primarily features of the modulation waveform. The inability of the nerve to follow constant amplitude pulses at relatively high rates apparently does not impair its ability to follow relatively low modulation frequencies in SAM pulse trains with high carrier rates. In general, higher carrier rates allow the faithful representation of higher modula-

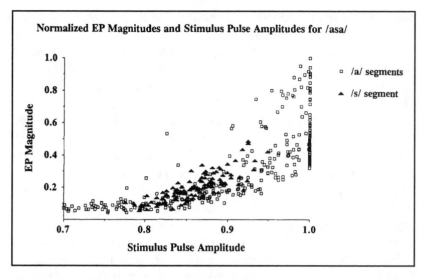

Figure 19-7. Scatter plot of normalized EP magnitudes versus normalized stimulus magnitudes for the speech token /asa/. Open squares show EP and stimulus magnitudes during the /a/ segments, and filled triangles show those magnitudes during the /s/ segment. The EP magnitudes are derived from recordings of neural responses in studies with Ineraid subject SR2 and correspond to the data also presented in Figures 19-5 and 19-6.

tion frequencies. Distortions and ambiguities appear when the modulation frequency is greater than 20 to 30% of the carrier rate. These results support the use of relatively high carrier rates in speech processors that use modulated pulse trains as stimuli.

DISCUSSION

Patterns of response to processed speech stimuli appear much as would be predicted from the patterns of response to simpler stimuli. For presentation of sequential pulses with identical or nearly identical amplitudes, one could predict that, for pulse rates approximating 1000/s, a large EP would be elicited by the first pulse in the series, a much smaller EP by the second pulse, a partial recovery of the EP for the third pulse, and so on.

Such patterns are observed during the vocalic segments of the example speech stimulus.

Also, responses to SAM pulse trains with high modulation depths (80 or 100%; see QPR 4:11) show a "peaking" of the neural response to a particular phase of the modulation waveform. Details other than the timing of that phase are represented poorly if at all in the response. In the example shown for the processed speech token, modulation depths approximate 40% or greater during the vocalic segments. As might be predicted from the results from studies with SAM pulse trains, the patterns of response to the processed speech stimulus show strong peaking in the responses, with peaks occurring at the fundamental frequency of the vocalic segments. Other details in the stimulus are not represented.

The fidelity of neural following to variations in pulse amplitudes might be improved through a change in the mapping function, for example, a more compressive mapping function as suggested in QPR 4:11. Such a compression would reduce depths of modulation that can (perhaps somewhat surprisingly) improve the representation of the modulation waveform (see patterns of responses for a 20% depth of modulation, as presented in Figures 3, 4, 6, and 7 of QPR 4:11). Also, successful application of any of the repair strategies outlined in Chapter 20 might be helpful. An observation for now is that temporal representations with implants are crude and highly limited, even for the best patients. Performance of these devices might be improved substantially with an amelioration or repair of such defects.

Acknowledgments. We thank subjects SR2, SR3, SR10, SR14, NP1, NP2, and NP4 for their participation in the studies described in this report.

Chapter 20

STRATEGIES FOR THE REPAIR OF DEFICITS IN TEMPORAL REPRESENTATIONS WITH COCHLEAR IMPLANTS[*]

Blake S. Wilson, Charles C. Finley, Mariangeli Zerbi, and Dewey T. Lawson

Results from the evoked potential studies described in Chapter 19 and even more thoroughly in QPR 4:7 have demonstrated limitations in the ability of the auditory nerve to follow electrical pulses at rates much above 200/s. In addition, the recorded responses to sinusoidally amplitude modulated (SAM) pulse trains have demonstrated various distortions in the neural representation of the modulation waveform, depending on carrier rate and modulation frequency.

In the present report we describe strategies to reduce or repair distortions in the neural encoding of repetitive electrical stimuli. Improvements in the fidelity of neural encoding might

---

*From QPR 4:9, August 1, 1994, through October 31, 1994.

allow patients to perceive a wider range of frequencies via their implants. Such improvements also might reduce uncertainties in judgments about certain stimuli, e.g., the perceptual ambiguities noted in QPR 4:7 for SAM pulse trains.

We note that temporal representations with implants are quite crude and limited in comparison with the representations found in normal hearing. In the normal case, a much higher level of asynchrony and stochastic independence is found among neurons in the auditory nerve (e.g., Abbas, 1993). This independence allows the nerve to follow acoustic stimulation frequencies up to several kHz in the population response to repetitive stimuli (e.g., Young & Sachs, 1979).

It may well be that improvements in temporal representations with implants could produce large improvements in speech reception. In addition, improvements in temporal representations might produce improvements in the "naturalness" of percepts for implant users, through a closer approximation to the patterns of responses found in the normal auditory nerve.

Possible ways to improve frequency following in electrically stimulated auditory nerves have been developed through use of our population model, described in QPR 4:7 and mentioned in Chapter 19. These possible ways have included: (a) adjusting pulse amplitudes so that an equal number of spikes is produced by each pulse in a train of pulses; (b) sharing stimulus pulses across electrodes, to distribute demand in conveying temporal information across subpopulations of neurons; (c) using stimulus waveforms that exploit the presence of membrane or synaptic noise; and (d) using high carrier rates for modulated pulse trains.

ADJUSTMENT OF PULSE AMPLITUDES

Improvement through the adjustment of pulse amplitudes is illustrated in Figure 20–1. Patterns of temporal response predicted by the population model are shown for our standard conditions without membrane noise (see QPR 4:7). The response for a train of constant amplitude pulses is presented in the left column and the response for a train of pulses with adjusted pulse

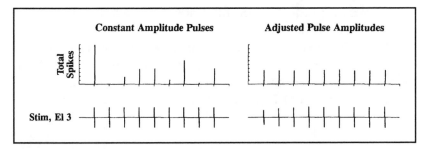

Figure 20-1. Predicted patterns of neural response to a train of constant amplitude pulses (*left column*) and to a train of pulses whose amplitudes have been adjusted to produce an equal number of spikes for each pulse (*right column*). The stimulus waveform is presented in the bottom panel of each column and the predicted pattern of neural responses in the top panel. Abbreviations include Stim for Stimulation and El for Electrode.

amplitudes is presented in the right column. The pulse rate is 1000/s for both columns.

Stimulation with the train of identical pulses produces a large number of spikes in response to the first pulse, none for the second pulse, and a variable number for subsequent pulses.

In contrast, a uniform pattern of responses across sequential pulses can be obtained through (relatively small) adjustments of pulse amplitudes. As indicated in the right column of Figure 20–1, the amplitude of pulse 1 is reduced so that the average of the responses for all pulses in the left column is produced. This lower pulse amplitude and correspondingly lower number of neural responses leaves a greater number of neurons available for the response to the second pulse. The amplitude of that pulse is adjusted to produce the same number of spikes again, as are the amplitudes of all subsequent pulses. The result is a set of afferent volleys from the auditory nerve at the rate of pulses in the stimulus and with equal numbers of spikes in each volley. If the central auditory system can make use of such an input, then pitch percepts produced by stimuli with adjusted pulse amplitudes might be higher than pitch percepts for stimuli without the adjustments. Also, the percepts with the adjusted pulse amplitudes may be purer inasmuch as the spectral structure of the afferent input to the central system is much simpler for the adjusted amplitudes case.

As a first step in evaluating this strategy, we have demonstrated that patterns of intracochlear evoked potentials (EPs) can be altered through manipulations in pulse amplitudes. Results for Ineraid subject SR2 are presented in Figures 20–2 and 20–3.

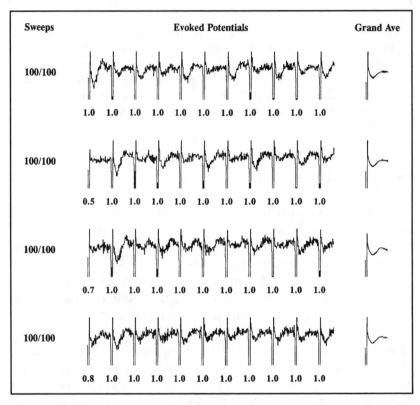

Figure 20–2. Recordings of intracochlear evoked potentials (EPs) for Ineraid subject SR2. Stimuli included 16.4 µs/phase pulses presented at 1000 pulses/s to electrode 3. The number beneath each pulse artifact indicates the relative amplitude of the corresponding pulse. Maximum pulse amplitude was 750 µA. The number of sweeps used in the recordings for each polarity of pulses is indicated in the left column for each condition. The average of EPs following each pulse for a given condition is shown in the right column, under the heading of "Grand Ave." Potentials were recorded differentially between electrode 4 and an external electrode at the ipsilateral mastoid.

In Figure 20–2 the amplitude of the first pulse was set at 1.0, 0.5, 0.7, or 0.8 times the amplitude of the (identical) remaining pulses. The pulse rate was 1000/s. The control condition, with all pulses of equal amplitude, produces the alternating pattern of EPs described before for this subject (e.g., see Figure 19–1). Reductions in the amplitude of the first pulse produce reductions in the magnitude of the EP following that pulse. No EP is detected for the 0.5 amplitude pulse (for the number of sweeps used in the present recordings), and a relatively small EP is seen for the 0.7 amplitude pulse. The 0.8 amplitude pulse produces an EP similar in magnitude to the grand average of EPs, across the 200 pulses in each 200-ms burst of pulses. With reductions in the magnitude of the first EP, we would expect that fewer neurons would be in refraction at the time of the second pulse. This idea is supported by the relatively large magnitudes of EPs following the second pulse for the three conditions of reduced amplitudes for pulse 1.

In a second experiment, iterative adjustments were made in the amplitudes of the first four pulses in the burst to produce approximately equal magnitudes of EPs. The result is shown in Figure 20–3.

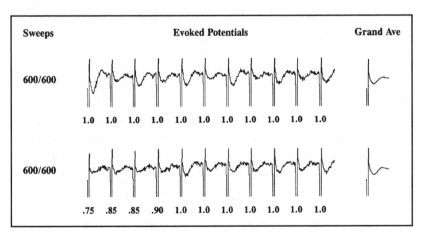

Figure 20–3. Recordings of intracochlear evoked potentials for Ineraid subject SR2. Organization for the figure is the same as that for Figure 20–2. The present figure shows results obtained with an adjustment of pulse amplitudes for the first four pulses in the burst.

Ultimately, we will want to produce equal magnitudes of EPs across all pulses in the 200-ms burst. Once that is accomplished, we will be in a position to conduct psychophysical experiments to compare pitch percepts elicited with a train of constant amplitude pulses versus a train of pulses with adjusted amplitudes. We plan to conduct such experiments under support of a separate project. If the outcome is positive, that is, if pitch percepts change in the hypothesized ways, then we will begin work to implement the approach in a speech processor design, either in that separate project or the present project, depending on availability of investigator time and other resources.

We note that such a positive outcome from the psychophysical experiments would have important implications for basic auditory theory.

SHARING OF PULSES ACROSS ELECTRODES

The strategy of sharing pulses across electrodes is illustrated in Figure 20–4. The left column shows a control condition, as in Figure 20–1, with stimulation of only one electrode using a train of constant amplitude pulses. The right column shows the predicted pattern of neural responses for pulses distributed across eight electrodes, spaced 4 mm apart, as in the Ineraid implant system. Electrode 1 receives the first pulse, electrode 4 the second, electrode 7 the third, and so on. The rate of stimulation on any one electrode is 125 pulses/s. As indicated in the model prediction, the local neural population can follow this low rate with high uniformity from pulse to pulse. The aggregate rate across electrodes is 1000 pulses/s. The afferent volley, summed across the entire auditory nerve, includes equal numbers of spikes at 1 ms intervals. If the central auditory system is able to integrate this input spatially across the auditory nerve, then a percept corresponding to a 1000 pulses/s stimulus might be produced.

To investigate this possibility, we conducted magnitude estimation experiments with two Ineraid patients (subjects SR2 and SR13) in which percepts elicited by stimulation of a single electrode were compared with percepts elicited by stimulation of multiple electrodes, in the "shared electrodes" paradigm outlined

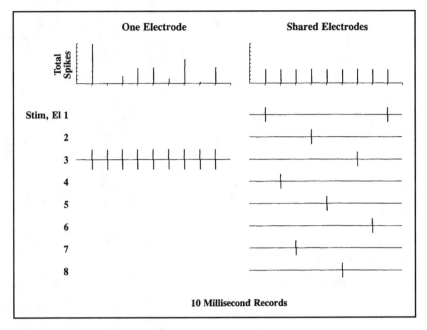

Figure 20–4. Predicted patterns of neural response to a train of constant-amplitude pulses delivered to a single electrode (*left column*) and to interleaved trains of constant-amplitude pulses delivered to eight electrodes (*right column*). The stimuli are presented in the bottom panels and predicted patterns of neural responses in the top panels. Abbreviations include Stim for Stimulation and El for Electrode.

above. The subjects were asked to nominate a pitch between 1 and 100 for each stimulus. The stimuli included 200 ms bursts of pulses presented singly to electrode 3 at the rates of 66.7, 133.3, 200, 266.7, 400, 600, and 800 pulses/s, or across three adjacent electrodes (electrodes 2, 3, and 4) at the aggregate rates of 200, 400, 600, 800, 1200, 1800, and 2400 pulses/s. The results for subject SR2 are shown in Figure 20–5. The open squares show the mean of pitch judgments for stimulation of electrode 3 alone, and the triangles show the mean of pitch judgments for stimulation across electrodes 2, 3, and 4. The open triangles show those results for the aggregate rate across electrodes and the closed triangles show the results for the rate on any one of the three electrodes. The results for subject SR13 were essentially identical to those shown in Figure 20–5 for SR2.

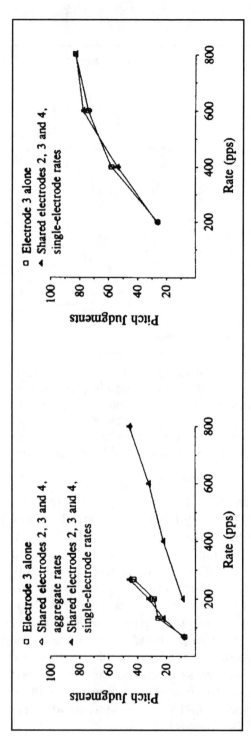

Figure 20-5. Results from a magnitude estimation experiment, in which the subject (SR2) was asked to nominate a pitch for each stimulus. The subject was instructed to nominate a low number for a low pitch and a high number for a high pitch. Stimuli included 200-ms bursts of 33 µs/phase pulses presented singly to electrode 3 at the rates of 66.7, 133.3, 200, 266.7, 400, 600, and 800 pulses/s, or across three adjacent electrodes (electrodes 2, 3, and 4) at the aggregate rates of 200, 400, 600, 800, 1200, 1800, and 2400 pulses/s. The pulse amplitude for each condition was adjusted to produce a most comfortable loudness (MCL) percept. Once the amplitudes for MCL percepts had been identified, the stimuli for the various conditions were played in sequence. Fine adjustments in pulse amplitudes were then made, and the sequence repeated, until the stimuli for all conditions were judged to be equally loud. In the experiments, the stimuli for the different conditions were presented in a randomized order according to the method of constant stimuli. The number of trials for each condition was 30. Results for conditions involving low rates are presented in the left panel and results for conditions involving high rates in the right panel. Abbreviations include pps for pulses/s.

As is evident from Figure 20–5, use of shared electrodes did not produce pitches higher than those elicited with stimulation of a single electrode. That is, the judgments for shared electrodes stimulation overlie the judgments for single electrode stimulation when the shared electrodes judgments are plotted according to the rate on any one electrode. The subjects apparently were able to separate the inputs from the different cochlear regions stimulated by the different electrodes in the shared electrodes paradigm in making judgments related to rate of stimulation. The central auditory system did not, at least in this case, integrate the different inputs spatially.

The 4-mm spacing of electrodes in the Ineraid implant may be too great to demonstrate such integration. Spatial integration of inputs by the central auditory system in normal hearing occurs within critical bands — corresponding to approximately 1 mm regions along the cochlear partition — for a wide range of tasks and behaviors.

In contrast to the present findings, a shared electrodes paradigm might produce higher pitch percepts if multiple electrodes could be placed within a critical band distance, and if those electrodes could stimulate different populations of neurons. As testing time permits, we hope to conduct studies with patients in our "Nucleus Percutaneous" series to evaluate what may be a closer approximation to that situation. The electrodes in the Nucleus array are spaced 0.75 mm apart, just within a critical band distance. If we identify a patient who can reliably discriminate adjacent electrodes on the basis of pitch judgments, then we will use those electrodes in a repetition of the experiment described above. The question will be whether the Nucleus subject perceives higher pitches with shared stimulation of the two adjacent electrodes than with stimulation of either electrode alone. A positive outcome would provide a strong incentive to develop new types of electrodes for cochlear implants, with a much greater number and density of contacts compared with present electrodes. Such an electrode might allow independent or quasi-independent stimulation of three or more populations of neurons within a critical band distance, especially if the contacts are placed in close proximity to the target spiral ganglion cells, to reduce overlaps in neural excitation fields associated with adjacent electrode positions.

Pending the availability of patient testing time and other resources, a positive outcome would be pursued by us in subsequent studies with Nucleus percutaneous subjects. In particular, we would incorporate the shared electrodes paradigm into a speech processor design and determine whether shared stimulation of pairs of adjacent electrodes may provide an advantage in recognizing speech.

SELECTION OF STIMULUS WAVEFORMS

Another of the strategies mentioned above is to use stimulus waveforms that exploit the presence of membrane or synaptic noise. The idea is illustrated in Figure 20–6, which compares simulations with and without membrane noise (further details about the simulations are presented in QPR 4:7). The stimuli include pulses presented at 500/s and 1000/s, with various pulse durations and amplitudes for each rate, as indicated in the left part of the figure. We note that, for the model with membrane noise, the simulation of responses to 30 μs/phase pulses presented at 1000 pulses/s is in excellent agreement with recorded patterns of intracochlear EPs for Ineraid subject SR2 for the same or similar stimulus conditions (see, e.g., the recorded pattern of responses in the middle panel of Figure 19–3).

Note that neural following of pulses presented at either rate is improved with the addition of membrane noise. For the conditions with membrane noise, magnitudes of neural responses are nearly uniform after pulse 2 for stimulation at 500 pulses/s. The high uniformity observed for 30 μs/phase pulses is slightly improved with increases in pulse duration. Responses for the pulse duration of 1000 μs/phase are essentially identical after pulse 2.

In contrast, following is not particularly good for the condition of stimulation with 30 μs/phase pulses presented at 1000 pulses/s. In particular, an alternating pattern of responses is observed over the duration of 50 (illustrated) or 200 ms bursts of pulses. For stimulation at 1000 pulses/s, an increase in pulse duration produces a large improvement in frequency following, as shown in the bottom panel of the left column of Figure 20–6. Some improvement also is observed for the model simulations

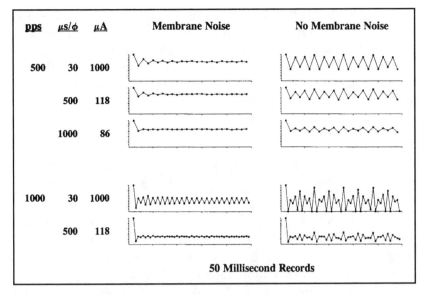

Figure 20–6. Predicted patterns of neural responses to trains of pulses presented at the rates of 500 or 1000 pulses/s. The durations and amplitudes of the pulses for various conditions are indicated in the table on the left side of the figure. Results from simulations using the standard conditions plus membrane noise are shown in the left column and results from simulations using the standard conditions only are shown in the right column. Abbreviations include pps for pulses/s and μs/φ for μs/phase.

without membrane noise, but this improvement is relatively modest. It appears that the presence of membrane noise may be exploited with the use of long-duration, low-amplitude pulses.

We plan to evaluate these predictions of the population model in magnitude estimation experiments with implant subjects. We will ask the subjects to report on pitches for a set of stimuli including bursts of pulses with various pulse durations and pulse rates. For example, the set would include 30 μs/phase pulses presented at 1000 pulses/s and 500 μs/phase pulses also presented at 1000 pulses/s. Amplitudes of initial pulses in the bursts will be ramped in a variation of the basic experiment to reduce or eliminate the initial transient in the neural response following pulse 1.

A positive outcome from these experiments, that is, a correlation of higher perceived pitch with longer pulse duration, would provide the basis for subsequent studies aimed at evaluating the use of long-duration pulses in speech processor designs. Obviously, use of such pulses would interact with other desirable attributes in a processor, such as use of relatively high rates of stimulation on single channels and use of nonsimultaneous stimulation across channels. Such tradeoffs could be evaluated in speech reception studies.

USE OF HIGH CARRIER RATES

A further possibility is that use of high carrier rates may improve substantially the neural representation of the modulation waveform for SAM pulse trains. This possibility is illustrated in Figure 20–7, which shows simulations for three carrier rates and for modulation frequencies of 100, 200, 300, and 400 Hz for each rate. Simulations both with and without membrane noise are shown. The simulations with noise for the 1000 pulses/s carrier are in close agreement with the patterns of intracochlear EPs recorded for Ineraid subject SR2 for the same or similar stimulus conditions (see, e.g., the recorded patterns of responses in the bottom two panels of Figure 19–3).

Note that the representations of the 300 and 400 Hz modulation waveforms are improved with increases in carrier rate. For the simulations with membrane noise, the complex pattern of neural response for modulation of a 1000 pulses/s carrier at 300 Hz is replaced by a uniform pattern that better reflects the periodicity of the modulation waveform when the carrier rate is increased to 5000 pulses/s. Also, the presence of two distinct intervals in the neural response to a 1000 pulses/s carrier modulated at 400 Hz is eliminated with an increase in the carrier rate to 5000 pulses/s.

A further increase in the carrier rate, to 10,000 pulses/s, produces further improvements in the predicted representation of the modulation waveforms. For example, responses to the cycles of the 400 Hz modulation waveform are essentially identical after the second cycle with the 10,000 pulses/s carrier, whereas those responses show an alternating pattern with the 5000 pulses/s carrier.

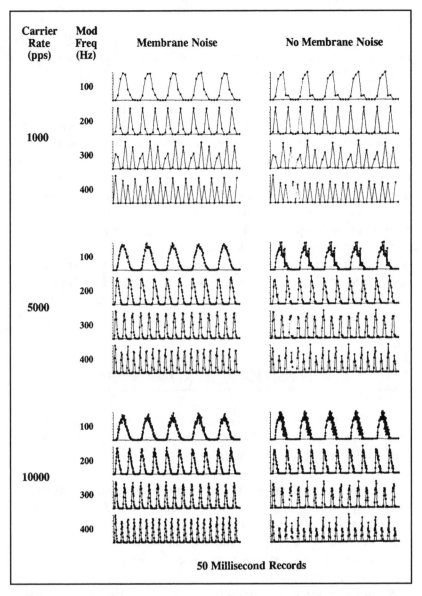

Figure 20–7. Predicted patterns of neural response to SAM pulse trains, for the indicated carrier rates and modulation frequencies. Results from simulations using the standard conditions plus membrane noise are shown in the left column and results from simulations using the standard conditions only are shown in the right column. The duration of the carrier pulses was 30 μs/phase and the depth of modulation was 100%. Abbreviations include pps for pulses/s, and Mod Freq for Modulation Frequency.

Improvements also are observed with increases in carrier rate for the simulations without membrane noise. However, the quality of the representations is higher for the simulations with membrane noise, especially for the 10,000 pulses/s carrier. For example, a strong alternating pattern of responses is seen for the 400 Hz modulation waveform in the simulation without membrane noise, whereas the pattern is uniform for that modulation waveform in the simulation with membrane noise. The use of relatively high carrier rates may represent an alternative to the use of long duration pulses as a way of exploiting the presence of membrane noise (in this case through temporal jitter in the responses of single neurons across any of several pulses, from cycle to cycle in the modulation waveform).

We plan to evaluate the use of high carrier rates in CIS processors. Special current sources, with the capability of delivering interleaved pulses at high rates, are under construction for support of these and other studies.

ADDITIONAL STRATEGIES

Additional strategies have been identified through further modeling studies and through discussions of model results with others. The additional strategies include:

- Exploiting the presence of membrane noise in another way, by designing stimuli that selectively address the neural nodes of Ranvier with the greatest amount of noise, presumably along the narrow-diameter peripheral processes of auditory neurons (see Verveen, 1962; Verveen & Derksen, 1968).
- Introducing a pharmacologic agent into the cochlea, for example, through an osmotic pump (Brown et al., 1993), that would increase the level of membrane noise (this suggestion was offered by Josef Miller in a conversation with Wilson on effects of membrane noise, 1994; also see Junge, 1992, Chapter 12, for a discussion of membrane noise and pharmacological manipulations of the noise).

- Presenting an external noise signal (or signals, on different electrodes) along with the deterministic stimulus, which might enhance effects of existing membrane noise.
- Use of alternating pulse polarities to address slightly different populations of neurons with successive pulses (this idea was suggested by Bryan Pfingst in a conversation with Wilson, 1994).

DISCUSSION

Recordings of intracochlear evoked potentials have shown that temporal representations with implants are crude and highly limited. Modeling studies, in conjunction with EP recordings, have provided insights into ways those representations might be improved. We expect to evaluate in at least a preliminary way some of these possibilities in the upcoming final three-quarters of the current project.

Acknowledgments. A brief description of strategies for the repair of deficits in temporal representations with implants was presented at the 25th Annual Neural Prosthesis Workshop, held in Bethesda, Maryland, October 18–21, 1994. The modeling studies described there and in this report were supported by Project IV of NIH Program Project Grant P01-DC00036. Studies with human subjects, including psychophysical tests and recordings of intracochlear EPs, were supported by the present project. We are grateful to the subjects for their enthusiastic participation and generous contributions of time. We also would like to thank Josef Miller and Bryan Pfingst for their helpful and highly insightful suggestions.

Chapter 21

HIGH RATE STUDIES, SUBJECT SR2*

Blake S. Wilson, Charles C. Finley, Mariangeli Zerbi, Dewey T. Lawson, and Chris van den Honert

Recordings of intracochlear evoked potentials (EPs) have allowed us to visualize temporal patterns of neural responses for a wide variety of electrical stimuli. Subjects for such recordings have been patients with percutaneous access to their implanted electrodes, that is, users of the Ineraid device or a research version of the Nucleus device. Stimuli to date have included: (a) trains of identical pulses with various pulse rates, pulse amplitudes, and burst durations; (b) pairs of identical pulses with a wide range of interpulse intervals; (c) pairs of pulses with several fixed interpulse intervals and various amplitudes for the first pulse; (d) sinusoidally amplitude modulated (SAM) pulse trains with various carrier rates, modulation frequencies, modulation depths, and burst durations; (e) the pulsatile outputs of a single-channel speech processor; and (f) a single-pulse probe following a masker consisting of a pulse train or a SAM pulse train. Use of a subtraction technique has allowed us to investigate responses to stimuli with pulse rates in excess of 1000/s, which otherwise would be difficult to interpret because of substantial overlaps among successive EP waveforms.

---

*From QPR 5:7, February 1, 1997, through April 30, 1997.

Studies also have been conducted to evaluate possible psychophysical correlates of the recorded patterns of neural responses for various stimuli. For example, we have evaluated scaling of modulation frequencies for SAM pulse trains with a relatively wide range of carrier rates.

In this report we present recordings for one subject of neural population responses to trains of identical pulses and SAM pulse trains, for pulse rates between 100 and 10,162/s. We also present preliminary results from psychophysical experiments in which the subject was asked to scale pulse rate for unmodulated pulse trains, and modulation frequency for SAM pulse trains, according to perceived pitch. Rates for the unmodulated pulse trains varied between 100 and 600 pulses/s, and modulation frequencies for SAM pulse trains varied between 100 and 600 Hz. Carrier rates for the SAM pulse trains varied between 504 and 10,162 pulses/s.

SYSTEM USED FOR RECORDINGS OF INTRACOCHLEAR EVOKED POTENTIALS

The system we use for recordings of intracochlear EPs is illustrated in Figure 21–1 (for further details, see QPR 4:7 and Wilson et al., 1997). Intracochlear potentials are measured differentially between an unstimulated electrode in the implant and an external electrode at the ipsilateral mastoid. Body potential is measured with a reference electrode at the wrist. Stimuli are delivered between an intracochlear electrode and a separate reference electrode implanted in the temporalis muscle (for monopolar stimulation) or between two intracochlear electrodes (for bipolar stimulation). A fast recovery amplifier is used to restore sensitivity of recording as soon as possible after saturation of the input by stimulus pulses. In addition, an equal number of sweeps for negative leading and positive leading biphasic pulses are summed to cancel components of the artifacts. With these techniques, the blanker circuit (shown as an optional component in Figure 21–1) generally is not necessary for clear separation of EPs from residual artifacts, and was not used in obtaining the data shown in this report.

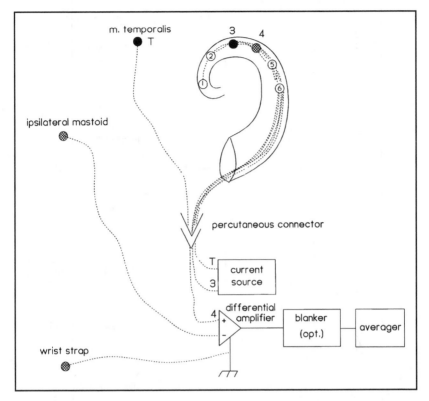

Figure 21-1. Apparatus for recording intracochlear evoked potentials.

This arrangement for recording intracochlear EPs can be used with implant systems having direct percutaneous access to the implanted electrodes, for instance the Ineraid system as shown in Figure 21–1. We also have made recordings with subjects implanted with a percutaneous connector version of the 22-electrode Nucleus array.

EXAMPLES OF RECORDINGS FOR RATES OF STIMULATION AT AND BELOW 1000 PULSES/S

Examples of recordings for three subjects, including subject SR2, are presented in Figure 21–2. The stimuli in these examples were 200-ms trains of identical 33 µs/phase pulses, with the

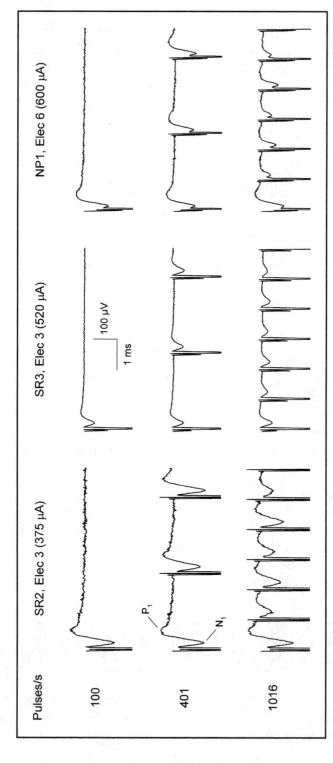

Figure 21–2. Intracochlear evoked potentials for subjects SR2, SR3, and NP1.

pulse rates of 100, 401, and 1016/s. Monopolar stimulation was used. For each subject, the amplitude of the pulses was adjusted to produce a most comfortable loudness (MCL) percept for the 1016 pulses/s condition. This amplitude was held constant for the lower rates, which produced percepts with lower loudnesses.

The figure shows the first 6 ms of the 200-ms records for each subject. The large downward "spikes" are residual (uncanceled) artifacts during and shortly after the presentations of stimulus pulses. (The lower parts of the artifacts are not shown in Figure 21–2.) Following these pulse artifacts are neural evoked potentials, with a negative peak (N_1) approximately 250 μs after each pulse onset and a positive peak (P_1) approximately 600 μs after the pulse onset. The magnitudes of the EPs, as measured by the absolute difference between the peak voltages at N_1 and P_1, range up to about 190 μV for the subjects and conditions of Figure 21–2.

For low rates of stimulation the EPs reflect the identical amplitudes of the pulses. For the 401 pulses/s conditions in Figure 21–2, for example, nearly equal EPs are observed across the three illustrated pulses for each subject. At the highest rate shown in the figure, 1016 pulses/s, an alternating pattern of response is observed, with a large EP following the first pulse, a much diminished EP following the second pulse, a partially recovered EP following the third pulse, another small EP following the fourth pulse, and so on. This pattern may at least in part be an expression of the refractory properties of auditory neurons. Presumably, many neurons are available for stimulation by the first pulse, when the nerve is at rest and the excitability of each neuron is at its maximum. Neurons stimulated by that pulse then become refractory to subsequent stimulation. At the time of the second pulse, approximately 1 ms later, those neurons would be in a period of relative refraction (Hartmann et al., 1984; Parkins, 1989), with reduced excitability. Thus, not as many neurons would be expected to respond to the second pulse. At the time of the third pulse, neurons stimulated by the first pulse but not the second will have recovered much (but not all) of their initial excitability. More neurons might be expected to respond to the third pulse than to the second. The alternation between relatively large and relatively small EPs can persist for hundreds of milliseconds at particular rates for a given subject and stimulating electrode (see, e.g., the middle panels of Figures 19–2 and 19–3).

The magnitudes of EPs and patterns of responses across rates of stimulation vary widely among subjects and often among electrodes within subjects (Wilson et al., 1997). These differences may reflect differences in refractory properties of the stimulated neurons, the number of neurons participating in the response, subthreshold integration of sequential pulses at neural membranes, the level of membrane noise at nodes of Ranvier, or some combination of these and perhaps other factors. Some of these possible contributors to the temporal patterns of neural responses to intracochlear electrical stimulation are discussed in detail later in this chapter.

SUBTRACTION TECHNIQUE FOR PULSE RATES HIGHER THAN 1000/S

Analysis of recordings for pulse rates above about 1000/s is complicated by the fact that the EPs for successive pulses overlap when the interval between the pulses is shorter than approximately 1 ms (see the EP waveforms in Figure 21–2). Thus, the waveform following a particular pulse in a train of pulses reflects not only the response to that pulse but also the trailing parts of the EPs to the prior pulse or pulses.

A way to derive the response to the Nth pulse in a recording containing overlapping EPs is illustrated in Figure 21–3. The effects of all prior stimuli and responses overlapping with the Nth response can be removed by subtracting a record for a burst with N-1 pulses, as shown in the right column of the figure. This method is time consuming, requiring N recordings for a train with N pulses, but it allows us to study responses to individual pulses for pulse rates exceeding 1000/s.

NEURAL REPRESENTATIONS OF UNMODULATED PULSE TRAINS

Results from studies with subject SR2 using both low and high rates of stimulation are presented in Figure 21–4. Patterns of

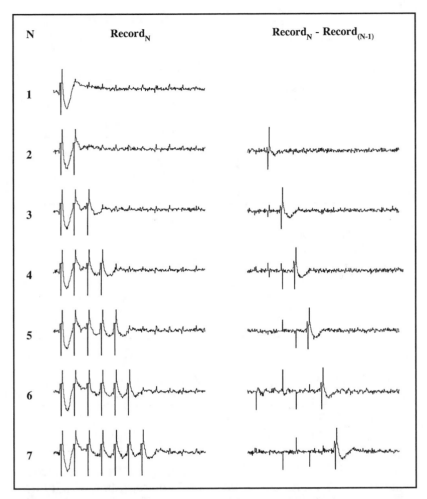

N	Record$_N$	Record$_N$ - Record$_{(N-1)}$
1		
2		
3		
4		
5		
6		
7		

Figure 21-3. Example of subtraction technique used for measurement of evoked potentials (EPs) to pulses presented at high rates. The three columns show the number of pulses (N), the record of the pulse artifact(s) and response(s) collected with that number of pulses (Record$_N$), and the derived EP obtained by subtracting a record collected with N-1 pulses from a record collected with N pulses (Record$_N$ – Record$_{(N-1)}$). Pulses were presented at the rate of 2033/s for conditions involving more than one pulse. Data are from studies with subject SR2.

responses for low rates of stimulation are presented in the left column and patterns of responses for high rates in the right column. The figure shows the magnitudes of the EPs following each

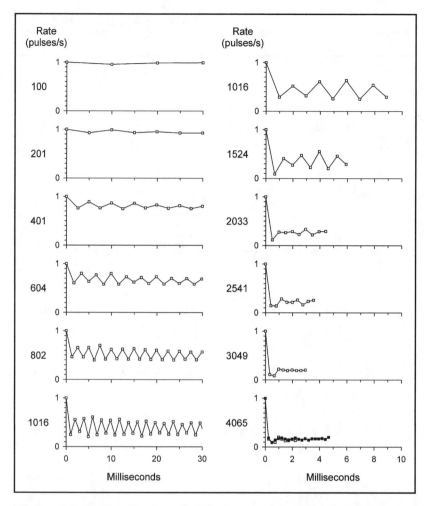

Figure 21-4. Magnitudes of evoked potentials (EPs) for stimulation of subject SR2's intracochlear electrode 3 and recording with intracochlear electrode 4. Patterns of EP magnitudes for relatively low pulse rates are shown in the left column and those for relatively high rates in the right column. Responses for the conditions in the right column were derived using the subtraction technique illustrated in Figure 21-3. The EP magnitudes are normalized to the magnitude of the EP following the first pulse for each condition. The pulse amplitude used across all conditions was 375 µA, and the pulse duration was 33 µs/phase. The filled symbols in the panel for 4065 pulses/s stimulation show results from a repeated measure collected during a separate visit to the laboratory by SR2. Note that different time scales are used for the left and right columns. (The first, third, and sixth panels in the left column represent the same conditions as those for the recordings shown in the left column of Figure 21-2.)

stimulus pulse. The magnitudes were measured as the absolute difference between the voltages at the N_1 and P_1 peaks in each EP waveform. These magnitudes then were normalized to the magnitude of the EP following the first pulse for each condition. The subtraction technique was used to derive EP magnitudes for the conditions in the right column (including the 1016 pulse/s condition). Stimulus pulses were delivered to electrode 3 in the subject's Ineraid implant, with reference to a remote electrode in the temporalis muscle, and intracochlear voltages were recorded with the adjacent electrode 4 in the implant, with reference to the external electrode at the ipsilateral mastoid. Note that different time scales are used for the left and right columns in Figure 21–4.

The figure shows that EPs for this subject and stimulating electrode reflect the identical amplitudes of the stimulus pulses with nearly identical magnitudes of response for the pulse rates of 100 and 201/s. At 401 pulses/s an alternating pattern of responses is observed, with relatively large responses for the odd-numbered pulses and relatively small responses for the even-numbered pulses. Alternating patterns of responses also are observed for the higher rates, with progressively greater decrements in the response to pulse 2 and progressively greater differences between responses for the odd- and even-numbered pulses as the rate is increased up to 1016 pulses/s. At somewhat higher rates, the alternating pattern is replaced by more complicated patterns of responses, for example, at 1524 pulses/s. At still higher rates, results for SR2 show a return to a simpler pattern of responses, with uniform magnitudes of sequential EPs for identical stimulus pulses after the first millisecond of stimulation. This uniformity is most evident in the patterns of responses for the 3049 and 4065 pulses/s conditions in Figure 21–4.

Modeling studies suggest that such uniform patterns beyond the first millisecond may be a result of a more stochastic response among neurons to the stimulus pulses (see, e.g., Figure 8 and the accompanying discussion in QPR 4:7). When pulses are presented at high rates, low levels of neural membrane noise at nodes of Ranvier may interact with the pulses to produce stochastic independence among neurons. Slight variations in neural threshold due to the membrane noise may introduce a "jitter" in firing times across neurons for rapidly presented pulses. The effect of such jitter would be expected to increase with time after the beginning of a train of pulses, as initially small differences in discharge histories among neurons grow. After a relatively short period, differences in discharge histories may produce a high level of stochastic independence among neurons.

Such a mechanism would allow different subpopulations of neurons in the excitation field to respond to sequential pulses (see QPR 4:7 and Parnas, 1996). The total number of neurons responding to any one pulse would in general be small compared to the number stimulated by single pulses at low rates of stimulation (or by the first pulse for high rates). Thus, one might expect relatively small EPs for high rates in conjunction with relatively uniform EPs from pulse to pulse for trains of identical pulses, following the "transient" events of the first millisecond.

Responses during that initial millisecond may reflect a response of many neurons to the first pulse, when excitability of the neurons is at its maximum, followed by a subsequent depression in response(s) when those same neurons are in a period of absolute refraction or early in a period of relative refraction. Responses during the initial millisecond also may reflect effects of temporal integration at neural membranes. In particular, note that responses to pulse 2 increase as the rate is increased from 1524 to 4065 pulses/s. For some neurons, stimulation with pulse 1 alone might not be sufficient for excitation. Integration of pulses 1 and 2, however, might be sufficient. In such cases, a neuron would respond to pulse 2.

The possibility of temporal integration effects is illustrated further in Figure 21–5, which shows patterns of response for rates up to 10,162 pulses/s. For rates at and above 5039 pulses/s, magnitudes of response for the second and third pulses are greater than the magnitudes of the responses to the subsequent pulses during the next 0.5 ms or thereabouts. These results suggest that, for the conditions of Figures 21–4 and 21–5, the population of neurons not stimulated by pulse 1 may be relatively small and that temporal integration of subthreshold pulses does not occur beyond about 0.5 ms. (The apparent temporal integration is strong for the 7622 and 10,162 pulses/s conditions in Figure 21–5, corresponding to interpulse intervals of 98 and 131 µs, respectively, and is progressively less strong as the rate is reduced to 2033 pulses/s, corresponding to an interpulse interval of 492 µs, which of course is close to 0.5 ms.)

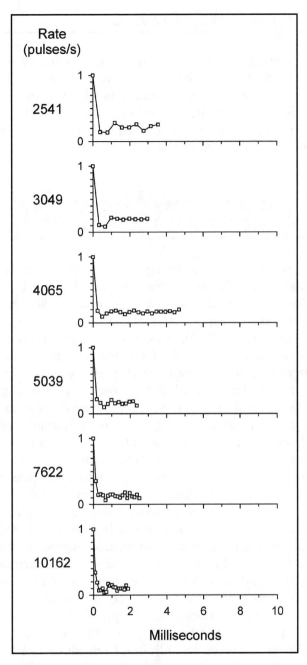

Figure 21-5. Magnitudes of evoked potentials, as in Figure 21–4, but here for higher rates of stimulation. The panels for the 2541, 3049, and 4065 pulses/s conditions are the same as those in Figure 21–4, and are repeated here to illustrate increases in the response to pulse 2 as rate is increased from 2541 to 10,162 pulses/s.

The alternating and more complex patterns of responses observed for SR2 at rates between about 400 and 2500 pulses/s (Figure 21–4) may indicate limitations in the transmission of stimulus information to the central nervous system. That is, such patterns appear to reflect the properties of the auditory nerve as well as properties of the stimulus.

NEURAL REPRESENTATIONS OF MODULATED PULSE TRAINS

A majority of the processing strategies in current clinical use, including the SPEAK and CIS strategies, use modulated pulse trains as stimuli. To obtain information on how such stimuli are represented in the population responses of the auditory nerve, we have recorded intracochlear EPs for SAM pulse trains with seven subjects. Studies with most of these subjects included wide ranges of modulation frequencies and various carrier rates up to 1016 pulses/s. Studies with SR2 have included the carrier rate of 4065 pulses/s.

A representative set of results for carrier rates at and below 1016 pulses/s is presented in Figure 21–6. The stimuli in this case were delivered to electrode 3 in subject SR3's Ineraid implant, with reference to a remote electrode in the temporalis muscle, and neural responses were recorded with electrode 4 in the implant, with reference to the external electrode at the ipsilateral mastoid. The stimuli were produced with a 16.4-μs sampling interval, and the number of samples between each sequential pulse was selected to produce close approximations to the carrier rates of 250, 500, and 1000 pulses/s. Those approximations were 251, 504, 1016 pulses/s, respectively. The modulation frequency for each condition was scaled by an equal amount and thus, for example, the precise modulation frequency for the lower right panel of Figure 21–6 is 406.4 Hz (400 Hz × the scaling factor of 1.016). The carrier level was adjusted to produce a MCL percept for the condition just mentioned, 406.4 Hz modulation of the 1016 pulses/s carrier. This level was held constant across all conditions, producing somewhat lower loudnesses for the remaining modulation frequencies for the 1016 pulses/s carrier and for all conditions with the 504 and 251 pulses/s carriers.

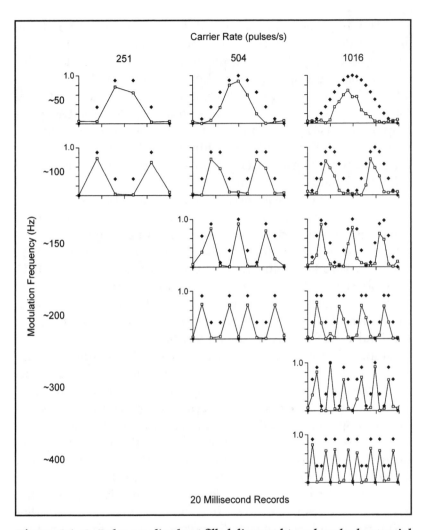

Figure 21-6. Pulse amplitudes (*filled diamonds*) and evoked potential (EP) magnitudes (*connected open squares*) for sinusoidally amplitude-modulated pulse trains. Normalized values are shown. Approximate modulation frequencies are indicated in the figure, and calculation of the exact frequencies is described in the text. The data are from studies with Ineraid subject SR3. The carrier level for all conditions was 600 μA, and the pulse duration was 33 μs/phase. Stimuli were delivered to intracochlear electrode 3 and recordings of neural responses were made with intracochlear electrode 4.

The amplitudes of the stimulus pulses for each condition are indicated by solid diamonds and the magnitudes of the EPs following each pulse by connected open squares. The pulse amplitudes are normalized to the maximum amplitude across all conditions, and the EP magnitudes are normalized to the maximum magnitude across all conditions as well. The peak amplitude was 600 μA and the pulse duration was 33 μs/phase (two 16.4-μs samples/phase). Although only the first 20 ms of the records are shown in Figure 21–6, the total duration of each SAM pulse train was 200 ms.

The patterns of responses appear to reflect both sampling of the modulation waveform by the carrier pulses and the nonlinear properties of auditory neurons. Examples of apparent refractory effects may be seen in the panels for 100.8 Hz modulation of the 504 pulses/s carrier and for 101.6 Hz modulation of the 1016 pulses/s carrier. The third and fourth pulses for the 504 pulses/s carrier have identical amplitudes and yet the neural response to the fourth pulse is substantially lower than the response to the third pulse. For the 1016 pulses/s carrier, the sixth pulse is higher in amplitude than the fifth pulse and yet the neural response to the second of those two pulses is again lower in magnitude.

Note also that when the modulation frequency is low compared to the carrier rate the pattern of EP magnitudes approximates the pattern of pulse amplitudes. For 50.4 Hz modulation of the 504 pulses/s carrier, for example, the pattern of neural responses looks almost sinusoidal, with a somewhat closer approximation to the stimulus pulses in the first half of the modulation cycle. As the modulation frequency is increased, the asymmetry of responses in each modulation cycle increases. For 100.8 Hz modulation of the 504 pulses/s carrier, for example, a "peaking" of the responses is observed in the first half of each modulation cycle.

Further increases in modulation frequency produce more complex patterns of responses. The pattern of responses for 151.2 Hz modulation of the 504 pulses/s carrier reflects the overall frequency of modulation but also shows large variations from cycle to cycle. The "sampling" of the sinusoidal modulation waveform becomes progressively sparser with increases in modulation frequency. The sparse sampling for the 151.2 Hz modulation condition only crudely reflects the modulation waveform. As the modulation frequency approaches one-half the carrier rate (the "Nyquist frequency," see Rabiner & Schafer, 1978), multiple intervals and other anomalies can appear in the stimuli and in the patterns of responses. Multiple intervals appear, for example, in the stimuli and pattern of responses for 201.6 Hz modulation of the 504 pulses/s carrier. The time between peaks in the response alternates between long (~6 ms) and short (~4 ms) intervals. Neither of these intervals corresponds to the period of the modulation waveform (~5 ms).

The effects just described for the 504 pulses/s conditions scale with carrier rate. For the 1016 pulses/s carrier, for example, a highly complex pattern of responses is observed at the modulation frequency of 304.8 Hz, and a pattern of responses with two distinct intervals is observed at the modulation frequency of 406.4 Hz. For the 251 pulses/s carrier, two distinct intervals are observed in the pattern of responses at the modulation frequency of 100.4 Hz, although the 20 ms segment of the record presented in Figure 21–6 is too short to show both intervals for this particular condition.

Percepts reported by subjects SR2 and SR3 when listening to these stimuli are consistent with the recorded patterns of responses. For the 504 pulses/s carrier conditions, the subjects report increases in pitch with increases in modulation frequency. The percepts elicited with relatively low modulation frequencies are described as smooth and tonal. However, the percept for the 151.2 Hz modulation condition is described as sounding rough and complex. Also, the percept for the 201.6 Hz modulation condition is described as combining at least two separate tones. For the 1016 pulses/s carriers, the percepts for the 152.4 and 203.2 Hz modulation conditions are described as relatively smooth and tonal, particularly the percept for the 203.2 Hz modulation condition. The percepts for the two lower modulation frequencies also are described as smooth and tonal, as before. For the higher modulation frequencies, however, a rough and complex percept is again reported, but this time at the modulation frequency of 304.8 Hz, and a multitonal percept is again reported, but this time at the modulation frequency of 406.4 Hz. These reports for the higher carrier rate are consistent with the scaling of neural response patterns with changes in carrier rate, as described above.

In broad terms, the results of Figure 21–6 suggest that the carrier rate in CIS and other processors should be 4 to 5 times higher than the highest frequency in the modulation waveforms for a smooth and unambiguous representation of those waveforms. Busby et al. (1993) have offered this same suggestion, based on results from their psychophysical studies with patients using the Nucleus device.

Additional studies have been conducted by us to evaluate effects of even higher carrier rates on neural representations of modulation waveforms (Wilson et al., 1996). Results for SR2 are presented in Figure 21–7. The stimuli were delivered to intracochlear electrode 3, with reference to a remote electrode in the temporalis muscle, and the neural responses were recorded with intracochlear electrode 4, with reference to the external electrode at the ipsilateral mastoid. The carrier level across all conditions was 475 µA, and the pulse duration was 33 µs/phase.

The comparison in Figure 21–7 is between the carrier rates of 1016 pulses/s and 4065 pulses/s, for the modulation frequencies of 100, 200, 300, 400, 500, and 600 Hz. Note that the combinations of carrier rate and modulation frequencies are somewhat different from those of the corresponding conditions in Figure 21–6, as the modulation frequencies were not scaled in the experiments of Figure 21–7. Note also that 30 ms records are presented in Figure 21–7, rather than the 20 ms records found in Figure 21–6. The EP magnitudes in Figure 21–7 are normalized to the maximum magnitude across all conditions.

Results for the 1016 pulses/s carrier show relatively simple representations of the modulation frequency for the 100- and 200-Hz modulation conditions. The pattern of responses becomes more complicated at the modulation frequency of 300 Hz. At 400 Hz the pattern is both complicated and no longer reflects the period of the modulation waveform. The first interval between major peaks in the response (between pulses 2 and 5) roughly approximates the period, but subsequent intervals are much longer than the period. (The difference between this pattern of responses and the pattern for the corresponding condition in Figure 21–6 is consistent with the slight difference in the combinations of modulation frequency and carrier rate.)

Close approximation of the modulation frequency to the Nyquist frequency, as with the 500 Hz modulation condition, produces a pattern of stimulation in which pulses of relatively high amplitudes alternate with pulses of relatively low amplitudes.

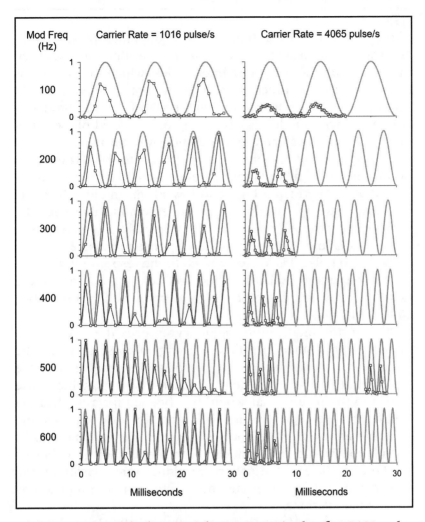

Figure 21-7. Evoked potential (EP) magnitudes for SAM pulse trains with the carrier rates of 1016 and 4065 pulses/s. EP magnitudes are normalized to the maximum value across all conditions. The modulation frequencies used in the studies of this figure are somewhat different from those used in the studies of Figure 21-6 and are exact for all conditions. Responses for the high rate carrier were derived using the subtraction technique illustrated in Figure 21-3. Data are from studies with subject SR2. The carrier level for all conditions was 475 µA, and the pulse duration was 33 µs/phase. Stimuli were delivered to intracochlear electrode 3 and recordings of neural responses were made with intracochlear electrode 4.

The difference between high and low amplitude pulses wanes and waxes at a "beat frequency" equal to the difference between the modulation and Nyquist frequencies, which in this case is 8 Hz. Modulation precisely at the Nyquist frequency would produce a series of alternating pulses with fixed amplitudes at two levels, with the levels depending on the fixed phase offset between the pulses and the modulation waveform.

The pattern of responses in Figure 21–7 for 500 Hz modulation of the 1016 pulses/s carrier reflects the pattern of stimulation, that is, alternating high and low EP magnitudes with the difference in high and low magnitudes diminishing over the half-period of the 8 Hz beat frequency. In addition, the response to pulse 4 is low compared to the response to pulse 2, and the response to pulse 8 is low compared to the response to pulse 6. This latter pattern probably reflects refractory properties of the neurons, as discussed before in connection with Figures 21–2, 21–4, and 21–6.

When the modulation frequency exceeds the Nyquist frequency a phenomenon called "aliasing" occurs, in which the pattern of stimulation for a given modulation frequency above the Nyquist frequency is identical (except for a possible phase offset) to the pattern that would be obtained for a modulation frequency below the Nyquist frequency by an equal amount. For example, with a 1000 pulses/s carrier, identical patterns of stimulation would be produced with modulation frequencies of 400 and 600 Hz (the pattern resulting from aliasing by the 600 Hz modulation is like the uncorrupted pattern produced by 400 Hz modulation).

For the present conditions the 400 and 600 Hz modulation frequencies are not quite equally distant from the Nyquist frequency (508 Hz). However, they are close enough to produce similarities in the patterns of stimulation and responses. A complicated pattern of response is again observed for the 600 Hz modulation condition that does not reflect the frequency of the modulation waveform.

Three regions of responses can be identified for the 1016 pulses/s carrier. At relatively low modulation frequencies, that is, 100 and 200 Hz, the responses simply represent the modulation waveform. At somewhat higher modulation frequencies complex patterns of response are observed. Those patterns do not correspond to any details of the modulation waveform and, indeed, at the modulation frequency of 400 Hz do not represent the modulation frequency. Severe sampling artifacts occur as the Nyquist frequency is approximated or exceeded by the modulation frequency. Results of such artifacts can be seen in the patterns of responses for the 500 and 600 Hz modulation conditions.

Patterns of responses for the 4065 pulses/s carrier show simple representations for all modulation frequencies included in the studies of Figure 21–7 (responses for this high carrier rate were derived using the subtraction technique of Figure 21–3). The patterns of responses follow closely the patterns of stimulation for the modulation frequencies of 400 Hz and lower. The distortions noted before for 300 and 400 Hz modulation of the 1016 pulses/s carrier are eliminated with the increase in carrier rate to 4065 pulses/s. At the higher modulation frequencies of 500 and 600 Hz, the patterns of responses for the 4065 pulses/s carrier show a shallow alternation between high and low peaks for successive cycles of the modulation waveform. For the 500 Hz condition this alternation may be damped or absent after the initial cycles, as suggested by the pattern of responses for two cycles beginning at about 24 ms after the onset of the burst.

Additional aspects of the responses for the 4065 pulses/s carrier are that: (a) the peak magnitudes are lower than those for the 1016 pulses/s carrier, and (b) the responses from pulse to pulse are smooth and continuous within modulation cycles. These aspects are consistent with the idea that high rate stimuli elicit a more stochastic pattern of responses within and among neurons than low rate stimuli, as described above in connection with responses to unmodulated pulses presented at high rates. However, the gradual increase in pulse amplitudes at the beginning of the burst for the SAM pulse trains may reduce or eliminate the initial "transient" response observed with unmodulated pulse trains.

PERCEPTION OF MODULATED PULSE TRAINS

Findings from recordings of intracochlear EPs led us to measure effects of carrier rate on psychophysical scaling of modulation frequencies. Results for subject SR2 are presented in Figure 21–8.

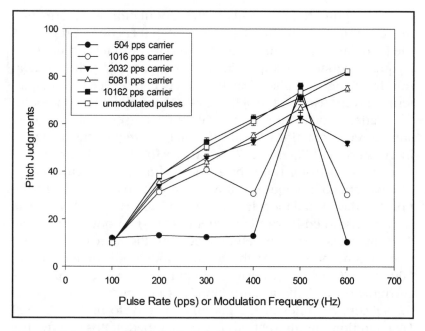

Figure 21-8. Scaling of pitch judgments for unmodulated pulse trains as a function of pulse rate, and for sinusoidally amplitude modulated (SAM) pulse trains as a function of modulation frequency. Data are from studies with subject SR2.

Electrode 3 was stimulated at MCL levels for all stimuli, which included 200 ms bursts of both SAM and unmodulated pulse trains. Six conditions were studied for each of five carrier rates and for the unmodulated pulse trains. The conditions for the SAM pulse trains included 100% modulation at frequencies of 100 through 600 Hz at 100 Hz intervals. The conditions for the unmodulated pulse trains included the corresponding pulse rates of 100 through 600/s, at 100 pulses/s intervals. Separate scaling experiments were conducted for each of the carrier rates and for the unmodulated pulse trains. The amplitudes of the stimuli were adjusted prior to each experiment as necessary to eliminate any differences in loudness across conditions. The subject was instructed to assign a number between 0 and 100 for each stimulus in the experiment according to perceived pitch. Thirty stimuli per condition were presented in random order across conditions for the experiments involving unmodulated pulses and the carrier rates of 2032, 5081, and 10,162 pulses/s. Sixty stimuli per condition were presented for the experiments involving the carrier rates of 504 and 1016 pulses/s.

Figure 21–8 shows the means and standard errors of the means of the judgments for each of the six conditions for each of the six experiments. As expected from the prior recordings of intracochlear EPs, carrier rate influenced the range over which pitch increased monotonically with increases in modulation frequency. For the 1016 pulses/s carrier, increases in modulation frequency beyond 300 Hz did not produce monotonic increases in pitch. In fact, judged pitch is not statistically different for the 200, 400, and 600 Hz modulation conditions. This finding is consistent with a predominance of 5-ms intervals between major peaks in the neural response patterns for these conditions, as shown in the left column of Figure 21–7. The judgment for 500 Hz modulation is substantially higher than the judgment for all other conditions. This finding also is consistent with the pattern of neural responses, which shows peaks separated by 2 ms. The increases in pitch up to the modulation frequency of 300 Hz may correspond to a progressive reduction in the intervals between principal peaks in the neural response patterns as the frequency is increased from 100 to 300 Hz.

Judgments for the 504 pulses/s carrier are highly similar for the modulation frequencies of 100, 200, 300, 400, and 600 Hz. In fact, the judgments for the lower four frequencies are statistically identical. Although this result may seem curious at first sight, plots of the stimuli show that each of these particular combinations of modulation frequency and carrier rate produces a predominance of 10 ms intervals between the major peaks.

The judgment for the 500 Hz modulation condition and the 504 pulses/s carrier shows a large increase in pitch compared with the judgments for the other modulation conditions. The close approximation of the modulation frequency to the carrier rate produces peaks in the stimuli at 2 ms intervals.

Pitch increases monotonically with increases in modulation frequency up to 500 Hz for the 2032 pulses/s carrier. Pitch is reduced for the 600-Hz modulation condition, and this judgment does not differ significantly from the judgment for the 400 Hz modulation condition.

For higher carrier rates, and for unmodulated pulses, pitch scales monotonically with increases in modulation frequency or pulse rate, respectively. The range of pitch judgments is greatest for the highest carrier rate and for the unmodulated pulses.

DISCUSSION

Results like those of Figure 21–8 show that increases in carrier rate can increase the range over which increases in modulation frequency produce monotonic increases in pitch. The question now is whether access to a greater range of pitches on single channels will be helpful in multichannel processors. One concern is that temporal channel interactions, due to summation at neural membranes of rapidly presented pulses from different electrodes, may be exacerbated with increased rates of stimulation. Such interactions may limit possible benefits of high rate stimuli. On the other hand, control or reduction of temporal channel interactions might remove this potential limitation. Work is in progress to develop novel stimulus waveforms specifically designed to leave neural membranes at their resting potential after delivery of a subthreshold pulse (e.g., Eddington et al., 1994). In this way, effects of sequential subthreshold pulses (from different electrodes) would not accumulate and cause an unwanted discharge of the neuron. In addition, parallel developments of new electrode designs (e.g., Kuzma, 1996; Kuzma et al., 1996; Seldon et al., 1994) may produce an electrode system with greater spatial specificity of stimulation and reduced interactions among electrodes compared to present designs. Use of such electrodes may reduce or eliminate the concern about temporal channel interactions.

A further alternative might be to separate pulses delivered to sequential electrodes by 130 μs or thereabouts. The data presented in Figure 21–5 suggest that this separation would reduce any temporal summation component of electrode interactions quite substantially, at least for SR2 and presumably for other patients as well. The extra time in the cycles of stimulation across electrodes in the array required for the temporal separation of the pulses might be compensated at least to some extent with the use of minimally short phase durations for the pulses. Also, use of an *n*-of-*m* processing strategy might be helpful in this respect, in that relatively few electrodes are selected in each cycle of stimulation and therefore more time can be interposed between sequential pulses while still maintaining a high stimulation rate at each of the (selected) electrodes. (The *n*-of-*m* strategy is described in Chapters 2 and 13.)

Implementation of high rate processors with multiple channels is technically demanding. Delivery of high rate stimuli within and across electrodes requires high bandwidth current sources capable of generating rectangular pulses with durations of 10 μs/phase or less. Also, for percutaneous connector systems, capacitive coupling among the leads in the cable to the connector can lead to "crosstalk" among channels for high frequency, high rate stimuli. New equipment has been developed in our laboratory (see QPR 5:4) and at the Massachusetts Eye and Ear Infirmary to support evaluations of high rate processors. In our system, for example, each of 24 current sources can generate pulses with phase durations as short as 5 μs, and capacitive cross-talk among the leads to percutaneous connectors has been reduced to insignificant levels through the use of "driven" shields for each of the leads. We will be using this equipment in future studies.

In the meantime, we have used equipment that can support lower rates of stimulation that are nonetheless higher than the typical rates used in the cochlear implant systems to date. That equipment was used, for example, in the studies with the subjects using the experimental version of the Nucleus device that includes a percutaneous connector. Those studies are described in Chapter 13 and included evaluation of a CIS processor that presented pulses to each of six electrodes at the rate of 2525/s. The control processor was the same in all other respects except for the pulse rate, which was 833/s for that processor. The cutoff frequency of the lowpass filters in the envelope detectors was 200 Hz for both processors.

As described in Chapter 13, the means of the scores across five subjects for the administered tests of consonant identification were not significantly different between the two processors. Among the subjects, two had marginally better scores with the higher rate processor (just attaining statistical significance) and two had marginally worse scores with that processor (also just attaining statistical significance), with respect to the control processor (see the "fst" row in Table 13–8).

These results did not indicate any clear benefit (or decrement) from use of the higher rate processor. However, that processor did not take advantage of the possibly higher frequencies that could be represented with the 2525 pulses/s rate at each electrode, as the cutoff frequency for the lowpass filters in the envelope detectors was held constant at 200 Hz. We now know from the present experiments that progressively higher frequencies can be represented and perceived unambiguously in the modulation waveforms as the carrier pulse rate is increased (see especially Figures 21–7 and 21–8). In particular, the present data suggest that frequencies as high as 500 Hz could have been represented unambiguously with the 2525 pulses/s processor if the cutoff frequency for the lowpass filters had been set at 500 Hz rather than at 200 Hz. Any such additional information might have been helpful to the subjects, and this possibility will also be evaluated along with even higher carrier rates in the future studies.

We note that results of studies by Brill et al. (1997), Brill & Hochmair (1997), and Kiefer et al. (1996, 1997) have provided indications of improved speech reception scores with processors using exceptionally high carrier rates. We have not seen improvements to date, as noted above. However, the conditions of the various experiments were different in multiple ways, and comparisons in a single laboratory among many carrier rates and at least several cutoff frequencies for the lowpass filters should provide a reliable indication of the value if any of the higher carrier rates. We have planned such studies.

POSTSCRIPT

The report on which this chapter is based was written in 1997. Since that time, additional related studies have been conducted by the RTI team and many others. The additional studies have included:

- Experiments like those of the present report, except with many more subjects, a broader repertoire of stimuli, and use of exactly the same stimuli in the electrophysiological and psychophysical measures (QPR 5:8)

- Development of the "conditioner pulses" concept and applications (e.g., Rubinstein et al., 1999)
- Evaluation of possible changes in speech reception over wide ranges in carrier rate and the cutoff frequency of the lowpass filters in the envelope detectors of CIS processors (QPRs 6:6 and 6:7)
- Further evaluations of carrier rate effects with CIS and other processors (e.g., Buechner et al., 2010; Friesen et al., 2005; Frijns et al., 2003; Fu & Shannon, 2000; Green et al., 2012; Kiefer et al., 2000; Loizou et al., 2000; Shannon et al., 2011)
- Further measures of intracochlear EPs in human subjects for electric pulses presented at high rates (Hughes et al., 2012)
- Further studies to evaluate possible relationships between temporal patterns of activity at the auditory nerve and pitch judgments for cochlear implant patients (e.g., QPR 5:8; Carlyon et al., 2002, 2010; Kong & Carlyon, 2010; Macherey & Carlyon, 2010; van Wieringen et al., 2003).

Several of these lines of investigation are still ongoing, as indicated in part by the recent dates for seven of the papers just cited.

The present report was the first to describe recordings of intracochlear EPs for pulse rates above 1000/s. It also was the first to describe correlates between perception and the temporal patterns of responses in the auditory nerve evoked by electrical stimuli, and it additionally presented new information on the distortions in those temporal representations for unmodulated and SAM pulse trains. The report provided a foundation for much subsequent research.

Acknowledgments. We thank subjects SR2 and SR3 for their participation in the studies described in this report.

PARTNERS IN RESEARCH

As noted in the Acknowledgments, the team at the Research Triangle Institute (RTI) was greatly augmented and enriched by participation in joint studies by many investigators from other organizations worldwide. The principal collaborations were with investigators at the University of California at San Francisco (UCSF) and the Duke University Medical Center (DUMC). We received spectacular help, advice, and partnership from Michael M. Merzenich, Dorcas K. Kessler, Patricia A. Leake, Stephen J. Rebscher, Robert A. Schindler, Robert V. Shannon, Lindsay Vurek, Mark W. White, David Wilkinson, and others from UCSF, and we received the same from Joseph C. Farmer, Jr., Nell B. Cant, John H. (Pete) Casseday, Leslie M. Collins, Warren M. Grill, William R. Hudson, Patrick D. Kenan, John T. McElveen, Jr., Patricia A. Roush, Debara L. Tucci, Bruce A. Weber, Robert D. Wolford (in the early years, before he joined the RTI team), and many others from DUMC. In addition, the RTI team conducted studies at UCSF up until mid-1985 and at DUMC from mid-1985 through the fall of 1995. Laboratory facilities were generously provided by UCSF and DUMC, and the investigators at those universities worked closely with us in the studies.

A partial listing of the many other investigators who worked alongside us over the years includes Sigfrid D. Soli, first with the 3M Company in Minnesota and later with the House Ear Institute in Los Angeles; Michael F. Dorman of Arizona State University; Philip Loizou, first with Arizona State University, then with the University of Arkansas at Little Rock, and then with the University of Texas at Dallas; James W. Heller and Ronald E. West of

Cochlear Americas Corp.; James F. Patrick of Cochlear Ltd. in Lane Cove, Australia; Jacques François of the Ecole d'Ingenieurs de Geneve in Geneva, Switzerland; Wolfgang K. Gstoettner, Jan Kiefer, Thomas Pfennigdorff, Jochen Tillein, Christoph A. von Ilberg of the J. W. Goethe Universität in Frankfurt, Germany; Stefan (Marcel) Pok, first with the J. W. Goethe Universität and later with the Medical University of Vienna in Vienna, Austria; Robert V. Shannon and John Wygonski of the House Ear Institute; Albert A. Maltan, first with the House Ear Institute, then with the MED-EL GmbH of Innsbruck, Austria, and then with the Advanced Bionics Corp. in Valencia, CA, USA; Artur Lorens of the International Center of Hearing and Speech in Kajetany, Poland; Joachim M. Müller and Franz Schön of the Julius Maximilians Universität in Würzburg, Germany; Josef M. Miller and Bryan E. Pfingst of the Kresge Hearing Research Institute at the University of Michigan; Martin P. O'Driscoll of the Manchester Royal Infirmary in Manchester, England; Peter Nopp of the MED-EL GmbH; Raymond Mederake of the MED-EL subsidiary in Starnberg, Germany; Colette Böex-Spano and Donald K. Eddington of the Massachusetts Eye & Ear Infirmary in Boston, MA, USA; William M. Rabinowitz of the Massachusetts Institute of Technology; Susan B. Waltzman of New York University; Sung June Kim of Seoul National University in Seoul, South Korea; Laurel J. Dent of Stanford University; David Calvert, Stephen Hutchison, and Gary Keibel of the Storz Instrument Company in St. Louis, MO, USA; Gerald E. Loeb, first as a guest researcher at the UCSF (on leave from the NIH), then with Queen's University in Kingston, Ontario, Canada, then with the Advanced Bionics Corp. (as its consulting Chief Scientist), and then with the University of California at Los Angeles; Oliver F. Adunka, first with the J. W. Goethe Universität and then with the UNC; Carol Higgins (now Carol Pillsbury) and Harold C. Pillsbury of the UNC; Marco Pelizzone of the Hôpital Cantonal Universitaire Geneva, in Geneva, Switzerland; Stefan Brill (before he became a member of the RTI team), Erwin S. Hochmair, Otto Peter, and Clemens M. Zierhofer of the University of Innsbruck in Innsbruck, Austria; Paul J. Abbas, Carolyn J. Brown, Bruce J. Gantz, Mary W. Lowder, Aaron J. Parkinson, Jay T. Rubinstein, and Richard S. Tyler of the University of Iowa; Korine Dankowski of the University of Utah; Christoph Arnoldner and Wolf-Dieter Baumgartner of the Medical University of Vienna in Vienna, Austria; Enrique A. Lopez-Poveda, first with the University of Castile — La Mancha and then with the University of Salamanca in Spain; and Margaret W. Skinner of Washington University in St. Louis, MO, USA. The affiliations for some of these people have changed (or changed further) since their active participation in the studies at RTI and Duke.

We also benefited from visits by many world leaders in the field of cochlear implants and related fields. A few among these visitors were Hugh J. McDermott from the University of Melbourne in Melbourne, Australia; Ingeborg J. Hochmair from the MED-EL GmbH; Erwin S. Hochmair from the University of Innsbruck (before his participation in studies at the RTI and DUMC); Deborah Ballantyne from the Universita Degli Studi di Roma "La Saienza" (Department of Otolaryngology) in Rome, Italy; Margaret (Margo) W. Skinner and A. Maynard Engebretson of Washington University (before Margo's participation in studies at RTI and Duke); Thomas Lenarz and Rolf D. Battmer from the Medizinische Hochschule Hannover in Hannover, Germany; Paul Carter from Cochlear Ltd. (while on leave at Cochlear Americas); Charles A. Miller from the University of Iowa; Matthew Bakke and Yifang Xu from Gallaudet University; Russell L. Snyder from UCSF; Kevin H. Franck from The Children's Hospital of Philadelphia in Philadelphia, PA, USA; Christopher W. Turner also from the University of Iowa; Craig A. Buchman from the UNC; and Peter S. Roland from the University of Texas Southwestern Medical Center. The discussions with these wonderful visitors were highly enlightening and in some cases suggested new questions for us to ask in our research.

TOPICS AND AUTHORS FOR THE RTI PROGRESS REPORTS

This Appendix includes tables of the topics and authors for the NIH progress reports produced as part of the projects at the Research Triangle Institute (RTI). There were seven projects in all, and the NIH numbers and exact dates for the projects are given in Table 1–2 in Chapter 1. The years during which each of the projects was conducted are indicated in the legends for the tables in this Appendix. The words "Quarterly Progress Report" are abbreviated in the tables by the acronym "QPR." Other organizations listed in the tables include the University of California at San Francisco (UCSF), the Duke University Medical Center (DUMC), Nucleus Ltd. (Nucleus), the Storz Instrument Company (Storz), MiniMed Technologies Incorporated (MiniMed), and MED-EL GmbH (MED-EL). Additional abbreviations in the tables include IP for "Interleaved Pulses"; CA for "Compressed Analog"; CIS for "Continuous Interleaved Sampling"; VCIS for "Virtual Channel Interleaved Sampling"; and TIMIT for "Texas Instruments and the Massachusetts Institute of Technology."

Table B–1. Progress Reports for Project 1 (1983–1985)

Report	Topic(s)	Authors
QPR 1	Development of plans for collaborative studies with UCSF; development of tools for such studies at UCSF; initial plans for an additional collaborative program with Duke University Medical Center	Wilson and Finley
QPR 2	Model of field patterns in the implanted cochlea; collaboration among UCSF, Storz, DUMC, and RTI; hardware interface for communication between an Eclipse computer and patient electrodes; design of software for a block-diagram compiler; discussion on the possibility of recording intracochlear evoked potentials	Wilson and Finley
QPR 3	Hardware interface; computer-based stimulator; Digital Control Unit (DCU) software for real-time communication between an Eclipse computer and stimulating hardware; incorporation of a Frankenhauser-Huxley description of node dynamics in an integrated field-neuron model	Wilson and Finley
QPR 4	Overview of first-year effort	Wilson, Finley, and Lawson
QPR 5	Further development and application of a field-neuron model	Finley and Wilson
QPR 6	Development of portable, real-time hardware; software for support of the RTI patient stimulator; software for support of basic psychophysical studies and speech testing; subject testing at UCSF	Wilson, Finley, and Lawson
QPR 7	Speech reception studies with a UCSF/Storz subject; present status and functional description of the block-diagram compiler	Wilson, Finley, and Lawson
QPR 8	Ensemble models of neural responses to intracochlear electrical stimulation	Wilson, Finley, and Lawson

Table B–1. continued

Report	Topic(s)	Authors
Final Report	Hardware interface; computer-based simulator of speech processors; integrated field-neuron model; ensemble models of neural responses evoked by intracochlear electrical stimulation; design of a portable speech processor; evaluation of processing strategies in tests with a USCF patient fitted with a percutaneous connector; reporting activity for the project	Wilson, Finley, and Lawson

Table B–2. Progress Reports for Project 2 (1985–1989)

Report	Topic(s)	Authors
QPR 1	Psychophysical and speech reception studies with an initial DUMC/Storz percutaneous subject	Wilson, Finley, and Lawson
QPR 2	Psychophysical and speech reception studies with a second DUMC/Storz percutaneous subject; further development of an interleaved pulses (IP) processor	Wilson, Finley, and Lawson
QPR 3	Initial development of a portable, real-time processor; measurements of intracochlear electric field patterns using a percutaneous cable	Finley, Wilson, and Lawson
QPR 4	Evaluation of idealized implementations of the processing strategy used in the Nucleus cochlear prosthesis	Wilson, Finley, and Lawson
QPR 5	Studies of loudness and pitch perception with monopolar or radial-bipolar stimulating electrodes	Wilson, Finley, and Lawson
QPR 6	Direct comparisons of analog and pulsatile coding strategies with six cochlear implant patients	Wilson, Finley, and Lawson

continues

393

Table B–2. continued

Report	Topic(s)	Authors
QPR 7	A portable processor for IP processing strategies	Finley, Wilson, and Lawson
QPR 8	Evaluation of two-channel "Breeuwer/Plomp" processors for cochlear implants	Wilson, Lawson, and Finley
QPR 9	Studies with 6 UCSF/Storz subjects	Wilson, Finley, and Lawson
QPR 10	Review of clinical trial results for 6 UCSF/Storz subjects, including learning effects with extended use	Wilson, Lawson, and Finley
QPR 11	Extension of cochlear implant laboratory capabilities; collaborative development of a next-generation auditory prosthesis	Wilson, Lawson, and Finley
QPR 12	Representations of speech features with cochlear implants	Wilson, Finley, and Lawson
QPR 13	Models of neural responsiveness to electrical stimulation	Finley, Wilson, and Lawson
QPR 14	Binary comparisons of speech processor performance	Lawson, Wilson, and Finley
Final Report	Direct comparisons of analog and pulsatile coding strategies; design and evaluation of a two-channel "Breeuwer/Plomp" processor; additional processor comparisons; psychophysical studies; development of a next-generation auditory prosthesis; reporting activity for the project	Wilson, Finley, and Lawson

Table B-3. Progress Reports for Project 3 (1989–1992)

Report	Topic(s)	Authors
QPR 1	Comparison of analog and pulsatile coding strategies for multichannel cochlear implants (6 UCSF/Storz subjects and 2 Ineraid subjects)	Wilson, Finley, and Lawson
QPR 2	New levels of speech perception with cochlear implants; computer interface for testing patients implanted with the Nucleus device	Wilson, Finley, and Lawson
QPR 3	Evaluations of alternative implementations of CIS, IP and Peak-Picker strategies; finite-element model of radial bipolar field patterns in the electrically stimulated cochlea	Wilson, Finley, and Lawson
QPR 4	Comparison of CA and CIS processors in tests with seven Ineraid subjects	Wilson, Lawson, and Finley
QPR 5	Further evaluation of CIS processors	Wilson, Finley, and Lawson
QPR 6	Parametric variations and the fitting of speech processors for single-channel brainstem prostheses	Lawson, Finley, and Wilson
QPR 7	A wearable speech processor platform for auditory research	Finley, Wilson, Zerbi, Hering, van den Honert, and Lawson
QPR 8	Importance of patient and processor variables in determining outcomes with cochlear implants	Wilson, Lawson, and Finley

continues

395

Table B–3. continued

Report	Topic(s)	Authors
QPR 9	Evaluation of a prototype for a portable processor; evaluation of components in the MiniMed cochlear prosthesis; evaluation of automatic gain control; preliminary studies of modulation perception; measures of dynamic range for a variety of pulse durations and rates	Wilson, Lawson, Finley, and Zerbi
QPR 10	Randomized update orders; slow rate CIS implementations; channel number manipulations; evaluation of other promising processing strategies; performance of CIS and CA processors in noise; use and possible development of new test materials	Wilson, Lawson, Finley, and Zerbi
QPR 11	Efficacy of CIS processors for patients with poor clinical outcomes	Wilson, Lawson, Finley, and Zerbi
QPR 12	Completion of "poor performance" series; summary of studies with 11 Ineraid subjects; auditory brainstem implant (ABI) studies	Wilson, Lawson, Zerbi, and Finley
Final Report	Comparisons of CA and CIS processors for multichannel cochlear implants; additional aspects of CIS performance; evaluation of other promising strategies; auditory brainstem implant; record of reporting activity for the project; suggestions for future research	Wilson, Lawson, Finley, and Zerbi

Table B–4. *Progress Reports for Project 4 (1992–1995)*

Report	Topic(s)	Authors
QPR 1	Virtual channel interleaved sampling (VCIS) processors: initial studies with subject SR2	Wilson, Lawson, Zerbi, and Finley
QPR 2	Single parameter variation studies for CIS processors	Lawson, Wilson, and Zerbi
QPR 3	Identification of virtual channels on the basis of pitch	Wilson, Zerbi, and Lawson
QPR 4	Representation of complex tones by sound processors for implanted auditory prostheses	Lawson, Zerbi, and Wilson
QPR 5	Transfer and dissemination of CIS processor technology; parametric and control studies with CIS processors	Wilson, Lawson, and Zerbi
QPR 6	Evaluation of VCIS processors	Wilson, Lawson, and Zerbi
QPR 7	Temporal representations with cochlear implants: modeling, psychophysical, and electrophysiological studies	Wilson, Finley, Zerbi, and Lawson
QPR 8	Further studies of complex tone perception by implant patients	Lawson, Wilson, and Zerbi
QPR 9	Strategies for the repair of distortions in temporal representations with implants	Wilson, Finley, Zerbi, and Lawson
QPR 10	A channel-specific tool for analysis of consonant confusion matrices	Lawson, Wilson, and Zerbi

continues

Table B–4. continued

Report	Topic(s)	Authors
QPR 11	Intracochlear evoked potentials for sustained electrical stimuli	Wilson, Finley, Lawson, and Zerbi
Final Report	Importance of the patient variable in determining outcomes with cochlear implants; parametric studies with CIS processors; importance of processor fitting; "Virtual Channel" and "Sharpened Field" CIS processors; Nucleus percutaneous study; design for an inexpensive but effective cochlear implant system; representation of complex tones by sound processors for implanted auditory prostheses; temporal representations with cochlear implants; record of reporting activity for the project; suggestions for future research	Wilson, Lawson, Zerbi, and Finley

Table B-5. *Progress Reports for Project 5 (1995–1998)*

Report	Topic(s)	Authors
QPR 1	Learning effects with extended use of CIS processors; review of results from studies with the first subject in the 22-electrode percutaneous study; upward extension of the CIS processed frequency spectrum	Lawson, Wilson, Zerbi, and Finley
QPR 2	Manipulations in spatial representations with implants	Wilson, Lawson, and Zerbi
QPR 3	22-electrode percutaneous study: results for the first five subjects	Lawson, Wilson, Zerbi, and Finley
QPR 4	New stimulator system for the speech reception laboratory	van den Honert, Zerbi, Finley, and Wilson
QPR 5	Bilateral cochlear implants controlled by a single speech processor	Lawson, Wilson, Zerbi, and Finley
QPR 6	Intracochlear evoked potentials in response to pairs of pulses: effects of pulse amplitude and interpulse interval	Finley, Wilson, van den Honert, and Lawson
QPR 7	High rate studies, subject SR2	Wilson, Finley, Zerbi, Lawson, and van den Honert

continues

Table B–5. continued

Report	Topic(s)	Authors
QPR 8	Relationships between temporal patterns of nerve activity and pitch judgments for cochlear implant patients	Wilson, Zerbi, Finley, Lawson, and van den Honert
QPR 9	Development of the evoked potentials laboratory	van den Honert, Finley, and Wilson
QPR 10	Effects of upward extension of the frequency range analyzed by CIS processors	Zerbi, Lawson, and Wilson
QPR 11	Design of new speech test materials and comparisons with standard materials	Lawson, Wilson, and Zerbi
Final Report	Summary of major activities and achievements for the project; new directions in implant design; summary of reporting activity for the project	Wilson, Lawson, Zerbi, Finley, and van den Honert

Table B–6. Progress Reports for Project 6 (1998–2002)

Report	Topic(s)	Authors
QPR 1	Pitch discrimination among electrodes for each of three subjects with bilateral cochlear implants; measurement of interaural timing and amplitude difference cues for those same subjects	Lawson, Zerbi, and Wilson
QPR 2	Measures of performance over time following substitution of CIS for CA speech processors	Lawson, Wilson, and Zerbi
QPR 3	Effects of manipulations in mapping functions on the performance of CIS processors	Wilson, Lawson, Zerbi, and Wolford
QPR 4	Speech reception with bilateral cochlear implants; update on longitudinal studies	Lawson, Wilson, Zerbi, and Finley
QPR 5	Comprehensive review of strategies for representing speech information with cochlear implants	Wilson, Lawson, Wolford, and Brill
QPR 6	Effects of changes in stimulus rate and envelope cutoff frequency for CIS processors	Wilson, Wolford, and Lawson
QPR 7	Further studies to evaluate effects of changes in stimulus rate and envelope cutoff frequency for CIS processors	Wilson, Wolford, and Lawson
QPR 8	Combined electric and acoustic stimulation of the same cochlea	Lawson, Wilson, Wolford, Brill, and Schatzer

continues

Report	Topic(s)	Authors
QPR 9	Binaural cochlear implant findings: summary of initial results with eleven subjects	Lawson, Brill, Wolford, Wilson, and Schatzer
QPR 10	New tools, including: (a) evaluation of the TIMIT Speech Database for use in studies with implant subjects, (b) processing of speech and other sounds using head-related transfer functions, and (c) an Access database of speech processor designs and study results	Cox, Wolford, Schatzer, Wilson, and Lawson
QPR 11	Further studies to evaluate combined electric and acoustic stimulation	Brill, Lawson, Wolford, Wilson, and Schatzer
QPR 12	Further studies regarding benefits of bilateral cochlear implants	Lawson, Wolford, Brill, Schatzer, and Wilson
QPR 13	Cooperative electric and acoustic stimulation of the peripheral auditory system—comparison of ipsilateral and contralateral implementations	Lawson, Wolford, Brill, Wilson, and Schatzer
Final Report	Summary of major activities and achievements for the project; some likely next steps in the further development of cochlear prostheses; summary of reporting activity for the project	Wilson, Brill, Cartee, Cox, Lawson, Schatzer, and Wolford

Table B–7. *Progress Reports for Project 7 (2002–2006)*

Report	Topic(s)	Authors
QPR 1	Pitch-matched and pitch-distinct electrode pairs in bilaterally implanted arrays	Lawson, Wolford, Wilson, and Schatzer
QPR 2	Longitudinal studies of improvement in performance with early experience using binaural cochlear implants	Lawson, Wolford, Wilson, and Schatzer
QPR 3	Additional perspectives on speech reception with combined electric and acoustic stimulation	Wilson, Wolford, Lawson, and Schatzer
QPR 4	Measurements of interaural timing differences; update on longitudinal studies of early performance improvements with binaural cochlear implants	Wolford, Lawson, Schatzer, Sun, and Wilson
QPR 5	Recent enhancements of the speech laboratory system	Schatzer, Zerbi, Sun, Cox, Wolford, Lawson, and Wilson
QPR 6	Signal processing strategy for a closer mimicking of normal auditory functions	Schatzer, Wilson, Wolford, and Lawson
QPR 7	Combined use of dual-resonance nonlinear (DRNL) filters and virtual channels	Wilson, Wolford, Schatzer, Sun, and Lawson

continues

Report	Topic(s)	Authors
QPR 8	Representation of fine structure or fine frequency information with cochlear implants	Wilson, Sun, Schatzer, and Wolford
QPR 9	Intracochlear potentials evoked by electrical stimulation with phase-separated balanced biphasic pulses	Cartee, Wilson, Cox, Wolford, and Lawson
QPR 10	Pitch ranking of electrodes for 22 subjects with bilateral implants; melody recognition tests for cochlear implant research	Lawson, Wilson, Wolford, Sun, and Schatzer
QPR 11	Laboratory interface for the new MED-EL PULSARCI[100] implant; further development of the streaming mode tools	Schatzer, Zerbi, Wilson, Cox, Lawson, and Sun
QPR 12	Initial studies with a recipient of the PULSAR implant	Lawson, Wilson, Schatzer, and Sun
QPR 13	Progress in Nucleus percutaneous studies	Lawson, Wilson, and Sun
QPR 14	Further progress in the Nucleus percutaneous studies	Lawson, Sun, and Wilson
QPR 15	Results from the Nucleus percutaneous studies	Lawson, Sun, and Wilson
Final Report	Major areas of research under this contract and suggested future directions	Wilson and Lawson

Appendix C

PUBLICATIONS RESULTING FROM THE RTI PROJECTS

Publications resulting from the RTI projects are listed in chronological order below. Some of the entries were published after the completion of the final project, but all of those and the other entries reported results from the projects, or were based at least in part on concepts or the experience gained from the projects.

REFERENCES

Wilson, B. S., Finley, C. C., Farmer, J. C., Jr., Lawson, D. T., Weber, B. A., Wolford, R. D., . . . Schindler, R. A. (1988). Comparative studies of speech processing strategies for cochlear implants. *Laryngoscope*, *98*, 1069–1077.

Wilson, B. S., Schindler, R. A., Finley, C. C., Kessler, D. K., Lawson, D. T., & Wolford, R. D. (1988). Present status and future enhancements of the UCSF cochlear prosthesis. In P. Banfai (Ed.), *Cochlear implants: Current situation* (pp. 395–427). Erkelenz, Germany: Rudolf Bermann GmbH.

Wilson, B. S., (moderator), Dent, L. J., Dillier N., Eddington, D. K., Hochmair-Desoyer, I. J., Pfingst, B. E., . . . Walliker, J. (1988). Round table discussion on speech coding. In P. Banfai (Ed.), *Cochlear implants: Current situation* (pp. 693–704)., Erkelenz, Germany: Rudolf Bermann GmbH.

Wilson, B. S., Finley, C. C., Lawson, D. T., & Wolford, R. D. (1988). Speech processors for cochlear prostheses. *Proceedings of the IEEE*, *76*, 1143–1154.

Finley, C. C., Wilson, B. S., & White, M. W. (1990). Models of neural responsiveness to electrical stimulation. In J. M. Miller & F. A. Spelman (Eds.), *Cochlear implants: Models of the electrically stimulated ear* (pp. 55–96). Berlin, Germany: Springer-Verlag.

Wilson, B. S., Finley, C. C., & Lawson, D. T. (1990). Representations of speech features with cochlear implants. In J. M. Miller & F. A. Spelman (Eds.), *Cochlear implants: Models of the electrically stimulated ear* (pp. 339–376). Berlin, Germany: Springer-Verlag.

Wilson, B. S., Lawson, D. T., Finley, C. C, & Wolford, R. D. (1991). Coding strategies for multichannel cochlear prostheses. *American Journal of Otology, 12*(Suppl. 1), 56–61.

Wilson, B. S., Finley, C. C., Lawson, D. T., Wolford, R. D., Eddington, D. K., & Rabinowitz, W. M. (1991). Better speech recognition with cochlear implants. *Nature, 352*, 236–238. (This paper is the most highly cited publication on studies involving cochlear implant subjects, with 442 citations as of February 17, 2011; the next most-highly cited publication has 240 citations as of the same date.)

Wilson, B. S. (1993). Signal processing. In R. Tyler (Ed.), *Cochlear implants: Audiological foundations* (pp. 35–85). San Diego, CA: Singular.

Wilson, B. S., Lawson, D. T., Finley, C. C., & Wolford, R. D. (1993). Importance of patient and processor variables in determining outcomes with cochlear implants. *Journal of Speech and Hearing Research, 36*, 373–379.

Lawson, D. T., Wilson, B. S., & Finley, C. C. (1993). New processing strategies for multichannel cochlear prostheses. *Progress in Brain Research, 97*, 313–321.

Wilson, B. S., Finley, C. C., Lawson, D. T., Wolford, R. D., & Zerbi, M. (1993). Design and evaluation of a continuous interleaved sampling (CIS) processing strategy for multichannel cochlear implants. *Journal of Rehabilitation Research and Development, 30*, 110–116.

Wilson, B. S., Lawson, D. T., Zerbi, M., & Finley, C. C. (1994). Recent developments with the CIS strategies. In I. J. Hochmair-Desoyer & E. S. Hochmair (Eds.), *Advances in cochlear implants* (pp. 103–112). Vienna, Austria: Manz.

Wilson, B. S., Lawson, D. T., Zerbi, M., Finley, C. C., & Wolford, R. D. (1995). New processing strategies in cochlear implantation. *American Journal of Otology, 16*, 669–675.

Wilson, B. S., Lawson, D. T., & Zerbi, M. (1995). Advances in coding strategies for cochlear implants. *Advances in Otolaryngology—Head and Neck Surgery, 9*, 105–129.

Gates, G. A., Daly, K., Dichtel, W. J., Dooling, R. J., Gulya, A. J., Hall, J. W., . . . Brown, J. (1995). Cochlear implants in adults and children.

Journal of the American Medical Association, 274, 1955–1961. (This is the NIH Consensus Statement on Cochlear Implants in Adults and Children, published in *JAMA*.)

Wilson, B. S. (1997). The future of cochlear implants. *British Journal of Audiology, 31,* 205–225. (This paper was an invited Guest Editorial in celebration of the journal's 30th anniversary.)

Lawson, D. T., Wilson, B. S., Finley, C. C., Zerbi, M., Cartee, L. A., Roush, P. A., . . . Tucci, D. L. (1997). Cochlear implant studies at Research Triangle Institute and Duke University Medical Center. *Scandanavian Audiology, 26*(Suppl. 46), 50–64.

Wilson, B. S., Finley, C. C., Lawson, D. T., & Zerbi, M. (1997). Temporal representations with cochlear implants. *American Journal of Otology, 18,* S30–34.

Wilson, B. S., Rebscher, S., Zeng, F.-G., Shannon, R. V., Loeb, G. E., Lawson, D. T., & Zerbi, M. (1998). Design for an inexpensive but effective cochlear implant. *Otolaryngology—Head and Neck Surgery, 118,* 235–241.

Lawson, D. T., Wilson, B S., Zerbi, M., van den Honert, C., Finley, C. C,. Farmer, J. C., Jr., . . . McElveen, J. T., Roush, P. A. (1998). Bilateral cochlear implants controlled by a single speech processor. *American Journal of Otology, 19,* 758–761.

Rubinstein, J. T., Wilson, B. S., Finley, C. C., Abbas, P. J. (1999). Pseudospontaneous activity: Stochastic independence of auditory nerve fibers with electrical stimulation. *Hearing Research, 127,* 108–118.

Wilson, B. S. (2000). New directions in implant design. In S. B. Waltzman & N. Cohen (Eds.), *Cochlear implants* (pp. 43–56). New York, NY: Thieme.

Tucci, D. L., Roush, P. A., Lawson, D. T., Wilson, B. S., Zerbi, M., & Farmer, J. C., Jr. (2000). Surgical experience with the modified percutaneous Nucleus cochlear implant. In S. B. Waltzman & N. Cohen (Eds.), *Cochlear implants* (pp. 167–169). New York, NY: Thieme.

Tyler, R. S., Parkinson, A., Wilson, B. S., Parkinson, W., Lowder, M., Witt, S., . . . Gantz, B. (2000). Evaluation of different choices of *n* in an *n*-of-*m* processor for cochlear implants. *Advances in Oto-Rhino-Laryngology, 57,* 311–315.

Niparko, J. K., & Wilson, B. S. (2000). History of cochlear implants. In J. K. Niparko, K. I. Kirk, N. K. Mellon, A. M. Robbins, D. L. Tucci, and B. S. Wilson (Eds.), *Cochlear implants: Principles and practices* (pp. 103–107). Philadelphia, PA: Lippincott Williams & Wilkins.

Cartee, L. A., van den Honert, C., Finley, C. C., & Miller, R. L. (2000). Evaluation of a model of the cochlear neural membrane. I. Physiological measurement of membrane characteristics in response to intrameatal electrical stimulation. *Hearing Research, 146,* 143–152.

Cartee, L. A. (2000). Evaluation of a model of the cochlear neural membrane. II: comparison of model and physiological measures of membrane properties measured in response to intrameatal electrical stimulation. *Hearing Research, 146,* 153–166.

Wilson, B. S. (2000) Cochlear implant technology. In J. K. Niparko, K. I. Kirk, N. K. Mellon, A. M. Robbins, D. L. Tucci, & B. S. Wilson (Eds.), *Cochlear implants: Principles and practices* (pp. 109–119). Philadelphia, PA: Lippincott Williams & Wilkins.

Wilson, B. S. (2000). Strategies for representing speech information with cochlear implants. In J. K. Niparko, K. I. Kirk, N. K. Mellon, A. M. Robbins, D. L. Tucci, & B. S. Wilson (Eds.), *Cochlear implants: Principles and practices* (pp. 129–170). Philadelphia, PA: Lippincott Williams & Wilkins.

Tyler, R. S., Gantz, B. J., Rubinstein, J. T., Wilson, B. S., Parkinson, A. J., Wolaver, A. A., . . . Lowder, M. W. (2002). Three-month results with bilateral cochlear implants. *Ear and Hearing, 23,* 80S–89S.

Tyler, R. S., Parkinson, A. J., Wilson, B. S., Witt, S., Preece, J. P., & Noble, W. (2002). Patients utilizing a hearing aid and a cochlear im-plant: Speech perception and localization. *Ear and Hearing, 23,* 98–105.

Tyler, R. S., Preece, J. P., Wilson, B. S., Rubinstein, J. T., Parkinson, A. J., Wolaver, A. A., & Gantz, B. J. (2002). Distance, localization and speech perception pilot studies with bilateral cochlear implants. In T. Kubo, Y. Takahashi, & T. Iwaki (Eds.), *Cochlear implants—An update* (pp. 517–521). The Hague, The Netherlands: Kugler.

Loeb, G. E., & Wilson, B. S. (2003). Prosthetics, sensory systems. In M. A. Arbib (Ed.), *Handbook of brain theory and neural networks* (2nd ed., pp. 926–929). Cambridge, MA: MIT Press.

Wilson, B. S., Lawson, D. T., Müller, J. M., Tyler, R. S., & Kiefer, J. (2003). Cochlear implants: Some likely next steps. *Annual Review of Biomedical Engineering, 5,* 207–249.

Wilson, B. S. (2004). Engineering design of cochlear implants. In F.-G. Zeng, A. N. Popper, & R. R. Fay (Eds.), *Cochlear implants: Auditory prostheses and electric hearing* (pp. 14–52). New York, NY: Springer-Verlag. (This book is Volume 20 in the highly acclaimed *Springer Handbook of Auditory Research,* and also may be cited as B. S. Wilson. [2004]. *Springer Handbook of Auditory Research, 20,* 14–52.)

Loeb, G. E., & Wilson, B. S. (2004). Cochlear prosthesis. In G. Adelman & B. H. Smith (Eds.), *Encyclopedia of neuroscience* (3rd ed.). Amsterdam, The Netherlands: Elsevier. (The *Encyclopedia* is available both in book and CD-ROM formats.)

Wilson, B. S., Sun, X., Schatzer, R., & Wolford, R. D. (2004). Representation of fine-structure or fine-frequency information with cochlear implants. *International Congress Series, 1273,* 3–6.

Dorman, M. F., & Wilson, B. S. (2004). The design and function of cochlear implants. *American Scientist, 92,* 436–445.

Wilson, B. S., Schatzer, R., Lopez-Poveda, E. A., Sun, X., Lawson, D. T., & Wolford, R. D. (2005). Two new directions in speech processor design for cochlear implants. *Ear and Hearing, 26,* 73S–81S.

Wilson, B. S. (2006). Speech processing strategies. In H. R. Cooper & L. C. Craddock (Eds.), *Cochlear implants: A practical guide* (2nd ed., pp. 21–69). Philadelphia, PA, and London, UK: Whurr.

Cartee, L. A., Miller, C. A., & van den Honert, C. (2006). Spiral ganglion cell site of excitation I: Comparison of scala tympani and intrameatal electrode responses. *Hearing Research, 215,* 10–21.

Cartee, L. A. (2006). Spiral ganglion cell site of excitation II: Numerical model analysis. *Hearing Research, 215,* 22–30.

Wilson, B. S., Schatzer, R., & Lopez-Poveda, E. A. (2006). Possibilities for a closer mimicking of normal auditory functions with cochlear implants. In S. B. Waltzman & J. T. Roland, Jr., (Eds.), *Cochlear implants* (2nd ed., pp. 48–56). New York, NY: Thieme.

Loeb, G. E., & Wilson, B. S. (2007). Cochlear prosthesis. In G. Adelman & B. H. Smith (Eds.), *Encyclopedia of neuroscience* (4th ed.). Amsterdam, The Netherlands: Elsevier. (The *Encyclopedia* is available both in book and CD-ROM formats; this paper in the 4th edition is a substantially revised and updated version of the paper in the 3rd edition.)

Wilson, B. S., & Dorman, M. F. (2007). The surprising performance of present-day cochlear implants. *IEEE Transactions on Biomedical Engineering, 54,* 969–972.

An, S. K., Park, S. I., Jun, S. B., Byun, K. M., Lee, C. J., Wilson, B. S., . . . Kim, S. J. (2007). Design for a simplified cochlear implant system. *IEEE Transactions on Biomedical Engineering, 54,* 973–982.

Buss, E., Pillsbury, H. C., Buchman, C. A., Pillsbury, C. H., Clark, M. S., Haynes, D. S., . . . Barco, A. L. (2008). Multi-center US bilateral MED-EL cochlear implantation study: Speech perception over the first year of use. *Ear and Hearing, 29,* 20–32.

Wilson, B. S., & Dorman, M. F. (2008). Interfacing sensors with the nervous system: Lessons from the development and success of cochlear implants. *IEEE Sensors Journal, 8,* 131–147.

Wilson, B. S., & Dorman, M. F. (2008). Cochlear implants: A remarkable past and a brilliant future. *Hearing Research, 242,* 3–21. (This paper is the lead article in the special issue on Frontiers of Auditory Prosthesis Research: Implications for Clinical Practice edited by Guest Editor Bryan Pfingst. It also has been among the most heavily downloaded articles from the *Hearing Research* Web site, and has been number 1, 1, 2, 4, 1, 2, 2, 5, 2, 3, and 4 on the download list in the eleven quarters since the article was published in September 2008.)

Wilson, B. S., & Dorman, M. F. (2008). Cochlear implants: Current designs and future possibilities. *Journal of Rehabilitation and Research Development, 45*, 695–730. (This paper is a feature article in the special issue on Cochlear Implants edited by Guest Editor Harry Levitt. The paper also was the most heavily downloaded article from the journal's Web site for at least part of 2011.)

Wilson, B. S., & Dorman, M. F. (2009). The design of cochlear implants. In J. K. Niparko, K. I. Kirk, N. K. Mellon, A. M. Robbins, D. L. Tucci, & B. S. Wilson (Eds.). *Cochlear implants: Principles and practices* (2nd ed., pp. 95–135). Philadelphia, PA: Lippincott Williams & Wilkins.

Wilson, B. S., & Dorman, M. F. (2009). Stimulation for the return of hearing. In A. Rezai, E. Krames, & H. Peckham (Eds.), *Neuromodulation: A comprehensive handbook* (pp. 713–722). Amsterdam, The Netherlands: Elsevier.

Loeb, G. E., & Wilson, B. S. (2009). Cochlear prosthesis. In L. R. Squire (Ed.), *Encyclopedia of neuroscience* (pp. 1051–1054). Amsterdam, The Netherlands: Elsevier.

Wilson, B. S., Lopez-Poveda, E. A., & Schatzer, R. (2010). Use of auditory models in developing coding strategies for cochlear implants. In R. Meddis, E. A. Lopez-Poveda, A. Popper, & R. R. Fay (Eds.), *Computational models of the auditory system* (pp. 237–260). New York, NY: Springer-Verlag. (This book is another volume in the highly acclaimed *Springer Handbook of Auditory Research*, and also may be cited as Wilson et al. [2010]. *Springer Handbook of Auditory Research, 35*, 237–260.)

Tucci, D. L., Merson, M. H, & Wilson, B. S. (2010). A summary of the literature on global hearing impairment: Current status and priorities for action. *Otology and Neurotology, 31*, 31–41.

Tyler, R. S., Witt, S. A., Dunn, C. C., Perreau, A., Parkinson, A. J., & Wilson, B. S. (2010). An attempt to improve bilateral cochlear implants by increasing the distance between electrodes and providing complementary information to the two ears. *Journal of the American Academy of Audiology, 21*, 52–65.

McElveen, J. T., Jr., Blackburn, E. L., Green, J. D., Jr., McLear, P. W., Thimsen, D. J., & Wilson, B. S. (2010). Remote programming of cochlear implants: A telecommunications model. *Otology and Neurotology, 31*, 1035–1040.

Wilson, B. S. (2010). Partial deafness cochlear implantation (PDCI) and electric-acoustic stimulation (EAS). *Cochlear Implants International, 11*(Suppl. 1), 56–66. (This paper is an invited keynote article for a special issue of the journal.)

Dorman, M. F., Yost, W. A., Wilson, B. S., & Gifford, R. H. (2011). Speech perception and sound localization by adults with bilateral cochlear implants. *Seminars in Hearing, 32*, 73–102.

Wilson, B. S. (2011). A "top down" or "cognitive neuroscience" approach to cochlear implant designs and fittings. *Cochlear Implants International, 12*, S35–S39.

Wilson, B. S., & Dorman, M. F. (2011). Remediation of severe or total losses of hearing with cochlear implants. In S. Ahuja (Ed.), *Usher syndrome: Pathogenesis, diagnosis and therapy* (pp. 327–345). Hauppauge, NY: Nova Science.

Wilson, B. S., Dorman, M. F., Woldorff, M. G., & Tucci, D. L. (2011). Cochlear implants: Matching the prosthesis to the brain and facilitating desired plastic changes in brain function. *Progress in Brain Research, 194*, 117–129.

Wilson, B. S., & Dorman, M. F. (2012). Signal processing strategies for cochlear implants. In M. J. Ruckenstein (Ed.), *Cochlear implants and other implantable hearing devices* (pp. 51–84). San Diego, CA: Plural.

Wilson, B. S. (in press). Treatments for partial deafness using combined electric and acoustic stimulation of the auditory system. *Journal of Hearing Science.*

Appendix D

CONTENTS OF THE RTI PROGRESS REPORTS SORTED BY TOPIC

This Appendix presents the contents of the progress reports according to topic. Major topics are indicated by the headings below, and subtopics are indicated by the bullets and the lines beneath the bulleted items. The report or reports corresponding to each topic are indicated by project number (1 to 7) and then by the report within that project. For Quarterly Progress Reports, the format for the presentation of this information is "X:Y," where X is project number and Y is the report number. For example, the third Quarterly Progress Report for Project 4 is represented as "4:3." For Final Reports, the format is "X:F," where X is again the project number and the letter "F" indicates that the report is the final report for that project. Thus, the code "5:F" would indicate that the report including a particular topic is the Final Report for Project 5. Abbreviations in the remainder of this Appendix are the same as those listed and used in Appendix B.

TOOLS AND TOOL BUILDING

- Block diagram compiler (1:2; 1:3; 1:4; 1:7)

    1:2   Design of software for a block-diagram compiler

    1:3   Computer-based simulator

413

1:4 Description of the use and application of a computer-based simulator of speech processors for multichannel auditory prostheses

1:7 Present status and functional description of the block-diagram compiler

■ Portable sound processors (1:6; 1:F; 2:3; 2:7; 3:7; 3:9)

1:6 Development of portable, real-time hardware; circuit diagrams and software for a portable F_0 extractor using the AMDF algorithm

1:F Design of a portable speech processor

2:3 Initial development of a portable, real-time processor

2:7 A portable processor for IP processing strategies

3:7 A wearable speech processor platform for auditory research

3:9 Evaluation of a prototype for a portable processor

■ Laboratory system for psychophysical and speech reception studies (1:2; 1:3; 1:6; 1:F; 2:11; 5:4; 7:5)

1:2 Hardware interface for communication between an Eclipse computer and patient electrodes

1:3 Hardware interface; Digital Control Unit (DCU) software for real-time communication between an Eclipse computer and stimulating hardware

1:6 Software for support of the RTI patient stimulator; software for support of basic psychophysical studies and speech testing

1:F Hardware interface; computer-based simulator of speech processors

2:11 Extension of cochlear implant laboratory capabilities

5:4 New stimulator system for the speech reception laboratory

- Access database of speech processor designs and study results (6:10)

    6:10 An Access database of speech processor designs and study results

- Streaming mode tool (7:5; 7:11)

    7:5 Recent enhancements of the speech laboratory system: streaming mode

    7:11 Further development of the streaming mode tools

DESIGN AND EVALUATION OF NOVEL PROCESSING STRATEGIES

- Interleaved pulses processors (1:7; 2:1; 2:2; 2:6; 2:9; 2:10; 2:12; 2:F; 3:1; 3:3)

    1:7 Speech testing studies with patient LP

    2:1 Psychophysical and speech reception studies with an initial DUMC/Storz percutaneous subject

    2:2 Psychophysical and speech reception studies with a second DUMC/Storz percutaneous subject; further development of an interleaved pulses (IP) processor

    2:6 Direct comparisons of analog and pulsatile coding strategies with six cochlear implant patients

    2:9 Studies with 6 UCSF/Storz subjects

    2:10 Review of clinical trial results for 6 UCSF/Storz subjects, including learning effects with extended use

    2:12 Representations of speech features with cochlear implants

    2:F Direct comparisons of analog and pulsatile coding strategies

    3:1 Comparison of analog and pulsatile coding strategies for multichannel cochlear implants (6 UCSF/Storz subjects and 2 Ineraid subjects)

7:7   Combined use of dual-resonance nonlinear (DRNL) filters and virtual channels

- "Closer mimicking" strategies (7:6; 7:7)

  7:6   Signal processing strategy for a closer mimicking of normal auditory functions

  7:7   Combined use of dual-resonance nonlinear (DRNL) filters and virtual channels

- Representation of "fine structure" or fine frequency information with implants (7:8)

  7:8   Representation of fine structure or fine frequency information with cochlear implants

- Additional strategies (e.g., Breeuwer/Plomp) (1:7; 2:8; 2:F; 3:10; 3:F; 6:5)

  1:7   Speech testing studies with patient LP (strategies included "*n*-of-*m*" designs using either analog or pulsatile stimuli, and strategies using multipulse excitation derived from the linear prediction residual signal)

  2:8   Evaluation of two-channel "Breeuwer/Plomp" processors for cochlear implants

  2:F   Direct comparisons of analog and pulsatile coding strategies; Design and evaluation of a two-channel "Breeuwer/Plomp" processor; additional processor comparisons

  3:10 Evaluation of other promising processing strategies

  3:F   Evaluation of other promising strategies

  6:5   Comprehensive review of strategies for representing speech information with cochlear implants

- Dependence of performance on parameter values (3:10; 4:2; 4:5; 4:F; 5:1; 5:2; 5:3; 5:7; 5:10; 6:3; 6:6; 6:7)

  - Multifaceted studies (4:2; 4:5; 4:F)

    4:2   Single parameter variation studies for CIS processors

- Compression (mapping) function (6:3)

    6:3   Effects of manipulations in mapping functions on the performance of CIS processors

- Channel update order (3:10)

    3:10 Randomized update orders

- Represented range of frequencies (5:1; 5:3; 5:10)

    5:1   Upward extension of the CIS processed frequency spectrum

    5:3   22-electrode percutaneous study: results for the first five subjects

    5:10 Effects of upward extension of the frequency range analyzed by CIS processors

- Importance of processor fitting (4:F)

    4:F   Importance of processor fitting

■ Learning effects and measures of performance over time (2:10; 5:1; 6:2; 6:4; 7:2; 7:4)

    2:10 Review of clinical trial results for 6 UCSF/Storz subjects, including learning effects with extended use

    5:1   Learning effects with extended use of CIS processors

    6:2   Measures of performance over time following substitution of CIS for CA speech processors

    6:4   Update on longitudinal studies (following the 6:2 report)

    7:2   Longitudinal studies of improvement in performance with early experience using binaural cochlear implants

    7:4   Update on longitudinal studies of early performance improvements with binaural cochlear implants

■ Music reception studies (4:4; 4:8; 4:F)

    4:4   Representation of complex tones by sound processors for implanted auditory prostheses

BILATERAL ELECTRICAL STIMULATION

COMBINED ELECTRIC AND ACOUSTIC STIMULATION (EAS) OF THE AUDITORY SYSTEM

AUDITORY BRAINSTEM IMPLANT (ABI)

INEXPENSIVE BUT STILL HIGHLY EFFECTIVE COCHLEAR IMPLANT SYSTEMS

BASIC PSYCHOPHYSICS

MODELS

TEMPORAL REPRESENTATIONS WITH COCHLEAR IMPLANTS

- Modeling studies (4:7)

  4:7   Temporal representations with cochlear implants: modeling, psychophysical, and electrophysiological studies

- Psychophysical studies (4:7)

  4:7   Temporal representations with cochlear implants: modeling, psychophysical, and electrophysiological studies

- Electrophysiological studies (4:7)

  4:7   Temporal representations with cochlear implants: modeling, psychophysical, and electrophysiological studies

- Strategies for repair of distortions in temporal representations (4:9)

  4:9   Strategies for the repair of distortions in temporal representations with implants

- Relationships between temporal patterns of nerve activity and pitch judgments (5:7; 5:8)

  5:7   High rate studies, subject SR2

  5:8   Relationships between temporal patterns of nerve activity and pitch judgments for cochlear implant patients

OTHER

- Technology transfer (4:5)

  4:5   Transfer and dissemination of CIS processor technology

- Cooperation with others (1:1; 1:2; 2:11; 2:F)

1:1 Development of plans for collaborative studies with UCSF; development of tools for such studies at UCSF; initial plans for an additional collaborative program with Duke University Medical Center

1:2 Collaboration among UCSF, Storz, DUMC and RTI

2:11 Collaborative development of a next-generation auditory prosthesis (with UCSF and MiniMed)

2:F Development of a next-generation auditory prosthesis

■ Interdependence of speech reception measures (3:4)

3:4 Comparison of CA and CIS processors in tests with 8 Ineraid subjects

■ Binary comparisons of speech processor performance (2:14)

2:14 Binary comparisons of speech processor performance

■ Importance of the patient variable in determining outcomes with cochlear implants (3:8)

3:8 Importance of patient and processor variables in determining outcomes with cochlear implants

■ Evaluation of other implant systems and processing strategies (2:4; 3:9)

2:4 Evaluation of idealized implementations of the processing strategy used in the Nucleus cochlear prosthesis

3:9 Evaluation of components in the MiniMed cochlear prosthesis

■ Evaluation of automatic gain control (3:9)

3:9 Evaluation of automatic gain control

■ Control of latency fields in electrically evoked hearing (1:8)

1:8 Ensemble models — suggested manipulations in latency profiles to code stimulus intensities and frequencies

■ Future directions (3:F; 4:F; 5:F; 6:F; 7:F)

   ▪ Summaries (3:F; 4:F; 7:F)

      3:F   Suggestions for future research

      4:F   Suggestions for future research

      7:F   Suggested future directions

   ▪ Full reports (5:F; 6:F)

      5:F   New directions in implant design

      6:F   Some likely next steps in the further development
            of cochlear prostheses

REFERENCES

Abbas, P. J. (1993). Electrophysiology. In R. S. Tyler (Ed.), *Cochlear implants: Audiological foundations* (pp. 317–355). San Diego, CA: Singular.

Armitage, P. (1957). Restricted Sequential Procedures. *Biometrika, 44*, 9–26.

Bess, F. H., & Townsend, T. H. (1977). Word discrimination for listeners with flat sensorineural hearing losses. *Journal of Speech and Hearing Disorders, 42*, 232–237.

Bilger, R. C., Black, F. O., Hopkinson, N. T., Myers, E. N., Payne, J. L., Stenson, N. R., Vega, A., & Wolf, R. V. (1977). Evaluation of subjects presently fitted with implanted auditory prostheses. *Annals of Otology, Rhinology, and Laryngology, 86*(Suppl. 38, No. 3, Part 2), 1–176.

Bogess, W. J., Baker, J. E., & Balkany, T. J. (1989). Loss of residual hearing after cochlear implantation. *Laryngoscope, 99*, 1002–1005.

Braida, L. D., & Durlach, N. I. (1972). Intensity perception II. Resolution in one interval paradigms. *Journal of the Acoustical Society of America, 51*, 483–502.

Brill, S., Gstöttner, W., Helms, J., von Ilberg, C., Baumgartner, W., Müller, J., & Kiefer, J. (1997). Optimization of channel number and stimulation rate for the fast CIS-strategy in the COMBI 40+. *American Journal of Otology, 18*(Suppl. 6), S104–106.

Brill, S., & Hochmair, E. S. (1997, May). *Speech understanding as a function of the number of active channels and stimulation rate in the CIS strategy as implemented in the Combi 40/Combi 40+.* Presented at the Vth International Cochlear Implant Conference, New York, NY.

Brimacombe, J. A., Arndt, P. L., Staller, S. J., & Beiter, A. L. (1994). Multichannel cochlear implantation in adults with severe-to-profound sensorineural hearing loss. In I. J. Hochmair-Desoyer & E. Hochmair (Eds.), *Advances in cochlear implants* (pp. 387–392). Vienna, Austria: Manz.

Bross, I. (1952). Sequential medical plans. *Biometrics, 8,* 188–205.

Brown, C. J., Abbas, P. J., & Gantz, B. (1990). Electrically evoked whole-nerve action potentials: Data from human cochlear implant users. *Journal of the Acoustical Society of America, 88,* 1385–1391.

Brown, J. N., Miller, J. M., Altschuler, R. A., & Nuttall, A. L. (1993). Osmotic pump implant for chronic infusion of drugs into the inner ear. *Hearing Research, 70,* 167–172.

Buechner, A., Frohne-Büchner, C., Gaertner, L., Stoever, T., Battmer, R. D., & Lenarz, T. (2010). The Advanced Bionics High Resolution Mode: Stimulation rates up to 5000 pps. *Acta Oto-Laryngologica, 130,* 114–123.

Busby, P. A., Tong, Y. C., & Clark, G. M (1993). The perception of temporal modulations by cochlear implant patients. *Journal of the Acoustical Society of America, 94,* 124–131.

Carlyon, R. P., Deeks, J. M., & McKay, C. M. (2010). The upper limit of temporal pitch for cochlear-implant listeners: Stimulus duration, conditioner pulses, and the number of electrodes stimulated. *Journal of the Acoustical Society of America, 127,* 1469–1478.

Carlyon, R. P., van Wieringen, A., Long, C. J., Deeks, J. M., & Wouters, J. (2002). Temporal pitch mechanisms in acoustic and electric hearing. *Journal of the Acoustical Society of America, 112,* 621–633.

Clark, G. M. (1987). The University of Melbourne-Nucleus multi-electrode cochlear implant. *Advances in Oto-Rhino-Laryngology, 38,* 1–189.

Davis, H., & Silverman, S. R. (1978). *Hearing and deafness.* New York, NY: Holt, Rinehart and Winston.

De Filippo, C. L., & Scott, B. L. (1978). A method for training and evaluating the reception of ongoing speech. *Journal of the Acoustical Society of America, 63,* 1186–1192.

Denes, P. B. (1963). On the statistics of spoken English. *Journal of the Acoustical Society of America, 35,* 892–904.

Dorman, M. F., Dankowski, K., & McCandless, G. (1990). Longitudinal changes in word recognition by patients who use the Ineraid cochlear implant. *Ear and Hearing, 11,* 455–459.

Dorman, M. F., & Gifford, R. H. (2010). Combining acoustic and electric stimulation in the service of speech recognition. *International Journal of Audiology, 49,* 912–919.

Dorman, M. F., Gifford, R. H., Spahr, A. J., & McKarns, S. A. (2007). The benefits of combining acoustic and electric stimulation for the recognition of speech, voice and melodies. *Audiology and Neurotology, 13,* 105–112.

Dorman, M. F., Hannley, M. T., Dankowski, K., Smith, L., & McCandless, G. (1989). Word recognition by 50 patients fitted with the Symbion multichannel cochlear implant. *Ear and Hearing, 10,* 44–49.

Dorman, M. F., Smith, L. M., Smith, M., & Parkin, J. L. (1996). Frequency discrimination and speech recognition by patients who use the Ineraid and continuous interleaved sampling cochlear-implant signal processors. *Journal of the Acoustical Society of America, 99,* 1174–1184.

Dowell, R. C., Brown, A. M., & Mecklenburg, D. J. (1990). Clinical assessment of implanted deaf adults. In G. M. Clark, Y.C. Tong, & J. F. Patrick (Eds.), *Cochlear prostheses* (pp. 93–205). Edinburgh, UK: Churchill Livingstone.

Dowell, R. C., Seligman, P. M., Blarney, P. J., & Clark, G. M. (1987). Evaluation of a two-formant speech-processing strategy for a multichannel cochlear prosthesis. *Annals of Otology, Rhinology, and Laryngology, 96*(Suppl. 128), 132–134.

Doyle, J. H., Doyle, J. B. Jr., & Turnbull, F. M. (1964). Electrical stimulation of eighth cranial nerve. *Archives of Otolaryngology, 80,* 388–391.

Dubno, J. R., & Dirks, D. D. (1982). Evaluation of hearing-impaired listeners using a nonsense syllable test. I. Test reliability. *Journal of Speech and Hearing Research, 25,* 135–141.

Dubno, J. R., Dirks, D. D., & Morgan, D. E. (1984). Effects of age and mild hearing loss on speech recognition in noise. *Journal of the Acoustical Society of America, 76,* 87–96.

Eddington, D. K. (1980). Speech discrimination in deaf subjects with cochlear implants. *Journal of the Acoustical Society of America, 68,* 885–891.

Eddington, D. K. (1983). Speech recognition in deaf subjects with multichannel intracochlear electrodes. *Annals of the New York Academy of Sciences, 405,* 241–258.

Eddington, D. K., Rubinstein, J. T., & Dynes, S. B. C. (1994). Forward masking during intracochlear electrical stimulation: Models, physiology, and psychophysics. *Journal of the Acoustical Society of America, 95,* 2904.

Eisen, M. D. (2006). History of the cochlear implant. In S. B. Waltzman & J. T. Roland, Jr. (Eds.), *Cochlear implants* (2nd ed., pp. 1–10). New York, NY: Thieme Medical.

Eisen, M. D. (2009). The history of cochlear implants. In J. K. Niparko, K. I. Kirk, A. M. Robbins, D. L. Tucci, & B. S. Wilson (Eds.), *Cochlear implants: Principles and practices* (2nd ed., pp. 89–93). Philadelphia, PA: Lippincott, Williams & Wilkins.

Finley, C. C., Wilson, B. S., & White, M. W. (1990). Models of neural responsiveness to electrical stimulation. In J. M. Miller & F. A. Spelman (Eds.), *Cochlear implants* (pp. 55–96). New York, NY: Springer-Verlag.

Finn, R., with the assistance of Hudspeth, A. J., Zwislocki, J., Young, E., & Merzenich M. (1998). Sound from silence: The development of cochlear implants. In *Beyond discovery: The path from research to human benefit* (pp.1–8). Washington, DC: National Academy of Sciences. Available online at http://www.beyonddiscovery.org/includes/DBFile.asp?ID=83.

Flanagan, J. L. (1972). *Speech analysis, synthesis and perception* (2nd ed.). Berlin, Germany: Springer-Verlag.

Frank, T., & Craig, C. H. (1984). Comparison of the Auditec and Rintelmann recordings of the NU-6. *Journal of Speech and Hearing Disorders, 49*, 267–271.

Frederickson, C. J., & Gerken, G. M. (1977). Masking of electrical by acoustic stimuli: Behavioral evidence for tonotopic organization. *Science, 198*, 1276–1278.

Friesen, L. M., Shannon, R. V., & Cruz, R. J. (2005). Effects of stimulation rate on speech recognition with cochlear implants. *Audiology and Neurotology, 10*, 169–184.

Frijns, J. H., Klop, W. M., Bonnet, R. M., & Briaire, J. J. (2003). Optimizing the number of electrodes with high-rate stimulation of the clarion CII cochlear implant. *Acta Oto-Laryngologica, 123*, 138–142.

Fu, Q. J., & Shannon, R. V. (2000). Effect of stimulation rate on phoneme recognition by nucleus-22 cochlear implant listeners. *Journal of the Acoustical Society of America, 107*, 589–597.

Gantz, B. J., & Turner, C. W. (2003). Combining acoustic and electrical hearing. *Laryngoscope, 113*, 1726–1730.

Gantz, B. J., Tyler, R. S., Knutson, J. F., Woodworth, G., Abbas, P., McCabe, B. F., . . . Brown, C. (1988). Evaluation of five different cochlear implant designs: Audiologic assessment and predictors of performance. *Laryngoscope, 98*, 1100–1106.

Gardi, J. N. (1985). Human brainstem and middle latency responses to electrical stimulation: A preliminary observation. In R. A. Schindler & M. M. Merzenich (Eds.), *Cochlear implants* (pp. 351–363). New York, NY: Raven Press.

Goetzinger, C. P. (1978). Word discrimination testing. In J. Katz (Ed.), *Handbook of clinical audiology* (2nd ed., pp. 149–158). Baltimore, MD: Williams & Wilkins.

Green, T., Faulkner, A., & Rosen, S. (2012). Variations in carrier pulse rate and the perception of amplitude modulation in cochlear implant users. *Ear and Hearing, 33*, 221–230.

Greenwood, D. D. (1990). A cochlear frequency-position function for several species—29 years later. *Journal of the Acoustical Society of America, 87*, 2592–2605.

Hannaway, C. (1996). *Contributions of the National Institutes of Health to the development of cochlear prostheses.* Report developed under contract for the National Institute on Deafness and Other Communication Disorders. Bethesda, MD: National Institute on Deafness and Other Communication Disorders.

Hartmann, R., & Klinke, R. (1990). Response characteristics of nerve fibers to patterned electrical stimulation. In J. M. Miller & F. A. Spelman (Eds.), *Cochlear implants: Models of the electrically stimulated ear* (pp. 135–159). New York, NY: Springer-Verlag.

Hartmann, R., Topp, G., & Klinke, R. (1984). Discharge patterns of cat primary auditory nerve fibers with electrical stimulation of the cochlea. *Hearing Research, 13,* 47–62.

Hochmair, I., Nopp, P., Jolly, C., Schmidt, M., Schösser, H., Garnham, C., & Anderson, I. (2006). MED-EL cochlear implants: State of the art and a glimpse into the future. *Trends in Amplification, 10,* 201–219.

Hodges, A.V., Schloffman, J., & Balkany, T. (1997). Conservation of residual hearing with cochlear implantation. *American Journal of Otology, 18,* 179–183.

Hughes, M. L., Castioni, E. E., Goehring, J. L., & Baudhuin, J. L. (2012). Temporal response properties of the auditory nerve: Data from human cochlear-implant recipients. *Hearing Research, 285,* 46–57.

Javel, E. (1990). Acoustic and electrical encoding of temporal information. In J. M. Miller & F. A. Spelman (Eds.), *Cochlear implants: Models of the electrically stimulated ear* (pp. 247–296). New York, NY: Springer-Verlag.

Jolly, C. N., Spelman, F. A., & Pfingst, B. E. (1994, February 6–10). Focusing potentials in the cochlea: Modeling and experimental data. In *Abstracts of the Seventeenth Midwinter Research Meeting, Association for Research in Otolaryngology* (p. 162). St. Petersburg Beach, FL.

Junge, D. (1992). *Nerve and muscle excitation* (3rd ed., pp. 210–226). Sunderland, MA: Sinauer Associates.

Kiefer, J., Pfennigdorff, T., Rupprecht, V., Huber-Egener, J., & von Ilberg, C. (1996, June). *The effect of stimulus rate and channel number on speech understanding with the CIS-strategy in cochlear implant patients.* Presented at the Third European Symposium on Paediatric Cochlear Implantation, Hannover, Germany.

Kiefer, J., von Ilberg, C., Rupprecht, V., Huber-Egener, J., Baumgartner, W., Gstöttner, W., & Stephan, K. (1997, May). *Optimized speech understanding with the CIS-speech coding strategy in cochlear implants: The effect of variations in stimulus rate and numbers of channels.* Presented at the Vth International Cochlear Implant Conference, New York, NY.

Kiefer, J., von Ilberg, C., Rupprecht, V., Hubner-Egner, J., & Knecht, R. (2000). Optimized speech understanding with the continuous interleaved sampling speech coding strategy in patients with cochlear implants: Effect of variations in stimulation rate and number of channels. *Annals of Otology, Rhinology, and Laryngology, 109,* 1009–1020.

Kong, Y. Y., & Carlyon, R. P. (2010). Temporal pitch perception at high rates in cochlear implants. *Journal of the Acoustical Society of America, 127,* 3114–3123.

Kuzma, J. A. (1996). Cochlear electrode implant assemblies with positioning system therefor. United States patent 5545219.

Kuzma, J. A., Seldon, H. L., & Brown, G. G. (1996). Self-curving cochlear electrode array. United States patent 5578084.

Lawson, D. T., Wilson, B. S., & Finley, C. C. (1993). New processing strategies for multichannel cochlear prostheses. *Progress in Brain Research, 97,* 313–321.

Lawson, D. T., Wilson, B. S., Zerbi, M., & Finley, C. C. (1995). Speech processors for auditory prostheses: Section on the 22 electrode percutaneous study. *First Quarterly Progress Report,* NIH project N01-DC-5-2103. Bethesda, MD: National Institutes of Health.

Lawson, D. T., Wilson, B. S., Zerbi, M., & Finley, C. C. (1996). Speech processors for auditory prostheses: 22 electrode percutaneous study—Results for the first five subjects. *Third Quarterly Progress Report,* NIH project N01-DC-5-2103. Bethesda, MD: National Institutes of Health.

Lawson, D. T., Wilson, B. S., Zerbi, M., van den Honert, C., Finley, C. C., Farmer, J. C., Jr., . . . Roush, P. A. (1998). Bilateral cochlear implants controlled by a single speech processor. *American Journal of Otology, 19,* 758–761.

Levitt, H. (2008). Cochlear prostheses: *L'enfant terrible* of auditory rehabilitation. *Journal of Rehabilitation Research and Development, 45,* ix–xvi.

Loeb, G. E., Byers, C. L., Rebscher, S. J., Casey, D. E., Fong, M. M., Schindler, R. A., . . . Merzenich, M. M. (1983). Design and fabrication of an experimental cochlear prosthesis. *Medical and Biological Engineering and Computing, 21,* 241–254.

Loizou, P. (2006). Speech processing in vocoder-centric cochlear implants. In A. Moller (Ed.), *Cochlear and brainstem implants* (pp. 109–143). Basel, Switzerland: Karger.

Loizou, P. C., Poroy, O., & Dorman, M. (2000). The effect of parametric variations of cochlear implant processors on speech understanding. *Journal of the Acoustical Society of America, 108,* 790–802.

Long, C. J., Eddington, D. K., Colburn, H. S., & Rabinowitz, W. M. (1999, August and September). *Bilateral cochlear implants: Fundamental psychophysics.* Poster presented at the 1999 Conference on Implantable Auditory Prostheses, Pacific Grove, CA.

Long, C. J., Eddington, D. K., Colburn, H. S., Rabinowitz, W. M., Whearty, M. E., & Kadel-Garcia, N. (1998). Speech processors for auditory prostheses. *Eleventh Quarterly Progress Report,* NIH project N01-DC-6-2100. Bethesda, MD: National Institutes of Health.

Macherey, O., & Carlyon, R. P. (2010). Temporal pitch percepts elicited by dual-channel stimulation of a cochlear implant. *Journal of the Acoustical Society of America, 127*, 339–349.

McDermott, H. J., McKay, C. M., & Vandali, A. E. (1992). A new portable sound processor for the University of Melbourne/Nucleus Limited multielectrode cochlear implant. *Journal of the Acoustical Society of America, 91*, 3367–3371.

McDermott, H. J., & Vandali, A. E. (1997). Spectral maxima sound processor. United States Patent 5,597,380.

Merzenich, M. M. (1985). UCSF cochlear implant device. In R. A. Schindler & M. M. Merzenich (Eds.), *Cochlear implants* (pp. 121–129). New York, NY: Raven Press.

Merzenich, M. M., Leake-Jones, P., Vivion, M., White, M., & Silverman, M. (1978). Development of multichannel electrodes for an auditory prosthesis. *Fourth Quarterly Progress Report*, NIH project N01-NS-7-2367. Bethesda, MD: National Institutes of Health.

Merzenich, M. M., Rebscher, S. J., Loeb, G. E., Byers, C. L., & Schindler, R. A. (1984). The UCSF cochlear implant project. State of development. *Advances in Audiology, 2*, 119–144.

Merzenich, M. M., & White, M. W. (1977). Cochlear implant: The interface problem. In F. T. Hambrecht & J. B. Reswick (Eds.), *Functional electrical stimulation* (pp. 321–340). New York, NY: Marcel Dekker.

Miller, G. A., & Nicely, P. E. (1955). An analysis of perceptual confusions among some English consonants. *Journal of the Acoustical Society of America, 27*, 338–352.

Minifie, F. D. (1973). Speech acoustics. In F. D. Minifie, T. J. Hixon, & F. Williams (Eds), *Normal aspects of speech, hearing and language* (pp. 235–284). Upper Saddle River, NJ: Prentice-Hall.

Moxon, E. C. (1971). *Neural and mechanical responses to electric stimulation of the cat's inner ear* [Doctoral dissertation]. Massachusetts Institute of Technology, Cambridge, MA.

Müller, J., Schön, F., & Helms, J. (2002). Speech understanding in quiet and noise in bilateral users of the MED-EL COMBI 40/40+ cochlear implant system. *Ear and Hearing, 23*, 198–206.

National Institutes of Health. (1988). Cochlear implants. *NIH Consensus Statement, 7*(2), 1–9. (This statement also is available in *Archives of Otolaryngology—Head and Neck Surgery, 115*, 31–36.)

National Institutes of Health. (1995). Cochlear implants in adults and children. *NIH Consensus Statement, 13*(2), 1–30. (This statement also is available in *JAMA, 274*, 1955–1961.)

Niparko, J. K., & Wilson, B. S. (2000). History of cochlear implants. In J. K. Niparko, K. I. Kirk, A. McConkey Robbins, D. L. Tucci, & B. S. Wilson (Eds.), *Cochlear implants: Principles and practices* (pp. 103–107). Philadelphia, PA: Lippincott, Williams & Wilkins.

Nuetzel, J. M., & Hafter, E. R. (1981). Discrimination of interaural delays in complex waveforms: Spectral effects. *Journal of the Acoustical Society of America, 69,* 1112–1118.

Owens, E., & Blazek, B. (1985). Visemes observed by hearing-impaired and normal-hearing adult viewers. *Journal of Speech and Hearing Research, 28,* 381–393.

Owens, E., Kessler, D. K., Raggio, M., & Schubert, E. D. (1985). Analysis and revision of the Minimal Auditory Capabilities (MAC) battery. *Ear and Hearing, 6,* 280–287.

Owens, E., & Raggio, M. (1987). The UCSF tracking procedure for evaluation and training of speech reception by hearing-impaired adults. *Journal of Speech and Hearing Disorders, 52,* 120–128.

Parkins, C. W. (1986). Cochlear prostheses. In R. A. Altschuler, D. W. Hoffman, & R. P. Bobbin (Eds.), *Neurobiology of hearing: The cochlea* (pp. 455–473). New York, NY: Raven Press.

Parkins, C. W. (1989). Temporal response patterns of auditory nerve fibers to electrical stimulation in deafened squirrel monkeys. *Hearing Research, 41,* 137–168.

Parnas, B. R. (1996). Noise and neuronal populations conspire to encode simple waveforms reliably. *IEEE Transactions on Biomedical Engineering, 43,* 313–318.

Pfingst, B. E. (1984). Operating ranges and intensity psychophysics for cochlear implants. *Archives of Otolaryngology, 110,* 140–144.

Pfingst, B. E., Glass, I., Spelman, F. A., & Sutton, D. (1985). Psychophysical studies of cochlear implants in monkeys: Clinical implications. In R. A. Schindler & M. M. Merzenich (Eds.), *Cochlear implants* (pp. 305–321). New York, NY: Raven Press.

Pfingst, B. E., & Sutton, D. (1983). Relation of cochlear implant function to histopathology in monkeys. *Annals of the New York Academy of Sciences, 405,* 224–239.

Rabiner, L. R., & Shafer, R. W. (1978). *Digital processing of speech signals.* Upper Saddle River, NJ: Prentice-Hall.

Rabinowitz, W. M., Eddington, D. K., Delhorne, L. A., & Cuneo, P. A. (1992). Relations among different measures of speech reception in subjects using a cochlear implant. *Journal of the Acoustical Society of America, 92,* 1869–1881.

Rabinowitz, W. M., Grant, K. W., & Eddington, D. K. (1988). Comparison of three sentence-level tests for evaluating audiovisual performance of subjects using a cochlear implant. *Journal of the Acoustical Society of America, 84,* S45.

Ranck, J. B., Jr. (1975). Which elements are exited in electrical stimulation of the mammalian central nervous system: A review. *Brain Research, 98,* 417–440.

Rizer, F. M. (1988). Postoperative audiometric evaluation of cochlear implant patients. *Otoloryngology—Head and Neck Surgery, 98,* 203–206.

Rubinstein, J. T., Wilson, B. S., Finley, C. C., & Abbas, P. J. (1999). Pseudospontaneous activity: Stochastic independence of auditory nerve fibers with electrical stimulation. *Hearing Research, 127,* 108–118.

Saoji, A. A., & Litvak, L. M. (2010). Use of "phantom electrode" technique to extend the range of pitches available through a cochlear implant. *Ear and Hearing, 31,* 693–701. Erratum in *Ear and Hearing, 32,* 143.

Schatzer, R., Wilson, B. S., Wolford, R. D., & Lawson, D. T. (2003). Speech processors for auditory prostheses: Signal processing strategies for a closer mimicking of normal auditory functions. *Sixth Quarterly Progress Report,* NIH project N01-DC-2-1002. Bethesda, MD: National Institutes of Health.

Schindler, R. A., & Kessler, D. K. (1987). The UCSF/Storz cochlear implant: Patient performance. *American Journal of Otology, 8,* 247–255.

Schindler, R. A., Kessler, D. K., Rebscher, S. J., Jackler, R. K., & Merzenich, M. M. (1987). Surgical considerations and hearing results with the UCSF/Storz cochlear implant. *Laryngoscope, 97,* 50–56.

Schindler, R. A., Kessler, D. K., Rebscher, S. J., Yanda, J. L., & Jackler, R. K. (1986). The UCSF/Storz multichannel cochlear implant: Patient results. *Laryngoscope, 96,* 597–603.

Schubert, E. D. (1985). Some limitations on speech coding for implants. In R. A. Schindler & M. M. Merzenich (Eds.), *Cochlear implants* (pp. 269–276). New York, NY: Raven Press.

Seitz, P. R. (2002). French origins of the cochlear implant. *Cochlear Implants International, 3,* 77–86.

Seldon, H. L., Daham, M. C., & Clark, G. M. (1994). Silastic with polyacrylic acid filler: Swelling properties, biocompatibility and potential use into cochlear implants. *Biomaterials, 15,* 1161–1169.

Shannon, R. V. (1983a). Multichannel electrical stimulation of the auditory nerve in man. I. Basic psychophysics. *Hearing Research, 11,* 157–189.

Shannon, R. V. (1983b). Multichannel electrical stimulation of the auditory nerve in man. II. Channel interaction. *Hearing Research, 12,* 1–16.

Shannon, R. V. (1993). Psychophysics. In R. S. Tyler (Ed.), *Cochlear implants: Audiological foundations* (pp. 357–388). San Diego, CA: Singular.

Shannon, R. V., Cruz, R. J., & Galvin, J. J. 3rd. (2011). Effect of stimulation rate on cochlear implant users' phoneme, word and sentence recognition in quiet and in noise. *Audiology and Neurotology, 16,* 113–123.

Shin, Y. J., Deguine, O., Laborde, J. L., & Fraysse, B. (1997). Conservation of residual hearing after cochlear implantation [in French]. *Revue de Laryngologie Otologie Rhinologie, 118*, 233–238.

Simmons, F. B., Epley, J. M., Lummis, R. C., Guttman, N., Frishkopf, L. S., Harmon, L. D., & Zwicker, E. (1965). Auditory nerve: Electrical stimulation in man. *Science, 148*, 104–106.

Singh, S., & Black, J. Y. (1966). Study of twenty-six intervocalic consonants as spoken by four language groups. *Journal of the Acoustical Society of America, 39*, 372–387.

Tobias, J. V. (1972). *Foundations of modern auditory theory II.* New York, NY: Academic Press.

Tong, Y. C., & Clark, G. M. (1985). Absolute identification of electric pulse rates and electrode positions by cochlear implant patients. *Journal of the Acoustical Society of America, 77*, 1881–1888.

Tong, Y. C., Lim, H. H., & Clark, G. M. (1989). Psychophysical and speech perceptual studies on cochlear implant-patients. In J. M. Miller & F. A. Spelman (Eds.), *Cochlear implants: Models of the electrically stimulated ear.* New York, NY: Springer-Verlag.

Townshend, B., Cotter, N., Van Campernolle, D., & White, R. L. (1987). Pitch perception by cochlear implant patients. *Journal of the Acoustical Society of America, 87*, 106–115.

Trautwein, P. (2006). *HiRes with Fidelity™ 120 sound processing: Implementing active current steering for increased spectral resolution in CII BionicEar® and HiRes90K users.* Technical Report. Valencia, CA: Advanced Bionics Corporation. Available at http://www.bionicear.com/userfiles/File/HiRes_Fidelity120_Sound_Processing.pdf.

Tyler, R. S., Preece, J. P., Lansing, C. R., Otto, S. R., & Gantz, B. J. (1986). Previous experience as a confounding factor in comparing cochlear-implant processing schemes. *Journal of Speech and Hearing Research, 29*, 282–287.

Tyler, R. S., Preece, J. P., & Lowder, M. W. (1983). *The Iowa cochlear-implant test battery.* Laboratory report. Iowa City, IA: University of Iowa at Iowa City, Department of Otolaryngology—Head and Neck Surgery.

Tyler, R. S., Preece, J. P., & Lowder, M. W. (1987). *The Iowa audiovisual speech perception laser videodisc.* Laser videodisc and laboratory report. Iowa City, IA: University of Iowa at Iowa City, Department of Otolaryngology—Head and Neck Surgery.

van den Honert, C., & Stypulkowski, P. H. (1987a). Single fiber mapping of spatial excitation patterns in the electrically stimulated auditory nerve. *Hearing Research, 29*, 195–206.

van den Honert, C., & Stypulkowski, P. H. (1987b). Temporal response patterns of single auditory nerve fibers elicited by periodic electrical stimuli. *Hearing Research, 29*, 207–222.

van Hoesel, R. J. M., & Clark, G. M. (1995). Fusion and lateralization study with two binaural cochlear implant patients. *Annals of Otology, Rhinology, and Laryngology, 104*(Suppl. 166), 233–235.

van Hoesel, R. J. M., & Clark, G. M. (1997). Psychophysical studies with two binaural cochlear implant subjects. *Journal of the Acoustical Society of America, 102*, 495–507.

van Hoesel, R. J. M., Tong, Y. C., Hallow, R. D., & Clark, G. M. (1993). Psychophysical and speech perception studies: A case report on a binaural cochlear implant subject. *Journal of the Acoustical Society of America, 94*, 3178–3189.

van Hoesel, R. J. M., & Tyler, R. (2003). Speech perception, localization and lateralization with bilateral cochlear implants. *Journal of the Acoustical Society of America, 113*, 1617–1630.

Van Tassell, D. J., Soli, S. D., Kirby, V. M., & Widin, G. P. (1987). Speech waveform envelope cues for consonant recognition. *Journal of the Acoustical Society of America, 82*, 1152–1161.

van Wieringen, A., Carlyon, R. P., Long, C. J., & Wouters, J. (2003). Pitch of amplitude-modulated irregular-rate stimuli in acoustic and electric hearing. *Journal of the Acoustical Society of* America, *114*, 1516–1528.

Verveen, A. A. (1962). Fibre diameter and fluctuation in excitability. *Acta Morphologica Neerlando-Scandinavica, 5*, 79–85.

Verveen, A. A., & Derksen, H. E. (1968). Fluctuation phenomena in nerve membrane. *Proceedings of the IEEE, 56*, 906–916.

von Ilberg, C., Kiefer, J., Tillein, J., Pfennigdorff, T., Hartmann, R., Stürzebecher, E., & Klinke, R. (1999). Electric-acoustic stimulation of the auditory system. *ORL: Journal for Oto-Rhino-Laryngology and Its Related Specialties, 61*, 334–340.

Wagener, K., Brand, T., & Kollmeier, B. (1999b). Development and evaluation of a German sentence test—part II: Optimization of the Oldenburg sentence test. *Zeitschrift für Audiologie, 38*, 44–56.

Wagener, K., Brand, T., & Kollmeier, B. (1999c). Development and evaluation of a German sentence test—part III: Evaluation of the Oldenburg sentence test. *Zeitschrift für Audiologie, 38*, 86–95.

Wagener, K., Kuehnel, V., & Kollmeier, B. (1999a). Development and evaluation of a German sentence test—part I: Design of the Oldenburg sentence test. *Zeitschrift für Audiologie, 38*, 4–15.

Wald, A. (1947). *Sequential analysis* (pp. 106–116). New York, NY: John Wiley and Sons.

Wang, M. D., & Bilger, R. C. (1973). Consonant confusions in noise: A study of perceptual features. *Journal of the Acoustical Society of America, 54*, 1248–1266.

Web of Knowledge, Version 5.3. (2011). New York, NY: Thomson Reuters.

White, M. W., Merzenich, M. M., & Gardi, J. N. (1984). Multichannel cochlear implants: Channel interactions and processor design. *Archives of Otolaryngology, 110,* 493–501.

Wilson, B. S. (1993). Signal processing. In R. S. Tyler (Ed.), *Cochlear implants: Audiological foundations* (pp. 35–85). San Diego, CA: Singular.

Wilson, B. S. (1997). The future of cochlear implants. *British Journal of Audiology, 31,* 205–225.

Wilson, B. S. (2000). New directions in implant design. In S. B. Waltzman & N. Cohen (Eds.), *Cochlear implants* (pp. 43–56). New York, NY: Thieme.

Wilson, B. S. (2004). Engineering design of cochlear implant systems. In F.-G. Zeng, A. N. Popper, & R. R. Fay (Eds.), *Auditory prostheses: Cochlear implants and beyond* (pp. 14–52). New York, NY: Springer-Verlag.

Wilson, B. S. (2006). Speech processing strategies. In H. R. Cooper & L. C. Craddock (Eds.) *Cochlear implants: A practical guide* (2nd ed., pp. 21–69). Hoboken, NJ: John Wiley & Sons.

Wilson, B. S. (2010). Partial deafness cochlear implantation (PDCI) and electric-acoustic stimulation (EAS). *Cochlear Implants International, 11*(Suppl. 1), 56–66.

Wilson, B. S., & Dorman, M. F. (2008a). Interfacing sensors with the nervous system: Lessons from the development and success of the cochlear implant. *IEEE Sensors Journal, 8,* 131–147.

Wilson, B. S., & Dorman, M. F. (2008b). Cochlear implants: A remarkable past and a brilliant future. *Hearing Research, 242,* 3–21.

Wilson, B. S., & Dorman, M. F. (2009). The design of cochlear implants. In J. K. Niparko, K. I. Kirk, A. M. Robbins, D. L. Tucci, & B. S. Wilson (Eds.), *Cochlear implants: Principles and practices* (2nd ed., pp. 95–135). Philadelphia, PA: Lippincott, Williams & Wilkins.

Wilson, B. S., & Dorman, M. F. (2012). Signal processing strategies for cochlear implants. In M. J. Ruckenstein (Ed.), *Cochlear implants and other implantable hearing devices* (pp. 51–84). San Diego, CA: Plural.

Wilson, B. S., & Finley, C. C. (1985). A computer-based simulator of speech processors for auditory prostheses. *Abstracts for the 8th midwinter research conference* (p. 209). Mt. Royal, NJ: Association for Research in Otolaryngology.

Wilson, B. S., Finley, C. C., Farmer, J. C., Jr., Lawson, D. T., Weber, B. A., Wolford, R. D., . . . Schindler, R. A. (1988a). Comparative studies of speech processing strategies for cochlear implants. *Laryngoscope, 98,* 1069–1077.

Wilson, B. S., Finley, C. C., Farmer, J. C., Jr., Weber, B. A., Lawson, D. T., Wolford, R. D., . . . Schindler, R. A. (1987, April). *Comparative studies of speech processing strategies for cochlear implants.* Presented at the

90th Annual Meeting of the American Laryngological, Rhinological and Otological Society, Denver, CO.

Wilson, B. S., Finley, C. C., & Lawson, D. T. (1986). Speech processors for auditory prostheses: Psychophysical and speech reception studies with a second DUMC/Storz percutaneous subject, and further development of an interleaved pulses (IP) processor. *Second Quarterly Progress Report*, NIH project N01-NS-5-2396. Bethesda, MD: National Institutes of Health.

Wilson, B. S., Finley, C. C., & Lawson, D. T. (1989). Speech processors for auditory prostheses: New levels of speech recognition with cochlear implants. *Second Quarterly Progress Report*, NIH project N01-DC-9-2401. Bethesda, MD: National Institutes of Health.

Wilson, B. S., Finley, C. C., & Lawson, D. T. (1990a). Speech processors for auditory prostheses: Section on evaluation of alternative implementations of the continuous interleaved sampler, interleaved pulses, and peak-picker processing strategies. *Third Quarterly Progress Report*, NIH project N01-DC-9-2401. Bethesda, MD: National Institutes of Health.

Wilson, B. S., Finley, C. C., & Lawson, D. T. (1990b). Representations of speech features with cochlear implants. In J. M. Miller & F. A. Spelman (Eds.), *Cochlear Implants: Models of the Electrically Stimulated Ear* (pp. 339–376). New York, NY: Springer-Verlag.

Wilson, B. S., Finley, C. C., Lawson, D. T., & Wolford, R. D. (1988b). Speech processors for cochlear prostheses. *Proceedings of the IEEE*, *76*, 1143–1154.

Wilson, B. S., Finley, C. C., Lawson, D. T., Wolford, R. D., Eddington, D. K., & Rabinowitz, W. M. (1991a). Better speech recognition with cochlear implants. *Nature, 352*, 236–238.

Wilson, B. S., Finley, C. C., Lawson, D. T., & Zerbi, M. (1997). Temporal representations with cochlear implants. *American Journal of Otology, 18*(Suppl. 6), S30–34.

Wilson, B. S., Finley, C. C., Lawson, D. T., Zerbi, M., & van den Honert, C. (1996, October). *High rate coding strategies*. Presented at the International Workshop on Cochlear Implants, Vienna, Austria.

Wilson, B. S., Lawson, D. T., Finley, C. C., & Wolford, R. D. (1991b). Coding strategies for multichannel cochlear prostheses. *American Journal of Otology, 12*(Suppl. 1), 56–61.

Wilson, B. S., Lawson, D. T., Finley, C. C., & Wolford, R. D. (1993). Importance of patient and processor variables in determining outcomes with cochlear implants. *Journal of Speech and Hearing Research, 36*(2), 373–379.

Wilson, B. S., Lawson, D. T., Müller, J. M., Tyler, R. S., & Kiefer, J. (2003). Cochlear implants: Some likely next steps. *Annual Review of Biomedical Engineering, 5*, 207–249.

Wilson, B. S., Lawson, D. T., Zerbi, M., & Finley, C. C. (1992). Speech processors for auditory prostheses: Virtual channel interleaved sampling (VCIS) processors—Initial studies with subject SR2. *First Quarterly Progress Report*, NIH project N01-DC-2-2401. Bethesda, MD: National Institutes of Health.

Wilson, B. S., Lawson, D. T., Zerbi, M., & Finley, C. C. (1994). Recent developments with the CIS strategies. In I. J. Hochmair-Desoyer & E. S. Hochmair (Eds.), *Advances in cochlear implants* (pp. 103–112). Vienna, Austria: Manz.

Wilson, B. S., Lawson, D. T., Zerbi, M., & Finley, C. C. (1995a). Speech processors for auditory prostheses: Section on the "Nucleus percutaneous study." *Final Report*, NIH project N01-DC-2-2401. Bethesda, MD: National Institutes of Health.

Wilson, B. S., Lawson, D. T., Zerbi, M., Finley, C. C., & Wolford, R. D. (1995b). New processing strategies in cochlear implantation. *American Journal of Otology, 16*, 669–675.

Wilson, B. S, Lopez-Poveda, E. A., & Schatzer, R. (2010). Use of auditory models in developing coding strategies for cochlear implants. In R. Meddis, E. A. Lopez-Poveda, A. Popper, & R. R. Fay (Eds.), *Computational models of the auditory system* (pp. 237–260). New York, NY: Springer-Verlag.

Wilson, B. S., Schatzer, R., & Lopez-Poveda, E. A. (2006). Possibilities for a closer mimicking of normal auditory functions with cochlear implants. In S. B. Waltzman & J. T. Roland, Jr. (Eds.), *Cochlear implants* (2nd ed., pp. 48–56). New York, NY: Thieme.

Wilson, B. S., Schindler, R. A., Finley, C. C., Kessler, D. K., Lawson, D. T., & Wolford, R. D. (1988c). Present status and future enhancements of the UCSF cochlear prosthesis. In P. Banfai (Ed.), *Cochlear implant: Current situation* (pp. 395–427). Erkelenz, Germany: Rudolf Bermann GmbH.

Young, E. D., & Sachs, M.B. (1979). Representation of steady-state vowels in the temporal aspects of the discharge patterns of populations of auditory-nerve fibers. *Journal of the Acoustical Society of America, 66*, 1381–1403.

Zeng, F. G., Rebscher, S., Harrison, W. V., Sun, X., & Feng, H. (2008). Cochlear implants: system design, integration and evaluation. *IEEE Reviews in Biomedical Engineering, 1*, 115–142.

INDEX

Note: Page numbers in **bold type** reference nontext material.